D1452590

Studies on the History of Society and Culture
Victoria E. Bonnell and Lynn Hunt, Editors

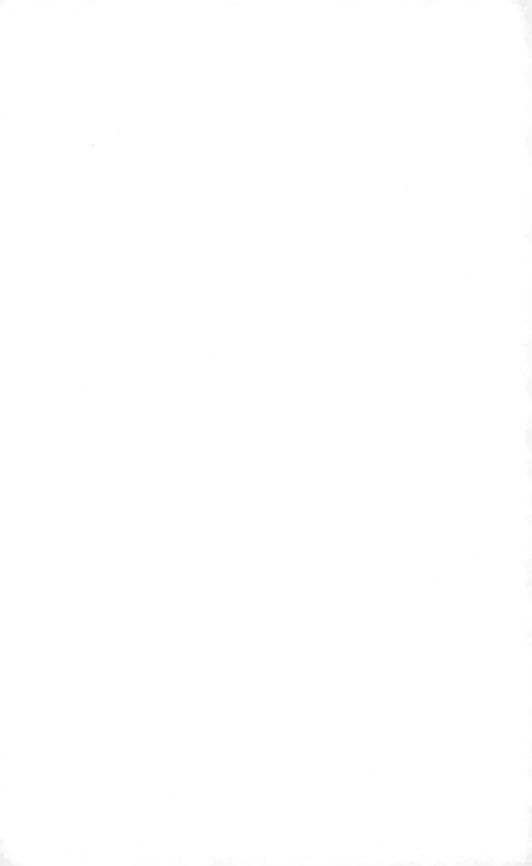

CHOLERA IN
POST-REVOLUTIONARY PARIS

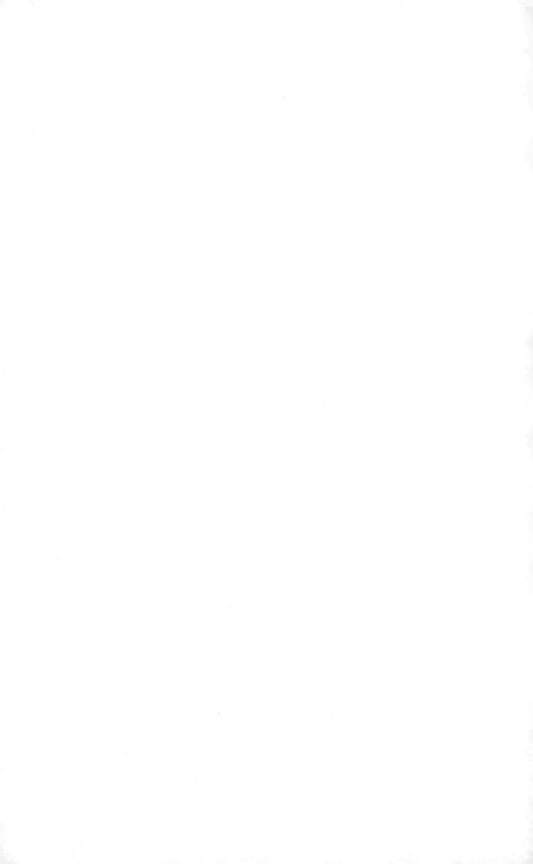

CHOLERA IN POST-REVOLUTIONARY PARIS

A CULTURAL HISTORY

CATHERINE J. KUDLICK

University of California Press
Berkeley · Los Angeles · London

University of California Press
Berkeley and Los Angeles, California

University of California Press, Ltd.
London, England

© 1996 by
Catherine J. Kudlick

Library of Congress Cataloging-in-Publication Data
Kudlick, Catherine Jean.
    Cholera in post-revolutionary Paris : a cultural history
/ Catherine J. Kudlick.
        p.   cm. — (Studies on the history of society and
culture; 25)
    Includes bibliographical references and index.
    ISBN 0-520-20273-2 (alk. paper)
    1. Cholera—France—Paris—History—19th
century.   I. Title.   II. Series.
    RC133.F9P334   1996
    614.5′14′09443609034—dc20   95-25418

Printed in the United States of America

9   8   7   6   5   4   3   2   1

The paper used in this publication meets the minimum
requirements of American National Standard for
Information Sciences—Permanence of Paper for Printed
Library Materials, ANSI Z39.48-1984.

Parts of Chapter 3 appeared in "The Culture of Statistics
and the Crisis of Cholera, 1830–1850," in *Re-creating
Authority in Revolutionary France,* ed. Bryant T. Ragan, Jr.,
and Elizabeth Williams (New Brunswick, N.J.: Rutgers
University Press, 1992). Parts of Chapter 4 appeared in
"Giving Is Deceiving: Cholera, Charity, and the Quest for
Authority in 1832," *French Historical Studies* 18, no. 2 (fall
1993): 457–81. © Society for French Historical Studies, 1993.

To my parents and doctors
and in memory of Walter Bazar
for the gift of sight
and to my teachers, colleagues, students,
and friends
for their gifts of insight

Contents

Illustrations

Table

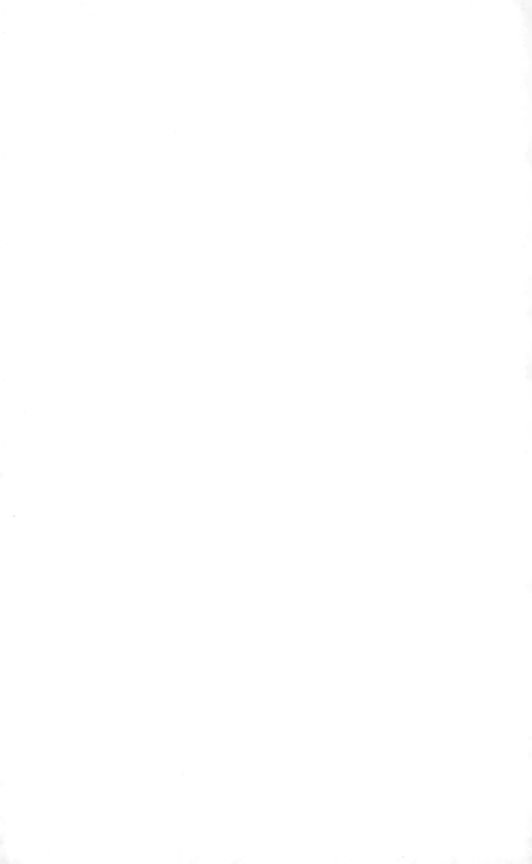

Acknowledgments

I would first like to thank Sheila Levine, my editor at the University of California Press, who stood by me and cholera, even in the roughest times. I think it is fair to say that, like me, she, her co-workers, and many of those I am about to name share the dubious distinction of being among the few in history who are genuinely glad to greet the arrival of cholera—in print.

The research and writing would not have been possible without money. Dissertation research was supported by a Bourse Chateaubriand from the French government, an International Doctoral Research Fellowship from the Social Science Research Council, a Tocqueville Foundation Grant from the Franco-American Foundation, and funds from the University of California, Berkeley. Awards from the National Endowment for the Humanities Travel to Collections program, the Bernadotte Schmitt Grant of the American Historical Association, and Faculty Research Grants from the University of California, Davis, enabled me to return to Paris in search of still more cholera. At a critical juncture in the project I received write-up support from a Faculty Development Grant and the Humanities Institute, both through the University of California, Davis.

The William Osler Library of the History of Medicine at McGill University in Montreal deserves a most special thanks. The library provided a stipend, as well as the luxury of wandering uninhibited (except by a leaky ceiling) through the stacks of their wonderful rare-book room. I am especially grateful to June Schachter and her staff, whose ingenuity, enthusiasm, and patience make me want to tailor all my future research to require a trip there. I am also indebted to professors Don Bates and George Weisz of McGill's Social Studies of Medicine Department for methodological and bibliographical suggestions.

Other libraries and archives also did much to facilitate "the march of cholera." In France, I wish to thank the staffs of the Bibliothèque Nationale, the Bibliothèque Historique de la Ville de Paris, the Archives Nationales, and the Archives de Paris et du Département de la Seine. The small staffs at the Archives de l'Archevêché de Paris, the Institut Catholique, along with the libraries of the Faculté de Médecine and the Académie Nationale de Médecine gave me much firsthand attention, a rare occurrence in the world of very big libraries. I am most grateful to the staffs at the Archives de l'Assistance Publique and the Archives de la Préfecture de Police, who made me feel welcome and provided many hours of help with everything from locating elusive documents to deciphering nineteenth-century doctor scrawl. In the United States, the staffs at the New York Academy of Medicine, the New York Public Library, the National Library of Medicine in Bethesda, and the libraries of the University of California at San Francisco and Berkeley all went out of their way to help me locate and reproduce documents. At the University of California, Davis, I want to extend special thanks to Jane Kimball, the most helpful and ingenious of research librarians.

I was very lucky to have had a number of different forums for presenting my work. Undergraduate students in my AIDS in Historical Context seminars over the past few years have provided an endless source of inspiration and a sense of real engagement. Graduate students in my seminars on "the new cultural history" helped me realize just how central bourgeois culture was to understanding cholera. Professionally, I am grateful for the opportunity to have presented work in progress to the following forums: the Humanities Institute at the University of California, Davis; the conference Re-creating Authority in Revolutionary France, sponsored by the Oklahoma Endowment for the Humanities and organized by Tip Ragan and Elizabeth Williams; the conference Re-reading the French Experience: New Approaches to Cultural Studies, organized by Rene Marion at the University of South Dakota; the Social History Workshop at the University of Chicago; the New York Area French History Seminar; the Stanford University History of Science Colloquium Series; the conference Violence and the Democratic Tradition in France, hosted by the History Department at the University of California, Irvine; and the History and Philosophy of Science Friday afternoon seminar at the University of California, Davis. I owe special gratitude to the History of Medicine and Culture Group (the "Med Heads") and the "French History Group," both at the University of California, Berkeley, for forcing me to stretch my mind and my imagination just that much further in an environment of fine wine and animated discussion.

As for people, I should first thank George Baer, Susanna Barrows, Jon Beecher, Louis Chevalier, Michel Foucault, Rick Gordon, and especially Arlette Farge for lighting the intellectual spark. Tom Laqueur taught the seminar that inspired this book and helped in the trying years of writing my dissertation. Lynn Hunt has always inspired (and sometimes forced!) me to think critically, to delve into the most interesting conceptual issues, and to write with a clarity of purpose. My colleagues from graduate school and junior faculty life—now intellectual playmates, conference buddies, and in several cases among my closest friends—were the best critics and champions I could ever hope for. Warm thanks to Andrew Aisenberg, Leora Auslander, David Barnes, Margie Beale, Rick Biernacki, Alice Bullard, Ian Burney, Josh Cole, Marianne Constable, Paul Friedland, Russ Geoffrey, Larry Glickman, Gabrielle Hecht, Anne Hyde, Sharon Marcus, Mary Odem, Charli Ornett, Lou Roberts, Lucy Salyer, Karen Sawislak, Sylvia Schafer, and Glennys Young. I owe an especially deep personal and intellectual debt to Tip Ragan, my grad school "brother," whose close companionship and careful scrutiny of every word I ever wrote about cholera made the hardest days in France and the United States just plain fun; everyone should be so lucky.

Colleagues in the field such as professors Ed Berenson, Richard Evans, Joby Margadant, Charles Rosenberg, Herb Sloan, and Elizabeth Williams all generously read the entire manuscript and discussed it with me. Only now as a busy academic can I fully appreciate the time they took to comment so seriously on my work. I also want to thank Patrice Bourdelais, Alain Corbin, and Patricia O'Brien for their encouragement and welcome bibliographical suggestions. As a reader for the University of California Press and now an intellectual friend, Colin Jones gave me some of the best advice and no doubt has saved me from some of the worst mistakes. I am also deeply indebted to Jan Goldstein, another reader for the Press, who believed in this project from the very beginning and whose tough but supportive commentary gave me the courage to keep going when I came within a hair's breadth of giving up.

The congenial environment of the Davis History Department has also been a source of intellectual and emotional support. I benefited from a number of excellent graduate student assistants. Diane Camurat, David Del Testa, Bridget Ford, Florence Lemoine, Tracy Miller, Joachim Roschmann, and Robin Walz may have learned more about the grueling side of writing a book than they had bargained for—many, many thanks. As for colleagues, I'd like to single out Bill Hagen, Karen Halttunen, Phyllis Jestice, Norma Landau, Roland Marchand, and Ted Margadant who endured multiple bouts with printed cholera and came up with invaluable suggestions for improvement in the process. Paula Findlen's comments on my rawest drafts (based, she claims, on her knowledge of French history from reading cereal boxes) made this a different and better book, and have also inspired a desperate search to discover what kind of cereal she eats. Clarence Walker fed me lamb, gossip, and provocative articles, while Mike Saler and I spent many hours in the most irreverent and intellectually engaging conversations about cholera's broader implications.

Abroad, my nonacademic friends taught me secrets about Paris and the Parisians without laughing too hard when I unknowingly used expressions from the nineteenth century in our daily banter. Anne Cancellièri, Catherine Defaux, Yann Gasnier, Françoise Robinet and her daughter Djamila, Matthew Tobin and his family kept me from loneliness, provided places to stay, fed me things I'd never tasted before, or kidnapped me for wild field trips to Turkish baths and beer-brewing Trappist monasteries when the documents stopped making sense. They made France magical and helped me know it better. Merci.

Finally, how to thank the people who put up with cholera even when they didn't quite see any use or end to it? I wish to acknowledge Nancy Ryan, whose sane outside perspective and emotional support during the fabulous meals we cook together helped me, especially at the end when my energy was flagging. My family also deserves special thanks. In particular, there is my Aunt Mary, whose deep, honest love has meant so very much. My sister Suz has cheered me on over the years. And last but not least are my parents, Mike and Jean Kudlick, who came around in every sense.

Introduction

The "Silence of 1849"

Cholera is not easily overlooked or forgotten. Remembering his service during the first Parisian epidemic in 1832, Dr. F. L. Poumiès de la Siboutie described the disease in his memoirs:

> Everything was strange and capricious about this disease. A neighborhood, a street, one side of a street, this or that house were ravaged; the rest were spared without any satisfactory reason for this sad preference. . . . A person was hit suddenly, without warning, even in the best state of health. . . . First there was vomiting and diarrhea. An icy coldness seized the entire body, which took on a bluish, almost purple color; the eyes retreated into their sockets, and the face acquired an ominous expression. . . . There was an abundance of pus, white and soapy in appearance. The decay after these discharges was so rapid that any victim who was fresh and healthy in the morning could die the same evening a mere skeleton.[1]

We now know that cholera is a water-born bacterium that lodges in the digestive tract and kills approximately half its victims through acute dehydration.[2] But in the early 1830s, when it first reached the West after being endemic for centuries in India, the disease quickly came to represent the most mysterious and terrifying killer in nineteenth-century Europe. Cholera's unknown causes, gruesome symptoms, and perceived preference for poorer neighborhoods made it a modern disease of unusual social significance. Not only did it ravage the human body in horrifying ways, but it also forced bourgeois residents and government officials to look beyond the physical, social, and political environment in which they lived to a mysterious world filled with misery, fear, and revolution.

As Paris climbed toward the most intense period of its urban and industrial growth, the first two great cholera epidemics ravaged the capital, one in 1832, the other in 1849. Official statistics reported that in 1832 approximately one in every nineteen inhabitants was diagnosed with the disease, and over eighteen thousand lives were lost;

seventeen years later one in every twenty-eight fell ill with cholera and nearly twenty thousand died.[3] Both epidemics hit the capital in March and lasted through the summer. Moreover, each one struck Parisians from all classes, occurred at a time when little was widely known about the disease, and followed periods of intense social unrest in the aftermath of revolutions in 1830 and 1848.

Despite these important similarities, however, the second outbreak received far less attention from contemporaries and thus, not surprisingly, has been virtually overlooked by historians.[4] For example, newspaper accounts of individual and government actions were strikingly fewer and less detailed in 1849. Whereas the official government organ, the *Moniteur universel*, published a total of 463 articles about cholera in 1832, only 40 appeared over the entire course of the second epidemic.[5] This discrepancy was also evident in nongovernment publications such as *L'Ami de la religion*. Like every other Parisian newspaper in 1832, the prominent Catholic organ hardly allowed a day to pass without a lengthy discourse on some aspect of either the disease or the epidemic; seventeen years later, however, the fascination with cholera did not reappear, and the triweekly paper printed one-fifth as many pieces about the disease as it had during the first outbreak.[6]

This quantitative silence was matched by a qualitative one. Consider, for example, the seemingly insignificant story of a new street name, a story given special resonance because of the particular circumstances of the first epidemic. Since the early thirteenth century, the rue de la Mortellerie in the center of Paris had been the neighborhood of stone masons (*morteliers*) and housed their guild.[7] With increased urbanization, filth, and overcrowding, however, the neighborhood and Parisian perceptions of the street had been transformed so that by the beginning of the nineteenth century it became impossible not to read the word *death* (*mort*) into the name *Mortellerie*. As early as 1808 residents of the street had petitioned the prefect of the Seine to change the name, finding the implicit association with death "disagreeable and troubling in and of itself." Landlords raised particularly strong objections, claiming it kept property values low.[8] The 1832 cholera epidemic confirmed residents' worst fears when, according to newspaper accounts, the short, narrow street emerged with the highest death rate in the entire capital.[9] The dramatic mortality received considerable public attention as health officials attempted to understand the cause of the outbreak, thus giving scientific legitimacy to what had once been a superstitious fear. Not surprisingly, in the years after the first cholera epidemic residents again approached the city administration, and on February 16, 1835, the ancient street unceremoniously became the rue de l'Hôtel de Ville by municipal decree.[10]

The story of the rue de la Mortellerie reveals that cholera's social significance in 1832 came both from the fact that responses to it reflected preexisting ideas about the Paris environment and from the fact that the outbreaks of disease served as a catalyst for reshaping attitudes about that environment. From the beginning of the nineteenth century, for example, residents of the rue de la Mortellerie had seen the decaying urban environment around them and implicitly understood its negative associations with the name of their street. It was not until the disproportionate deaths from cholera, however, that the problems accompanying urbanization—overcrowding, dirt, poverty—received enough publicity and scientific attention to warrant changing a name that had existed for centuries. Seen in this way, the new epidemic did not create the association between the street and death but rather provided a context in which it developed into something urgent and terrifying for both residents and government officials.

The city administration's ultimate willingness to change the name of the rue de la Mortellerie was thus bound up with how Parisians experienced and interpreted their encounters with cholera in 1832, an epidemic that seemed to capture almost every aspect of the public imagination. In long daily newspaper articles the government publicized the creation of neighborhood first-aid stations along with elaborate mortality figures and the names of charitable donors. Contemporary observers engaged in lively public debates over the capital's religious well-being and its relationship to the arrival of the mysterious new disease. On a more intimate level, personal letters and diaries of bourgeois Parisians described the horrifying spectacle of close relatives turning into living corpses and of bodies piling up in the streets. Few failed to remark upon what one historian has called "the inability of the city to absorb its dead."[11]

Most significantly, the arrival of cholera in 1832 reinforced the fears with which the ruling bourgeoisie and the lower classes viewed one another in the changing Paris environment. Because cholera ravaged the popular neighborhoods with great intensity and provoked brutal social unrest at the beginning of the epidemic, everyone believed it to be a disease of only the less fortunate, even though it would soon spread through all classes in the capital. Meanwhile, medical professionals, administrators, and journalists wrote of poorer neighborhoods, like the people who lived in them, as somehow being predisposed to cholera, and they also argued that fear itself might contribute to this predisposition. They concentrated their investigations on the dark, filthy, crowded districts in the center of the city, providing lurid descriptions of the masses, whom they saw as an animal-like horde living in dank, fetid hovels. For their part, the lower classes rose up in bloody riots against what they perceived to be a massive assassination plot by doctors in the service of the state. Believing that the wealthy had invented cholera as a pretext for poisoning them, they took to the streets and literally tore apart the bodies of several suspected poisoners. The grisly disturbances further confirmed the worst fears of bourgeois Parisians. One daily newspaper characteristically complained that "Paris resembles a village of savages," arguing that "these acts of fury that bloody our streets with hideous scenes are no remedy for the sickness, they are nothing but one more sickness [on the heels of revolution]."[12] In 1832 cholera could easily become fused with France's violent revolutionary past, while threatening to propel the capital into a perhaps even more terrifying revolutionary future.

By 1849 a remarkable and puzzling change had occurred in how Parisians understood and approached the epidemic crisis. Despite cholera's significant mortality rate and its arrival less than a year after the bloody 1848 revolution, residents seemed to greet the outbreak with a strange silence. Images of bodies and hearses, elaborate descriptions of first-aid stations, detailed mortality statistics, and lists of charitable donors were absent from accounts in diaries and newspapers alike. Notwithstanding the considerable social unrest in the aftermath of the previous year's bloody "June Days," in which as many as three thousand Parisians died on the barricades,[13] conservative bourgeois commentators did not discuss cholera very much, even as retribution for the sins of the 1848 revolution. Nor was there a revival of the ugly poison riots among the populace. Most strikingly, metaphors of urban and social pathology had largely disappeared from medical reports and public commentary. The question then becomes one of explaining a paradox: how is it that during the late 1840s, the very time when class had become the dominant framework for interpreting social experience in France, cholera was no longer understood in these terms?

Another way to frame the problem is by explaining it in terms of a "silence" that greeted the second epidemic. Used by most contemporaries who contrasted the two epidemics, the word *silence* also serves as a rhetorical shorthand for an intricate set of cultural responses that cast both the disease and reactions to it in a new light. Not the result of a deliberate policy of censorship or even a literal stifling of sentiment, the silence refers to the greater restraint displayed in virtually all responses to the second epidemic in the press, memoirs, medical reports, government circulars, and the behavior of the poor. Parisians discussed cholera less frequently and in less detail and at the same time stopped relying upon a vocabulary of social pathology to do so. At one level, this silence suggests actual quantitative gaps in documentation and the problem of trying to reconstruct a history from negative fragments. From this perspective, responses to cholera in 1849 appear to be but a pale, negative version of what came before, such as Parisians *failing* to riot or *not* describing the poor as barbarians. But, on another level, the silence had a distinctive character. The second epidemic established its own reality, one that both reflected and shaped prevailing attitudes about disease and the Paris environment. In 1849, for example, a clearer sense of cooperation among city administrators, doctors, and Church officials replaced the tensions and conflicts that had characterized their interactions during the first outbreak. Moreover, a public rhetoric of compassion and calls for granting the urban poor a certain respect replaced the angry, bitter words that had condemned victims of the disease only seventeen years before.

This silence was largely the responsibility of the Parisian bourgeoisie. The medical professionals, administrators, and journalists who spoke, whether consciously or unconsciously, in the name of their class left the vast majority of the documents depicting the epidemics.[14] Through such diverse means as pamphlets, case reports, newspaper articles and editorials, statistics, works of literature, and official correspondence written at the time of each outbreak, these people created cholera's historical record. At the same time, however, because they occupied positions that either required or compelled them to write about the outbreaks, they participated in shaping what I shall call a distinct epidemic reality—the responses to and perceptions of the outbreak—influenced by their own sense of class identity. Not always hegemonic actors seeking to impose a particular view of the disease and its consequences, theirs was what I call an "unwitting agency." Although they sought to depict an objective truth and produce a neutral recounting of events, for example, they in fact could not help presenting a highly subjective portrait of cholera based on their background, training, and experiences as members of the Parisian ruling classes.

By contrasting the vivid reactions in 1832 with the apparent silence in 1849, this book explores the complex process by which a disease acquired vastly different social and cultural meanings over a relatively short period of time. In taking such an approach, I have built on a rich and diverse literature that discusses the 1832 cholera epidemic in France. Because earlier works have already related the narrative of events,[15] medical policies,[16] demography,[17] and responses in the provinces,[18] I have been free to employ an interdisciplinary, sometimes eclectic, approach in the pages that follow. Earlier studies have tended to view cholera either as a catalyst for bringing social change or as a focal point for understanding government policy and urban social relations. For example, in *Une Peur bleue: Histoire du choléra en France* Patrice Bourdelais and Jean-Yves Raulot use cholera to analyze epidemiological data, to indicate trends in professionalization, and to map the complex hierarchical structure of medical administration throughout France in the 1832 and 1854 epidemics.[19] Similarly, George Sussman gauges the subtle shifts in medical ideas and administration policies during the early nineteenth century by looking at yellow fever and cholera.[20] Both of these important works consider urban social relations as peripheral to the significance of cholera.

Because of the class dimension of my analysis, I have been most directly engaged in a scholarly debate with Louis Chevalier and François Delaporte, both of whom have made significant—and controversial—contributions to the field. Writing in the late 1950s, Chevalier argued that the Paris environment produced particular pathological behaviors among the city's lower classes, behaviors that resulted ultimately from a form of biological determinism. By focusing on the "importance of biological facts in the description of social facts," he asserted that, especially during the 1832 cholera epidemic, class antagonisms were articulated in biological terms.[21] When the "dangerous classes" took to the streets in times of revolution or cholera, they did not do so out of political or even personal motivations; rather, according to Chevalier, the Parisian workers of the early nineteenth century were motivated by base instincts generated by the pathological Paris environment.

While Chevalier provided valuable analytic tools, he also put forth a highly disturbing thesis, which I challenge in this book. Juxtaposing a close reading of literary texts by such writers as Victor Hugo, Eugène Sue, and Honoré de Balzac with the more "objective," "scientific" statistical studies of urban investigators such as Louis René Villermé and A.-J. B. Parent-Duchâtelet, Chevalier created a richly documented and chilling portrait of the deepest fears of an anxious Parisian bourgeoisie under the Restoration and the July Monarchy. But even as a careful and resourceful chronicler of bourgeois opinion, he did not subject these views or their purveyors to critical scrutiny. As a result, we are left with the impression that Chevalier accepted the bourgeois verdict of the pathological, barbaric state of the poor at face value and that these views had emerged from the definitive voice of a wholly unified class of Parisian men. A closer look at the groups who shaped perceptions of the epidemics reveals that they were engaged in a variety of internal struggles that ultimately shaped how they approached cholera and the problem of the urban poor. Moreover, we need only look to the silence of 1849 to challenge Chevalier's assertions that the bourgeois views of the lower classes remained essentially unchanged in the middle of the nineteenth century; since his study stopped just short of the 1848 revolution, he did not have to address such questions as why the lower classes failed to misbehave when cholera returned, and what this new behavior meant for bourgeois opinion.

Published nearly thirty years after Chevalier's work, Delaporte's *Disease and Civilization* relied upon a similar class dichotomy, but Delaporte asserted that "practices" in fact defined cholera more than any objective reality of the disease.[22] For Delaporte, urban social relations emerged as an intricate web among the medical community, the government, and the lower classes during the 1832 outbreak. Unlike Chevalier, Delaporte saw these interrelationships as power relations aimed specifically at controlling the lower classes. As a result, he offered a valuable critique of the French medical establishment at the time of the first epidemic, one that makes a convincing case for reading between the lines of any official pronouncement about cholera. Unfortunately, Delaporte frequently went too far by presenting the Parisian bourgeoisie as conspiratorial villains, such as when he claimed they saw the epidemic as "a eugenic solution to a pressing social problem."[23] But even if the upper classes' social and political agenda shaped their interpretations of disease and popular responses to it, I argue that the motives and actions were not as clearly defined nor as blatantly oppressive as Delaporte implied.

To move beyond Chevalier and Delaporte, this study draws upon the ideas and methodology of social and cultural history, along with the histories of medicine, religion, politics, and institutions. In bringing these various fields together, it does not claim to offer a definitive history of either epidemic, nor does it fully respect traditional disciplinary boundaries. Instead, cholera serves as an opportunity for exploring larger issues: the cultural aspects of class formation, the unanticipated role of medicine in the creation of France's revolutionary tradition, and the process by which a particular set of ideas and values came to shape a unique sense of bourgeois identity in the mid-nineteenth century. Rather than take the bourgeoisie as an unproblematic category, as both Chevalier and Delaporte have done, I want to show the vital interplay between the epidemics and the creation of a bourgeois sense of identity. Using the insights of Michel Foucault and "the new cultural history," I see bourgeois Parisians more critically than Chevalier, yet more sympathetically than Delaporte.

Though Foucault never wrote anything about cholera per se, his work offers many conceptual and methodological insights.[24] First, he provided a new perspective on how medicine played a key role in establishing the dynamics of urban social relations in post-revolutionary France. By introducing the concepts of "bio-power" and "noso-politics," Foucault opened the way for seeing medical knowledge as a potentially invidious form of unplanned social and cultural domination.[25] For example, his sensitivity to the primacy of medical discourse in creating the population as a subject of clinical investigation helps explain how class could be defined in biological as well as social terms. Essentially, while other scholars showed how medicine and politics (in the form of parliamentary participation or defending liberal economic interests) were inseparable, Foucault carried this idea further to argue that medicine was itself a form of political discourse. Seen in this way, not only could an event such as cholera alter the position of doctors in French government and society, but it also could influence the very nature of their relationship.

Second, Foucault offered important conceptual tools for exploring the formation of bourgeois identity in Paris. One of his major underlying concerns was to examine the mechanisms of normalization in Western society through such topics as criminality, deviance, and sexuality.[26] While he did not set out to write a history of the European bourgeoisie, his preoccupation with how society elicits conformity made the dissemination of bourgeois values a cornerstone of his analysis. In order to understand the process of normalization at work, Foucault argued, one needs to go to the very heart of what a given culture takes for granted and subject these underlying assumptions to rigorous scrutiny. In the case of modern Europe, this analysis requires acknowledging the Enlightenment's darker side by suggesting that sacred positivist concepts such as "objectivity," "facts"—and even "truth" itself—are inherently subjective. By unraveling the complex process of normalization and by questioning the foundations of bourgeois values, Foucault helped open the way for increasing our awareness of the many ways in which bourgeois Parisians both knowingly and unknowingly created different perceptions of cholera and urban social relations.

Foucault also contributed to our understanding of bourgeois identity formation by offering a fresh way of seeing and defining power.[27] Rather than viewing it as something concrete that can be exchanged, fought over, or lost, Foucault saw power more abstractly as grounded in a complex grid of relations that often operates at the most banal level of daily life. Every human exchange, from those with government officials to family dynamics, suggests the workings of power. Being both intentional and nonsubjective, power is exercised internally and not always consciously as opposed to being imposed by a willful outside agent. In other words, power does not come from the "top down" or even from the "bottom up" because it flows from no central place that would be easy to pinpoint. The decentralized, fragmented, unstable, yet pervasive aspects of Foucault's definition of power suggest ways that we might move beyond seeing bourgeois Parisians as willfully oppressive, coercive, and greedy by offering a theoretical guide for understanding the exercise of bourgeois domination in all its complexity.

As a work in the new cultural history, this book departs from previous studies of responses to epidemic disease by placing greater emphasis on the role of language and discourse as forms of cultural expression.[28] The study of symbolic actions such as poison riots or the juxtaposition of disease and revolution, for example, supplement close readings of written documents such as medical reports and newspaper accounts. To this end, I have chosen to rely upon some seemingly obscure literary documents and memoirs rather than upon the more frequently cited works by writers such as Hugo and Sue, who used cholera as a plot device years after the actual outbreaks. Because works such as Eugène Roch's *Paris malade* and Jules Janin's *Paris depuis la révolution de 1830* were produced and appeared at the height of the epidemic crisis, they serve as good complements to the medical, administrative, religious, and journalistic sources from the same period. Only by juxtaposing so many diverse historical voices can we gain a full understanding of the complex reasons behind the different responses to each epidemic.

Likewise, scholarly developments in postmodernism, combined with the experience of writing this book during the AIDS epidemic, have suggested the need to pay particularly close attention to the *process* by which cholera acquired various meanings. The works of Foucault, Joan Scott, and Edward Said, along with the revolution in scholarship they inspired, present a compelling case for never taking cultural outcomes for granted.[29] After deconstructing the complex process by which language, institutional frameworks, educational structures, and other forms of discourse shape such monolithic Givens as sexuality, gender, and race, I found that the idea of treating cholera in analogous terms came naturally. Moreover, as an unfolding drama, the AIDS epidemic constantly reminded me to approach social responses to cholera as a dynamic rather than a static process. The early AIDS activists who challenged the mainstream media's depictions of the disease and of gay men not only made the mechanisms constructing an epidemic reality more visible but also made the working of the mechanisms themselves a central aspect of the epidemic story. While the Parisian press of the 1830s and 1840s bears almost no resemblance to that of my own day, the constant critique of the media and its depiction of AIDS could not help but make me read nineteenth-century representations with some of the same questions in mind.

Finally, unlike other studies of the Parisian epidemics, my book consciously explores the complex question of how historical agency functions. Through the idea of unwitting agency, I argue for a subtle understanding of "social control." Responses to cholera and urban social relations were shaped as much by unintended actions, experiments, and accidents as they were by self-conscious actors who successfully managed to impose their ideas. As I observed the medical professionals, administrators, and journalists who struggled to make sense of both outbreaks, I realized that even though few individuals significantly changed the course of a given epidemic, all of them nonetheless contributed to shaping that reality by acting in their own interests, which on the surface may have had little to do with cholera. The real targets and avenues of power were not always obvious to contemporaries or historians; some individuals could exercise power without being aware of this fact, just as they could believe themselves to be wielding it while ultimately contributing very little. Put another way, while a coherent image of cholera and bourgeois culture surfaced in the wake of each outbreak, no privileged voice emerged to tell the epidemic story.

Cholera itself enjoyed undeniable historical agency, simultaneously influencing and being defined by the history that surrounded it. As the historian Chantal Beauchamp observed, "Behind disease, there is always something else. More precisely, disease is always and at the same time itself and something different. Collective disease is the part and the whole, the origin and the outcome, the fact and the symbol, inextricably mixed together."[30] Cholera enjoyed historical agency as a killer that inspired fear and hatred. Moreover, cholera prompted important developments such as the creation of new institutions, unprecedented forms of collaboration between government and the medical community, as well as new ways of seeing and describing the Paris environment. But, as demonstrated by the silence of 1849, cholera was also molded by its potential victims. Cholera was a concept that could be shaped and reshaped to serve the needs of whoever sought to depict it, whether in the simple act of sketching a caricature that represented the disease or in the more abstract creation of an epidemic reality in the pages of the popular press. Seen in this way, cholera provides an especially fruitful opportunity for studying a complex form of historical agency, one where the actor and the acted upon not only coexisted but also influenced one another in fundamental ways.

—ʍ—

At first glance, many obvious factors might explain the silence of 1849. Scientific breakthroughs, an improved environment in Paris, government controls, or even a more blasé attitude on encountering cholera a second time—all offer possible reasons why inhabitants of the French capital approached the epidemic so differently. Although some of these factors may have contributed to altering contemporary perceptions of cholera, a critical analysis of them will show that they do not account for the silence. In this analysis, we can gain a sense of what contemporaries actually knew about the disease and what options they perceived they had for fighting it. Moreover, a close look at these factors provides valuable background for understanding the historical context for each epidemic.

Cholera remained a medical mystery well into the early 1850s. The official report, issued in 1850, a year after the second Parisian outbreak, captured the awe that many contemporaries still felt:

> Seeming so independent, [is cholera caused by] variations in temperature and the direction of the wind, [or] is it the result of some sort of electrical phenomena? Does it come from an imbalance of elements in the air we breathe? Should it be explained by the presence of thousands of tiny insects carried by the wind, or by the development of putrid miasmas? Will the future settle our doubts in this regard? Or, as with other diseases, must cholera disappear, after running its more or less long course, taking with it the secret of its cause as well as that of its disappearance?

The report concluded on a note of bittersweet optimism by observing that "the imagination can fear everything just as it can hope for anything."[31] Scientific impressions of cholera in fact appeared to have changed little from the first encounters in 1832. "Where does the cause of cholera reside?" Dr. C. P. Tacheron, a member of the sanitary commission in the Luxembourg quarter, paused to ask midway through his detailed statistical analysis of the first epidemic:

> Is it in the air, in emanations from the earth, in atmospheric influences? Who can point to it? How does it work? Does it come from overexciting the internal organs of the splenetic cavities? From altering the blood? Who can answer [these questions] in a satisfactory and positive manner? . . . The only thing we know for sure is that the disease is new for us, its effects are terrible, its causes and mode of action impenetrable.[32]

As one of the most prominent medical journals succinctly confessed in 1849, "Medicine is as powerless today against cholera as it was during the first epidemic."[33]

This is not to say, however, that scientists remained in complete ignorance.[34] Influenced by traditions of Greek and Roman medicine, French doctors in the first part of the nineteenth century tended to see cholera as the result of an imbalance within the humors of the body as well as between the body and its environment. Oppositional relationships between moisture (wet/dry) and temperature (hot/cold) created a state that determined whether an individual was healthy. For someone perceived to be ill, treatment consisted of attempts to redress an imbalance of these elements with measures such as changes in diet, change in location, raising or lowering body temperature, purging, or starving.

By the time of the first epidemic, when Paris had been the acknowledged capital of the Western medical world for nearly a generation, health officials had begun modifying these classical ideas in several important respects. Most significant for our story, they approached disease less from the standpoint of the individual body and more in relation to its broader environment.[35] This new emphasis had important implications for Parisians' understanding of cholera. First, it focused attention on the problems of the urban milieu, inspiring officials to prescribe preventive measures such as ventilating dwellings and throwing them open to light. Together, the critique of a blighted urban environment and the abandonment of a fatalistic view of disease in favor of one that emphasized avoidance and prevention constituted the core of a public health movement dedicated to fighting cholera. Second, the modified approach to disease created divisions within the nascent medical profession between contagionists (who believed disease was transmitted through direct contact with the body of an infected person) and anticontagionists (who believed it traveled in the air, emanating from the putrid miasmas of the squalid urban environment). While anticontagionism, or "environmentalism," would dominate official responses to epidemics during the middle third of the nineteenth century, contagionism also played a meaningful part, notably in the widely accepted belief that fear predisposed individuals to disease. Officials warned that cholera and panic fed one another as they spread from person to person, reducing a person's ability to resist whatever organism caused the disease.[36]

Scientific advancements later in the century would ultimately prove that both the contagionist and anticontagionist positions had some validity for understanding the mechanisms that transmitted cholera. The discoveries of John Snow (1854) and Robert Koch (1883) would reveal that the disease was carried by the bacillus *vibrio cholerae*, which thrives in warm, humid places, particularly water.[37] Because it strikes the human digestive tract, the only way to catch the disease is by ingesting it directly into the mouth, which can be easily done with infected hands or by eating tainted foods. The bacteria survives up to two weeks in feces; a week in ordinary dust, clothing, or bed linens of former patients; up to three weeks in butter and milk; and several days in fruits and vegetables that have been rinsed with contaminated water.[38] Before medical professionals understood these basic facts about the cause and spread of cholera, however, they arrived at explanations and possible cures based on what was known to them at the time. Because more elaborate ideas about contagion would begin to filter down into common understanding and practice only after the 1849 epidemic, new medical knowledge cannot account for the different responses in 1849.

Nor can the silence be explained by dramatic changes in the Paris environment. Despite a few noteworthy attempts at improvements, such as the extension of the rue Rambuteau during the mid-1840s, the physical quality of life for many in the French capital actually declined between 1832 and 1849. Baron Georges-Eugène Haussmann would not undertake his massive public works projects to rebuild the city until the mid-1850s. In the meantime, the poorer neighborhoods in the center and to the east, areas devastated by the highest number of cholera deaths in both epidemics, seemed to

Table 1   Population and Population Density
of Paris, 1801–1846

	Number *of Inhabitants*	*Density* (per square hectare)
1801	546,856	159
1817	713,966	208
1831	785,866	229
1846	1,053,897	307

SOURCE: Compiled from Louis Chevalier, *Laboring Classes and Dangerous Classes* (Princeton, 1973), 182, 193.

epitomize the dismal conditions of Parisian life. Often described as medieval in character, they were crowded, dark, and dirty. A labyrinth of narrow, winding streets acted as above-ground sewers, carrying a constant stream of slop and human waste. To the west, the wealthier districts suffered similar, though less extreme, overcrowding and uncleanliness.[39]

Perceptions of the city's decline were often linked to concerns about what many believed to be a dramatic increase in the number of people living in misery.[40] The mayor of the twelfth arrondissement in 1849 was especially outspoken about his neighborhood's ongoing deterioration. Writing in a daily newspaper, he complained that it was "troublesome to see concentrated in one place such a large number of inhabitants lodged in hovels tumbling down with decay, when by putting up new buildings one could provide this population with cleaner, more comfortable dwellings."[41] Most of these people were immigrants from the provinces, lured to Paris in search of jobs.[42] As a result, the population of the capital nearly doubled in the first half of the nineteenth century, leaving most inhabitants cramped within the city's unyielding fortifications. Although probably somewhat conservative, the official census figures in table 1 provide a general idea of the size of the city.

Such numbers reflect only an *average* of population density for the entire capital; in some of the older (and poorer) districts of the city, density and cholera mortality ran even higher. Maps accompanying the official government report issued after the 1849 epidemic made the point in particularly graphic terms (see figures 1 and 2). The dramatic influx of poor immigrants from the provinces

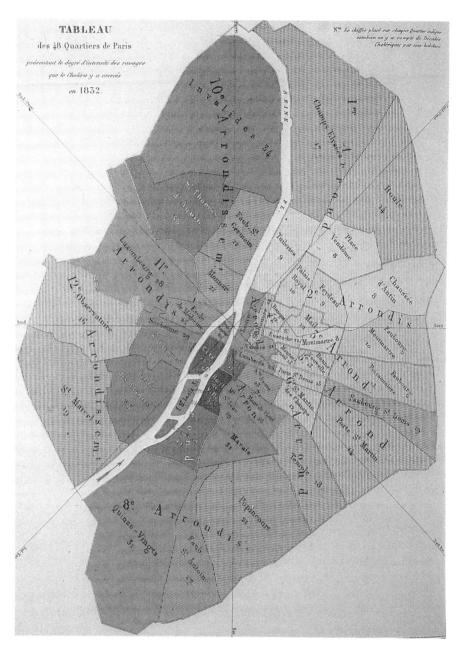

Figure 1. The official map of the 1832 cholera epidemic in Paris. Source: Administration Générale de l'Assistance Publique, *Rapport sur l'épidémie cholérique de 1853–54* (Paris, 1855). Dark portions indicate high cholera mortality.

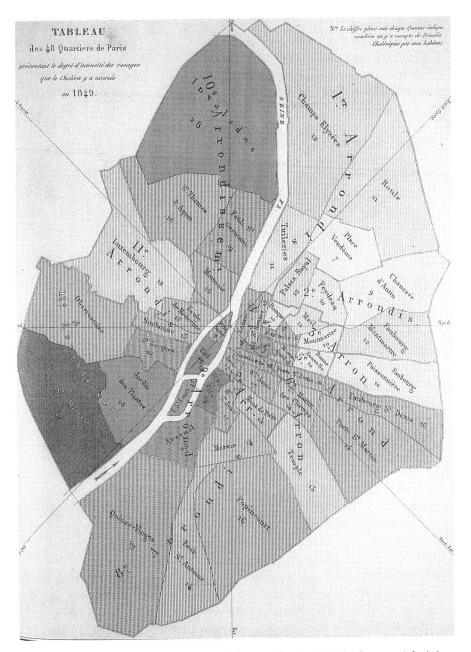

Figure 2. The official map of the 1849 cholera epidemic in Paris. Source: Administration Générale de l'Assistance Publique, *Rapport sur l'épidémie cholérique de 1853–54* (Paris, 1855). Dark portions indicate high cholera mortality.

taxed the capital's already faltering charitable and public-assistance resources, bringing overcrowding to hospitals.[43] The cholera epidemic of 1849 thus hit a city that was overpopulated and poorly equipped to handle an increasing population. Surprisingly, however, this terrifying environment, which was volatile enough to produce a revolution in 1848, did not drive impoverished Parisians into the streets with the arrival of cholera the following year. Even if the ferment in 1848 indicated that people did not quietly accept their lot, their calm in the face of cholera indicated that the disease was no longer threatening in the same way it had been in 1832.

Having eliminated scientific knowledge and the quality of urban life as possible reasons for the silence of 1849, let us next consider the patterns of each outbreak. Charting the actual progress of both epidemics, the government retrospective *Rapport sur les épidémies cholériques de 1832 et 1849* (one of the most explicit comparisons of the two outbreaks, published in 1850) found striking similarities as well as important differences.[44] Both started at almost exactly the same time of the year (March 26, 1832, and March 18, 1849), and both ended the following October. In 1849, as in 1832, the outbreak had a period of strong intensity, followed by relative calm and then a second, though much less extreme, phase of high mortality. But while noticeable, the relatively modest differences between mortality figures explored in the report could not account for the distinct reactions to each epidemic. Even within the context of the city's increasing population, the discrepancy would not warrant such a dramatic change in tone.

Discernible differences become apparent only by examining the impact of cholera on a day-by-day basis. Figures compiled after both epidemics indicated that the largest number of deaths in 1832 occurred within the first three weeks of the outbreak, while seventeen years later mortality was more evenly spread over a longer period.[45] Thus, at the outset, contemporaries were given the impression that, as the bourgeois *Journal des débats politiques et littéraires* put it in April 1849, "it is evident to everyone that the terrible scourge is not what it once was."[46] More important, the longer period of time between the first cases and the peak of the 1849 epidemic gave authorities valuable time to prepare first-aid stations, hospitals, body-removal procedures, and burial facilities. This potential readiness, combined with the fact that some minor improvements had been made in the city's hospitals, meant that officials believed that they needed relatively few extra supplies, services, or government expenditures in 1849.[47] With better facilities and the patient load spread out over a longer period, the administration might have been more adept at handling the crisis posed by the second epidemic. In reality, however, as we shall see, the administration was not well prepared once the second epidemic hit the capital with full force.

And even if the pattern of the epidemics diverged, the average Parisian had no way of knowing or understanding that the second epidemic would be different from the one that preceded it. "Anyone who saw the bacchanals of blood and death will never forget them," wrote a theater critic at the end of the 1832 epidemic. "Anyone who saw insurrection and cholera embracing one another like brother and sister, and running through the streets of the disheveled city will never forget them."[48] Neither officials nor private citizens could predict when or how the outbreak would end in 1849. Thus, the silence cannot be dismissed casually by asserting that Parisians had been through it all before, that experience had somehow made them blasé. Even if authorities had acquired some expertise in organizing and distributing relief, undoubtedly many residents of the capital still carried vivid impressions from their nightmarish encounters with the disease seventeen years earlier.[49] Or, put another way, if a revolutionary tradition associated with 1789 and the guillotine could excite old fears in 1830 and 1848, how could Parisians forget an epidemic tradition so easily?

Some might argue that a new, more repressive government helped Parisians "forget" through the imposition of censorship or other controls. As regimes that came to power in the wake of revolutions, the July Monarchy and Second Republic shared both differences and similarities. An experiment in constitutional monarchy, the regime known as the July Monarchy of Louis Philippe (1830–48) brought a limited segment of the French population into the political process. Meanwhile, its successor, the Second Republic (1848–51), at least paid lip service to incorporating a much broader segment of the population. At the same time, however, the president of the new republic, Louis Napoleon, was much more savvy about manipulating public opinion than Louis Philippe had been. Playing off his family name, which he used to promise order and promote stability, Napoleon's nephew made himself all things to all people.[50] Through propaganda that relied on such instruments as the popular press, the government self-consciously created an image of itself while attempting to tame the masses who had taken to the streets in 1848. President Louis Napoleon aggressively manipulated public opinion, a fact that might have influenced the regime's strategy in regard to cholera.

A careful look at how each regime approached censorship and the popular press, however, reveals that these policies cannot account for the silence that greeted the second epidemic. In fact, during the spring of 1849, newspapers may have actually enjoyed more freedom than they did in 1832, despite the powerful rhetoric supporting a free press used by the July Monarchy. Coming to power after the 1830 revolution, which had been sparked by the repressive censorship policies of the previous Restoration government, the July Monarchy openly defended freedom of the press, even actively incorporating it into its public image. Journalists had fought on the barricades in 1830 and had goaded a reluctant Louis Philippe into accepting the crown.[51] At the same time, however, anxious officials, including the king himself, were deeply ambivalent about the press, an institution that they believed openly fomented opposition. In the wake of frequent incidents of social unrest during its turbulent early years, the regime quickly became one of the most zealous persecutors of the press.[52] Between 1830 and 1833 Parisian newspapers had a record 150 condemnations "for offenses against political order"; 1832 was a particularly lively year for trials in the cour d'assises, with sixty-nine cases involving the press alone.[53] Despite its public rhetoric defending an open and free press, then, the July Monarchy in fact responded defensively, particularly during its early years, a period that coincided with the first outbreak.

In the case of the 1849 epidemic, numerous obstacles prevented the Second Republic from controlling news of cholera completely. Even if critics of the regime complained that officials had deliberately chosen to downplay the 1849 outbreak,[54] no archival evidence indicates the existence of a deliberate policy of tampering with cholera news.[55] Moreover, beginning in late March and continuing throughout the epidemic, a battery of large advertisements for remedies, reminiscent of those that appeared in 1832, were displayed prominently in newspapers that carried little other information about the disease. This commercial subtext suggests that Parisians at some level had to know that an epidemic was ravaging their city, and thus the apparent silence could not be wholly attributed to an administrative cover-up that kept them in ignorance. In fact, the regime, which had grown increasingly conservative and repressive during the months since Louis Napoleon's election as president in December 1848, imposed its most restrictive censorship policies on June 13, 1849—that is, only *after* the second epidemic had peaked.[56] And even if officials had consciously sought to downplay the epidemic by relegating it to the back pages of newspapers, much of the news in the 1840s was still transmitted orally, particularly among the lower classes, who would be most likely to riot. Given the relatively high cost and poor availability of many Parisian dailies even after 1848 and given the lack of leisure time available to workers for reading newspapers, stories about cholera were likely to spread as easily and quickly by word of mouth as they were by the printed page.[57] In fact, if the same popular attitude toward cholera had persisted from the first epidemic, it seems likely that the discrepancy between the official silence and the unofficial cures would itself have provoked major riots. Censorship, then, cannot account for the subdued response to the second epidemic either.

—⚑—

Since neither scientific breakthroughs, a changed Parisian environment, a blasé attitude, political machinations, nor censorship can explain the silence of 1849, we must look at broad issues unique to French society and culture in the first half of the nineteenth century. To understand the qualitative differences between how Parisians responded in 1832 and in 1849, I shall argue, we must look beyond the epidemics themselves to the capital's revolutionary tradition and the development of bourgeois identity over the course of the July Monarchy. The combination of these two elements played a powerful role in shaping attitudes toward cholera and class, which enabled Parisians to see the disease's arrival differently in 1849. Medical documents, government circulars, and accounts in the popular press all made class *the* salient point about the first outbreak, while playing it down during the second. Descriptions of cholera's apparent preference for the poor easily blended with discussions of social unrest and revolution to create the image of a disease defined as much in social terms as biological or medical ones.

The historical context of revolution, France's "revolutionary tradition," was central to all Parisians' understanding of both class and cholera during each outbreak.[58] While it is not within the scope of this book to engage fully with the historical debates between Marxists and revisionists over whether the French Revolution was driven principally by class conflict, I use the basic notion of class and class conflict ignited in 1789 and growing over the nineteenth century as a point of departure for understanding responses to both cholera epidemics.[59] The struggle between a newly empowered, extremely defensive bourgeoisie and a newly liberated "people" would continue to be played out over the course of the nineteenth century, with the bourgeoisie eventually achieving dominance. Broadly speaking, by dismantling seigneurialism, abolishing privilege, and ultimately overthrowing the monarchy, the revolution of 1789 had helped bring bourgeois Parisians to power politically and economically, while the revolutions in 1830 and 1848 solidified their social position. At the same time, the revolutionary events created a rhetoric as well as a historical precedent that allowed the less-fortunate classes to play an increasingly active, visible, and even self-conscious political role that threatened the still-precarious hold of the Parisian bourgeoisie.[60] But because the first revolutionary experiment had quickly dissolved into the Terror and bloodshed of 1793–94, perceptions of popular rebellion in Paris became closely linked with irrational violence.

Such a backdrop of revolutionary turmoil dominated social relations in the capital throughout much of the nineteenth century, particularly since images and ideas from 1789 and 1793–94 often appeared explicitly in the rhetoric of subsequent revolutions. This phenomenon was especially apparent during the first cholera outbreak, when contemporaries so readily conflated the epidemic with social unrest. But even in 1849, when few commented on the connections between disease and revolt, the fear of revolution helped inspire a more patronizing approach to the arrival of cholera. Hoping not to ignite new violence after the bloodshed of 1848, officials consciously backed away from inflammatory language and accusations against the lower classes. In effect, by creating a universalist language of rights in a context that was socially and economically inegalitarian, 1789 and its ensuing revolutionary tradition produced deep-rooted social antagonisms that would influence responses in both 1832 and 1849.[61]

The mysterious disease and the social unrest that accompanied it also helped reinforce a sense of identity, albeit a fragmented one, among the bourgeois Parisians who wrote about the events. But before exploring this identity, it is first necessary to have some basic understanding of who was "bourgeois" and what it meant to be one in Paris at the time of cholera. While I do not claim to provide the simple definition that has eluded both historians and contemporaries, I would like to devote the remainder of this chapter to introducing some basic assumptions and ideas that will enable us to consider the formation of Parisian bourgeois identity and its relationship to cholera.[62]

Because of Karl Marx's influential writings on the origins of capitalism and the French Revolution, both Marxist and non-Marxist scholars have framed the bourgeoisie more in economic and social terms than in cultural ones.[63] Seen in this way, the bourgeois Parisian might be characterized as someone who earned an income that enabled him to pay a certain amount in rent and taxes, employ servants, and enjoy a comfortable standard of material living—an income that would ultimately permit him to pay for a respectable funeral. According to these criteria, the Parisian bourgeoisie was dominated by bankers, industrialists, and financial speculators, as well as by members of the liberal professions and civil service. Using tax records and inventories collected after deaths, the foremost historian of the Parisian bourgeoisie estimated that approximately 15 percent of the city's total population fell within this group.[64]

In addition to basic economic and material criteria, the bourgeois of the July Monarchy were defined by a common social and political heritage that distinguished them from the country's declining aristocracy. Having emerged triumphant in the revolution of 1830, for example, they enjoyed the power and privileges of a group newly liberated from the temporary political exclusion imposed on them by the Restoration monarchy (1815–30). During this time the bourgeoisie had devoted their frustrated ambitions to areas of little interest to the aristocracy such as capital investment, manufacture, and education for professional careers. Their financial supremacy would eventually provide the economic advantage that would enable them to supplant the aristocracy in French politics and society. This was not a "hostile takeover" however; bourgeois Parisians also absorbed willing aristocrats into their ranks through marriage. This arrangement further strengthened bourgeois credibility, power, and social standing at the same time that it enhanced the position of the declining nobility.[65]

While an economic and social approach to defining the Parisian ruling classes provides a valuable initial portrait of the men who responded to the cholera epidemics, we need to look closely at other factors that might explain how they saw themselves and their class. In order to broaden the definition, we must recognize an intriguing paradox: a highly fragmented (and, as we have seen, relatively small) group understood itself as having a universalizing role in French society. This paradox lies at the center of what it meant to be bourgeois. Perhaps Henri Gisquet, the prefect of police during the 1832 cholera epidemic, put it best. "The bourgeoisie is too numerous [and] consists of too many [diverse] elements to enable me to offer any statistics," he explained in his memoirs, displaying uncharacteristic insight. "Besides," he added, "this work would be superfluous: everyone knows what is the bourgeoisie; it represents the vast majority of the population."[66] Or, according to one historian, the concept of a middle class itself was both pervasive and elusive, being elusive precisely because it was so pervasive.[67] Many contemporaries used terms such as "bourgeois" and "middle class" interchangeably with phrases such as "the intermediate classes," "the better-off classes," "the fortunate classes," or "the privileged persons of the capital." Thus (as with many scholars today), some writers saw implicit differences among the concepts, while others used them synonymously, a fact that makes it extremely difficult to arrive at a clear understanding of how contemporaries viewed their own social standing or class identity.

As Gisquet also pointed out, the term covered a vast and diverse number of people who defied easy categorization.[68] Within the ranks of the middle classes themselves, for example, there existed a discernible social hierarchy. The elite group, which I shall call "bourgeois," contained the professional segment of the middle classes most likely to play a significant role in defining and perpetuating values in mid-nineteenth-century Paris: members of liberal professions such as law and medicine, bankers, upper-level government employees, social commentators, men of letters, and legislators.[69] Here could be found the medical professionals, administrators, and journalists who would play such an important part in shaping perceptions of cholera. Below them were men engaged in trade and commerce, shop owners, office workers, bookkeepers, petty functionaries, and highly skilled artisans, to name but a few.[70] For purposes of clarity, the term *middle classes* is used here in the broadest and most inclusive sense and includes anyone who did not belong to the aristocracy or to the working classes.[71] The definition is further complicated by the fact that not all middle-class Parisians held the same values, and even if they did, the countless varieties of human experience prevented any two people from defining or living them in the same way.[72] As we shall see, for example, not all members of the intermediate classes supported the policies of the July Monarchy, the regime whose early critics sarcastically dubbed it "bourgeois," the very label it later embraced so proudly.[73] Many middle-class Parisians had thrived during the later years of the Restoration, which had made its own concessions to bourgeois interests with the creation of a constitutional monarchy that would offer some, albeit limited, inspiration for its successor.[74] The July Monarchy and the Second Republic, meanwhile, often angered bourgeois citizens.

So many differences encouraged an almost desperate search for common ground and ultimately a drive to make bourgeois values universal, just as Gisquet baldly claimed. This push to universalize helps us arrive at a sketch of the shared ingrained assumptions, values, and "collective emotions" that emerged in reactions to cholera and the establishment of bourgeois identity.[75] At the most intimate level, cholera helped articulate bourgeois attitudes about the human body, bodily functions, and personal cleanliness by providing a truly repulsive challenge.[76] The very symptoms of the disease undermined ideas of bourgeois decorum in the ongoing "civilizing process" that reached an apogee in the nineteenth century. Just when bourgeois Parisians were seeking most self-consciously to distance themselves from the physicality associated with the barbarous underworld of the poor, cholera made it a very public part of lived experience. For a proper bourgeois, the thought of dying from the dehydration caused by incessant vomiting and diarrhea just like some poor artisan or homeless person took on nightmarish qualities.[77] By providing an opportunity to articulate these horrors, the outbreak of cholera in 1832 helped underscore a sense of identity among bourgeois Parisians by revealing exactly how their lives differed from other victims of the epidemic.

More publicly, bourgeois Parisians displayed a common set of values that originated in the Enlightenment, got filtered through the French Revolution, and were pushed even further by positivist thinkers such as Auguste Comte. Faith in science and the human ability to reason, the importance of education and learning to interpret facts for oneself, as well as skepticism regarding religious authority and institutions could be traced to the writings of the philosophes. Representative government, the importance of private property, the need for order, balance, and moderation, and the rhetoric of equality also became a part of bourgeois culture in the nineteenth century. Finally, bourgeois Parisians saw themselves as participants in transforming a public sphere that gave them an increasing voice in government.[78] As members of the professions, they claimed responsibility for running the machinery of a state they would shape according to their values of order, rationality, equality, and transparency. Put another way, during the July Monarchy Enlightenment values became widespread among members of the Parisian bourgeoisie.[79]

The French Revolution provided an environment in which many of these Enlightenment ideas could be put into practice.[80] Events begun in 1789 affected the bourgeois response to cholera in three major ways. First, the Revolution created a climate in which bourgeois occupations such as medicine, administration, and journalism could thrive and become central to telling the epidemic story. As we shall see, revolutionary changes would not only nurture the development of these professions but would also redefine the ways in which their work was carried out. Second, the decline of the aristocracy as the dominant, dynamic force in France after 1789, and especially after 1830, helped place bourgeois Parisians in a bipartite social structure that pitted them against the poor. Less concerned with wresting power from their superiors, they now sought to maintain it in the face of their inferiors. Finally, because the promise of 1789 so quickly deteriorated into the Terror of 1793–94 and because the events liberated the *whole* of the Third Estate (the poor as well as the middle classes), bourgeois Parisians would have an ambivalent relationship to revolution through much of the following century. Put simply, the event that had given them power constantly reminded them that it could be easily taken away.

Such shared values and history brought the Parisian bourgeoisie together through a unique process of identity formation that accompanied each outbreak.[81] During the 1832 epidemic middle-class Parisians forged a sense of who they were through opposition. At the most immediate level, the crisis required doctors and administrators to work together in a way they never had before. Faced with an emergency of unprecedented magnitude, these men came to rely upon one another while creating and perpetuating a common set of assumptions about how the disease should be seen and treated.

Furthermore, by stimulating medical professionals and government officials to address problems in the urban environment, cholera made the lives of the poor dramatically visible to many middle-class Parisians for the first time. The increasingly large numbers of immigrants from the provinces who made their way to the capital in search of jobs during the 1820s and 1830s frequently lived in extreme poverty. According to some estimates, one in three Parisians died after a life very much on the margin of subsistence, while as many as one in ten of the city's inhabitants wandered the streets indigent and begging.[82] Even if the majority of those fortunate enough to find jobs worked in small-scale shops in the textile and building industries, the proliferation of *petits métiers* such as street musicians, ragpickers, pet groomers, water porters, and street hawkers became a source of concern to police officials, who viewed them as disturbing the peace or even as potential threats to social order.[83] With as much as 79 percent of the population consisting of individuals living in poverty,[84] medical investigations, police reports, and newspaper accounts highlighted a growing gulf between the haves and the have-nots, while providing the qualitative data that made bourgeois Parisians see the poor in new ways.

In other words, the 1832 epidemic helped foster a sense of identity among bourgeois Parisians by highlighting the vast differences that separated them from those beneath them on the social ladder. French middle-class men (like their American[85] and British[86] counterparts) were more likely to articulate who they were *not*. When these Parisians described their society as being divided into two basic camps, they emphasized the "them" more than the "us" in the relationship. For example, few of the documents about cholera ever used the pronoun "we" to refer to collective action taken by or for the middle classes.[87] Rather, they focused attention squarely on the habits and habitats of people unlike themselves, using contrast to develop a refracted sense of who they were.[88] Seen in this way, bourgeois identity in 1832 came more from facing a common enemy than from celebrating a shared sense of consciousness comparable to the one scholars have traced among the working classes.

Such a refracted sense of identity could be articulated in both conscious and less conscious ways. As we shall see, for example, medical documents, government circulars, newspaper articles, and statistical reports all portrayed responses to cholera as a battle between the haves and the have-nots (be it in reference to disease or to wealth), concepts shaped by bourgeois experience. Moreover, individual actions such as charitable contributions that were conspicuously publicized in the pages of the bourgeois press helped further to delineate class differences; such gestures were directed at the poor but also benefited the wealthy. Even acts not directly related to cholera such as serving in the bourgeois enclave of National Guard troops brought bourgeois men together in the face of a common enemy. The Guard, which often helped maintain order in the absence of a professional police force during the early years of the regime, was called upon to put down insurrections and generally to maintain public order during the social unrest that accompanied the 1832 outbreak.[89]

Bourgeois Parisians could forge a basic sense of identity by defining themselves against a "them" in 1832 for two reasons. First, even when they seemed to be on the defensive, these citizens, more than those either above or below them, tended to take themselves and their culture for granted. As Gisquet's understanding of the bourgeoisie demonstrated, the group viewed its world as a universalizing one in the nineteenth century. Believing themselves at the pinnacle of civilization, they seldom considered that other ways of life or other values might be preferable to their own. In a sense, bourgeois Parisians pictured their values as a "default setting" so universal and so obvious that they required little explanation or justification.[90] Second, this emphasis on the "them" helped resolve an apparent paradox by providing a sense of cohesion for a group whose principal underlying ideology stressed the importance of individual initiative.[91] By defining themselves by who they were not, bourgeois Parisians could maintain their cherished status as individuals because they did not have to actively embrace a collective identity that might threaten their individuality. Put linguistically, this group held onto the "I" by creating an identity based on "they" rather than "we." Because they saw their culture as a given, and because they derived a principal part of their identity by looking outward at who they were *not,* bourgeois Parisians developed a sense of affinity more than a true sense of identity or consciousness during the first epidemic.

By 1849, I shall argue, bourgeois Parisians had a stronger sense of who they were and had internalized the rhetoric, along with the confidence, for expressing it. The years between the two epidemics saw the growing consolidation of economic, political, and social power among the Parisian middle classes. The July Monarchy's emphasis on laissez-faire economics and encouragement of capitalist investment, epitomized by Prime Minister François Guizot's famous invitation to "get rich," created a climate conducive to bourgeois economic domination. Politically, the constitutional monarchy accepted representative government, acknowledging the right of the property-owning citizen to share power with the crown. In addition to enjoying a growing voice in the legislative assembly, members of the Parisian bourgeoisie were increasingly drawn into government power by being called upon as experts during the 1830s and 1840s. Meanwhile, after years of limited circulation and having only a back seat in political affairs, the press became a powerful mouthpiece for bourgeois values as it expanded during the July Monarchy. Socially, the middle classes had also begun to take control, as evidenced by the consolidation and growing influence of numerous professions such as medicine, law, and psychiatry during the 1830s and 1840s.[92]

While the events of 1848 enhanced the terrifying portrait of revolution, bourgeois Parisians were shaken but remained in control. With the establishment of a republic, the working classes had been brought more directly into the political process through universal male suffrage and thus were spared some of the overt criticisms they had once endured. While their increased political participation represented an important gain for the disaffected lower classes, it did not mean that members of the bourgeoisie fully accepted them as equal partners or even that they no longer feared the Parisian crowd.[93] On the contrary, this very fear inspired bourgeois politicians, administrators, and others to test a more conciliatory strategy for winning over their enemies. As the chapters that follow will show, a concrete sense of bourgeois identity would be essential in shaping responses to cholera and the lower classes in 1849.

—ɷ—

The following chapters are organized thematically rather than chronologically so that we might focus more directly on the processes by which bourgeois Parisians created perceptions of the epidemics and their own sense of identity. The first chapter places responses to cholera in a historical and social context. To offer a point of comparison for the early nineteenth century, the first part describes the role of epidemic diseases and attitudes toward them during the old regime. The remainder introduces the relationship between disease and revolution during the 1832 epidemic to demonstrate the deepest fears of bourgeois Parisians. Chapter 2 looks more closely at "cholera's messengers," the three groups that shaped perceptions of disease and the Paris environment during both epidemics: medical professionals, administrators, and journalists. It explores the forces that enabled these representatives of bourgeois culture to paint themselves and the epidemics in the particular way they did. Turning to the actual responses to each outbreak, Chapter 3 looks closely at the distribution of preventive instructions, the establishment of first-aid stations, and the reporting of statistical data to the Parisian public to understand how cholera's messengers collaborated and competed amongst themselves. Chapter 4 takes up the question of what happened when these groups confronted a fundamental outside challenge to their authority in the form of the Catholic Church and describes the complex synthesis of cultural authority that emerged as a result. The fifth chapter tests the hypotheses about bourgeois culture put forth in the rest of the book by offering a close reading of the responses to urban social unrest that accompanied each epidemic. The revolt of the ragpickers, the poison riots, and the unrest that accompanied the funeral of General Maximilien Lamarque in 1832 offer intriguing contrasts with the insurrection of June 13, which coincided with the period of peak mortality, and the strange silence that greeted cholera just seventeen years later.

1

The Epidemic
and Revolutionary
Traditions of Paris

When cholera first arrived during the spring of 1832, bourgeois
Parisians not only had to confront the epidemic and its causes but
also had to face a set of hard realities about life in the capital. For
over three decades Paris had been attracting an ever-increasing
number of restless immigrants from the provinces who settled principally in the poorer outer districts such as the faubourg Saint-
Antoine and the faubourg Saint-Jacques as well as in the center of
the city around Notre Dame and Les Halles. Finding little or no
work, many crowded into small apartments and spilled onto the
streets, where they forced medical professionals, administrators,
and—eventually—journalists to explore the terrifying dark side of
progress. Cholera seemed to confirm bourgeois Parisians' worst
nightmares by giving their anxieties an almost haunting visibility.
Accounts of the epidemic provided lurid descriptions of the city's
filthiest, most congested neighborhoods and of the "barbarians"
who inhabited these "hotbeds [*foyers*] of infection." These fears in
turn helped to shape perceptions of the epidemic reality in 1832.

Most significantly, during the first outbreak growing anxieties
about the decaying urban environment merged with the capital's
revolutionary tradition. Events in 1789, 1793–94, and 1830 had left
powerful legends of bloodshed and death that provided a core narrative against which all catastrophes could be measured. Once the
social and political landscape had been completely transformed by
the willful creation of a republic and the concomitant rethinking
of all aspects of public life in 1789–94, it would be impossible to
interpret any significant social event without at least raising the
question of how it related to the country's revolutionary past. Thus,
when cholera arrived on the heels of the 1830 revolution, it seemed
almost inevitable that contemporaries should willingly seize upon

the tradition as a means for making sense of a mysterious new epidemic.

This chapter explores the depths of bourgeois anxiety during the July Monarchy by looking at the historical context that gave cholera special significance. I begin with a brief discussion of attitudes toward epidemic disease and attempts to combat it during the old regime to offer a point of comparison for the later horror in the face of cholera. Next, the chapter examines the fusion of disease into the French revolutionary tradition, which culminated in the 1832 epidemic. Beginning with a discussion of how bourgeois Parisians came to see Paris as a "sick city" even before the arrival of cholera, this second section concludes with an analysis of the ways in which Parisians constantly compared the disease to revolution. Rather than juxtapose geographic maps of cholera mortality with those of political discontent in search of direct lines of causation, I explore the historical context to suggest how and why disease and revolution had become fused not just chronologically but also metaphorically in the minds of bourgeois Parisians. More revealing than quantitative links in this regard is how contemporaries perceived the relationship, how they used it to make sense of subsequent historical developments, as well as how these interpretations affected government policy, class relations, and the role of medicine in the development of modern society. The final section of the chapter examines how cholera exacerbated sharp distinctions between the haves and the have-nots, which had been growing since 1789. By focusing on medical discourse, official pronouncements, and discussions in the popular press, I want to show just how far bourgeois Parisians could go in attempting to create distance between themselves and the poor, and how this distance in turn could affect perceptions of the new disease in 1832.

DISEASE AND POVERTY
IN THE OLD REGIME

Endemic and epidemic disease were integral parts of life in early-modern France, particularly in the rural areas inhabited by the large majority of the country's population. Outbreaks of "enteric fevers" (typhoid), typhus, smallpox, scarlet fever, dysentery, syphilis, measles, diphtheria, and influenza regularly ravaged local towns and villages, as did epidemics of cattle plague, which had dire economic consequences during the eighteenth century. Weather and crop failure further compounded the effects of disease. Such occurrences were both routine and devastating, thus investing human life with a precarious quality that geared it toward immediate survival.[1]

Subjected to such whims of nature, the majority of people living in the old regime—regardless of their social standing—did not instinctively look to far-away government officials for help with diseases or their consequences. If they had money, they turned to local practitioners, few of whom had any training. More likely, they sought out "irregular healers," such as remedy vendors, *maiges* (an old word for physicians), witches, midwives, mountebanks, and other charlatans.[2] Alternatively, they might seek spiritual solutions by praying to appropriate saints, consulting the parish curé, or, if they had scrofula, appealing to the king himself. Significantly, these potential healers did not involve the secular authority of government in any way, for even the king originally possessed more healing power by virtue of his divine right than he did as head of the French state.[3]

Until the second half of the eighteenth century, the French government took only limited steps to promote itself as the permanent and established guardian of the public's health. To be sure, since the seventeenth century monarchies throughout Europe, including France, had sought to compile crude data on population size. Known as "political arithmetic," this accounting of life and death relied on clergy and other local officials to record the basic data of births, baptisms, marriages, and deaths.[4] At a time when human bodies were considered the state's primary military, tax, and labor resource, the size and vigor of a population became one of the principal measures of a mercantilist government's prosperity and promise. But the reality of life in the old regime prevented even an expanding and centralizing state like that inspired by Louis XIV from instituting a "medical police" comparable to that emerging in parts of Germany, Italy, and central Europe. Absolutist regimes lacked the administrative know-how and bureaucratic spirit to count the population accurately, let alone to assess the medical personnel and skills needed to ensure its health. Moreover, the Paris Medical Faculty's unreceptiveness to new ideas, combined with semi-autonomous local administrative structures, hindered the establishment of formal health commissions comparable to those set up in towns elsewhere on the continent.

Perhaps because of these obstacles, "health" remained something local, even private, a matter not intrinsically tied to the central government of the French state.[5] Even in the face of the most fearsome threat to public health—the outbreak of epidemic disease, frequently described as *maladies populaires*—the government of the old regime played a limited role. The Marseille plague in 1720–21, for example, reveals the somewhat restricted and temporary nature of official responses to epidemics before cholera.[6] During this crisis, which occurred before the advent of a mass popular press, residents formed their impressions of the plague from health instructions, sermons, broadsheets that were posted and read by local healers (many with dubious reputations), or simply by word of mouth. Apart from concerns about avoiding panic, no one—not even city officials—appears to have thought systematically about consciously creating and manipulating a particular epidemic reality.

Those who confronted epidemics during the old regime also were likely to have a different attitude toward the victims of disease from their nineteenth-century counterparts. Writers such as local priests and administrators acknowledged the disproportionate hardships of disease for the poor, and understood poverty as a special test in a Christian land. In early Catholic doctrine it was less a matter of "deserving" or "undeserving" poor; rather, all were God's children and ideally should be treated with kindness and respect. As with disease, fate placed these people in miserable circumstances that required the more fortunate to show their own humility through their voluntary distribution of alms, which would help assure them a place in heaven. "The poor in a State are rather like shadows in a painting," Dr. P. Hecquet observed in 1740; "they provide a necessary contrast about which humanity sometimes groans, but which honors the decree of Providence."[7] Moreover, even in the face of frequent mobility among the poor during the old regime, it was more possible (though not necessarily a given) that wealthier residents actually knew a pauper, a fact that might make potential donors less suspicious or less aloof. Seen in this way, old regime poverty had a certain immediacy, one with greater possibilities for personal links between the more and less fortunate members of a community.[8]

By the second half of the eighteenth century important intellectual and social changes recast the roles of government and medicine in relation to the French population at the same time that they altered attitudes toward the poor. The Enlightenment promoted ideas of progress, reason, and skepticism regarding religion, as well as faith in human science and inquiry. Following these precepts, it gave a key voice to trained experts, while it delineated a new sense of public welfare that focused on the health and happiness of the population. The viewpoint was essentially an optimistic one that placed humans at the center as both investigators and objects of investigation. In a lengthy article on "Population," for example, the *Encyclopédie*, the major culmination of Enlightenment ideas, discussed all the natural, cultural, and political forces that might influence the size of a population—forces that could and should be studied by humans.[9] Meanwhile, as part of their many attacks on the Church, philosophes such as Montesquieu and Rousseau began to challenge what they considered to be the indiscriminate charitable giving that encouraged too many unfortunates to remain poor and—by increasing implication—lazy. By shifting attention from the holiness of poverty, secular thought opened it to new forms of criticism, particularly from members of a bourgeoisie increasing its financial clout.[10]

By altering attitudes toward the population and poverty, Enlightenment thought opened the theoretical door for greater government intervention into the lives of citizens and helped define the form that such intervention might take during a crisis such as an epidemic. Nowhere were these ideas more clearly articulated than in the Royal Society of Medicine, founded in 1776 and given a royal charter two years later.[11] Bridging the gap between government officials and medical professionals, the Society collected an impressive quantity of data, mostly on rural life, through its investigations of epidemics that afflicted plants, animals, and humans, as well as through extensive exchanges with correspondents throughout France. These reports appeared under the rubric of "medical topographies," a loose genre of professional literature geared toward stimulating discussion among relative specialists. Before the Royal Society of Medicine could bring about a truly workable synthesis between the theory and practice of public health, however, the Revolution outlawed all privileged bodies of the old regime. In effect, the slate had been wiped clean for establishing a new relationship among medicine, society, and politics.

Ironically, even though the concepts "public" and "health" were each central to the Enlightenment, the term *public health* did not come into wide general use until the early decades of the nineteenth century. Despite its frequent theorizing about the importance of a large, satisfied population and the need for responsible government, for example, the *Encyclopédie*, contained no entry on public health per se.[12] Rather, scattered articles on subjects such as political arithmetic, epidemics, hospitals, cholera, hygiene (one paragraph), and health contributed important insights, without delineating a concrete theory about the relationship among politics, medicine, and society. The *Encyclopédie*'s discussions of "epidemic" and "cholera," elements that would be central to the conceptualization of public health less than fifty years later, contained virtually nothing about their potential social impact. It described an earlier variant of cholera as a disease of the human body in the most literal sense, affecting the balance of the four humors.[13] Epidemic, meanwhile, was an entity unto itself, a force in its own right, as opposed to the form a disease might take; the article suggested a blanket cure for all epidemics, regardless of the particular disease.[14] Whether described broadly or specifically, then, during the old regime diseases had an impact on society because they depleted a principal resource, the population. As we shall see, this population would soon become part and parcel of the epidemic itself as revealed in the idea of Paris's being a "sick city."

PARIS MALADE
AND ITS REVOLUTIONARY PAST

Perhaps no work about cholera made the links between the diseased individual and urban bodies more forcefully than Eugène Roch's *Paris malade* ("Sick Paris") published in 1832.[15] The two-volume, eight-hundred-page epic play repeatedly drove home the point of its title by describing the deaths of countless Parisians, linking their individual fates to that of the capital itself by juxtaposing death scenes with grander laments. Maybe without realizing it, the playwright attempted, in this long and detailed work, to produce an objective literary portrait of the epidemic that would ultimately give credibility to his critique of urban life. For Roch, as for many of his contemporaries, cholera was but one of a series of symptoms, all part of the city's general decay. "Ah! Paris! Look at you cured of cholera," one worker in the play characteristically uttered, returning from the riots that had accompanied the epidemic in June 1832; "but now you're gripped by civil war. You are still very sick indeed."[16] As the play's title suggested, the fusion between the individual and the urban bodies could hardly be more complete; after all, Roch could have easily called it *Parisiens malades*. By evoking the capital as an urban body rather than the bodies of its inhabitants, Roch enhanced the drama of the epidemic; his title, in effect, moved the work beyond depicting the ordinary realm of daily life experienced by individual human victims to depicting something much larger, more abstract, and terrifying.

Roch's play was in fact indicative of a remarkable change that occurred in bourgeois perceptions of Paris between 1730 and 1830. While many travelers to the capital in the eighteenth century complained that it contained "dirty, stinking alleys, ugly black houses, an air of filth and poverty, beggars, carters, [and] mending women" as opposed to "superb streets, palaces of marble and gold," the city's image remained fluid enough for a more optimistic, picturesque view to emerge.[17] In fact, many accounts described districts that would become the most dirty and dangerous in the nineteenth century as vital, prosperous, and luxurious. "It is the richest and most populous neighborhood on earth," wrote one observer of the area around Les Halles in 1724. "It has an abundance of everything: vegetables, market-garden produce and orchard fruit, sea and freshwater fish, all that contributes to the comforts and luxuries of life, all that is most excellent, most exquisite, most rare in the air and on earth."[18] Thus, while observers of urban life until the end of the eighteenth century understood that Paris contained its significant share of poverty, crime, and depravity, they could also see a certain beauty and hope. Here the horror remained distant, sometimes almost quaint.

When eighteenth-century critics did discuss problems in the Parisian environment, they tended to present them as distinct from the city itself. Writers such as Restif de la Bretonne, for example, described urban crime as part of an intriguing underworld of the Paris poor, a world apart, one interesting to upper-class readers, not unlike a travel account of a voyage in the New World.[19] Such problems as the spread of crime and begging could be explained as coming from somewhere else, the result of the immigration of rootless vagabonds from outside the capital rather than an intrinsic part of its indigenous population. Moreover, external forces such as geographic conditions, elevation, or weather explained the prevalence of hazards in the urban environment that lay well beyond human control. Such appraisals placed the blame for the city's ills on forces foreign to the social body; such evils were seen as an attack from beyond the borders of urban life.

A play such as Roch's *Paris malade* captured the essence of a new view that was taking hold by the time of the first epidemic, that of Paris as a sick city. Because of its brevity and broad implications, I have borrowed Roch's title to connote a language of social pathology specific to bourgeois Parisians during the 1820s and 1830s. "Paris malade" refers to contemporaries' literal (as opposed to figurative or metaphorical) understanding of the capital's poverty, filth, and overcrowding as a disease that had distinct affinities with the city's less-fortunate inhabitants and any individual symptoms of misery they displayed. While French doctors and social commentators would draw freely upon metaphors of disease throughout the nineteenth century and well into the twentieth to highlight specific social pathologies,[20] those who created Paris malade saw disease as emanating from the city's decrepit buildings and narrow streets as well as from the individuals who inhabited these places. Paris malade, then, signaled bourgeois Parisians' understanding that a complete and literal fusion of the diseased urban and human bodies had occurred.

Several different factors contributed to creating the idea of Paris malade by the 1820s. The drama of revolutionary events, which focused most intensively on Paris, helped strengthen the perception that a large gulf separated the city from the rest of France. Revolution, along with some of the most shocking proclamations and stories associated with terror and murder, had begun there. After all, it had been Parisian crowds that cheered the beheading of the king and queen. Moreover, the city's unchecked physical expansion and population explosion in the early part of the nineteenth century made Parisian growth seem beyond human control. Between 1801 and 1817, for example, the population officially increased from 546,856 to 713,966; it climbed even more dramatically from 785,866 in 1831 to 899,313 just five years later.[21] Not only was Paris beginning to demand the bulk of the country's provisions, but it also started to drain laborers from the surrounding countryside at an alarming rate.

By the 1820s these factors contributed to a more terrifying image of the capital and its inhabitants, which began to emerge in works from medical treatises to fiction. "To be born in Paris is to come into a world of filthy streets and poorly ventilated buildings," announced the introduction to one of the volumes of the *Nouveau tableau de Paris,* published in 1835. "It means having had a dirty stairway, a dank courtyard to play in; it [means] recognizing the sun only by hear-say, the springtime by accident, and the summer by the police ordinances against rabid dogs."[22] Writers and investigators of urban space became obsessed with the stench of the poor, the filth of cesspools, and the need to improve the means of removing waste from the city.[23] While old regime Paris obviously contained many dangers, the city that emerged during the first half of the nineteenth century redefined these perils, making them particularly frightening for bourgeois observers. Not only was an ever-increasing population threatening to explode beyond the city's ancient fortifications, but the new arrivals were seen as potential carriers of poverty and disease.

More than a simple superficial change in emphasis, this shift represented a fundamental restructuring of how Parisians perceived the nature of their city in the 1820s. Now, Paris suffered from a kind of internal imbalance rather than from externally imposed conditions of geography and climate; the city was plagued by forces of its own making. Implicit in this view was a moral judgment: not only was the capital becoming sick, but the sickness was part of the very fabric of urban existence and resulted from human activity rather than mysterious natural forces. In some sense this new awareness represented a discovery of the Enlightenment's darker side, a realization that humankind could be equally capable of creation and destruction. Such an evaluation would have far-reaching implications for the future of urban social relations in the capital.

The arrival of cholera in 1832 invested the sick city with both a literal and a metaphorical meaning, for it both confirmed and symbolized the extent of urban decay unmasked in the 1820s. When the epidemic decimated the capital without first claiming victims anywhere else in the country, the city became even more of an anathema. "Today just look at [the cholera epidemic] that oozes into Paris without having passed through our provinces," exclaimed one religious newspaper. "It isn't anywhere else in France—no one saw it at the borders. With a single jump it arrived in the capital and established itself in this den of iniquity, revolution, and impiety."[24]

Such views seemed especially compelling to provincials. Somehow, it was only fitting that Paris "the city of revolution, the birthplace of political tempests, the center of all vices" would produce a mysterious epidemic. "Unseen, [cholera] lurked in the atmosphere," gloated *La Gazette d'Auvergne;* "it stopped in this home of corruption; it swooped like a vulture on this city of strife, surprising it in the midst of all its pleasures, harvesting especially those unrestrained men who surrender to excessive passions and brutal pleasures."[25] The view that Paris represented "the scourge of France" sometimes even translated into quarantine policy in the provinces.[26] For those outside the city, the outbreak symbolized the capital's general decline, a message that Parisians were quickly coming to internalize as well.

The belief that cholera represented symptoms of a greater urban malady had a particularly strong influence on bourgeois Parisian writers and commentators. Perhaps because of their close proximity to the problems of city life and cholera, they readily conflated the ailing individual and social bodies. Writing in the popular *Livre des cent-et-un,* Charles Duveyrier described the capital as a "city that boils furiously like a copper cauldron, a city much like your people, pale and disfigured!"[27] In the preface to his *Description naturelle, morale et politique du choléra-morbus à Paris,* published a year after the first epidemic, Dr. Antoine Métral offered a similar image. "Paris, with its [sickly] constitution, would have suffered only mildly from cholera had it not so many narrow, filthy streets, had it not been thrown into the deepest misery torn apart by internal swelling, and if, as a result, it did not find itself resembling a sad, agitated, anxious, unhappy fellow ravaged by grief."[28] Such diagnoses blamed the patient and the way the victim lived rather than the disease.

By the time of cholera's arrival, then, contemporaries had come to perceive their capital as a "home of infection" as well as a sick urban body in which decay replaced growth as the dominant descriptive metaphor. While not responsible for this change in attitude, the arrival of cholera in 1832 did in fact give it credence by appearing to push the concept of decline one step further. To be sure, the thousands of victims who perished in the early days of the epidemic presented the capital with a real and immediate threat as administrators, medical professionals, and police tried to cope with practical matters such as body disposal and preventing panic. At a deeper level, such a crisis also prompted Parisians to raise critical questions about the nature of urban life, for by ultimately attacking all districts of the capital the epidemic made it impossible to ignore what were quickly coming to be seen as problems intrinsic to the entire urban body.

However, it was not only the biological aspects of the outbreak per se that terrified bourgeois Parisians but also the fact that the crisis drew attention to a larger set of social concerns embedded in the capital's revolutionary tradition. Any nineteenth-century discussion of Paris—be it a medical treatise, a diary, a play, or a novel—somewhere addresses the problem of revolution, for the issue rests at the root of how Parisians conceptualized their city. "For fifty years Paris has been the scene of distressing events," the official medical report for the 1832 cholera epidemic noted; "the violence of the [political] parties has armed citizens against one another; their blood has flowed in the streets, and horrible battles have created a spectacle."[29] Recounting events from the epidemic, playwright Roch suggested a revolutionary tradition so deeply embedded in French (that is, Parisian) culture that it had become inextricably bound with foreign perceptions of France itself, in effect confirming Metternich's famous dictum: "When Paris sneezes, Europe catches cold." At one point in the epic *Paris malade*, for example, a politician speaks of "the contagiousness of the French disease, this sort of cerebral fever that one also contracts through contact."[30] Responding to the archbishop of Paris, who had proclaimed the epidemic a consequence of the July Revolution, one writer pointed out that other major cities in Europe such as Berlin, Vienna, St. Petersburg, and London all had been ravaged by the epidemic, yet they did not experience revolutions.[31] Meanwhile, even countries such as Belgium and Poland that had mounted revolutions in 1830 did not mimic the French experience, though a close examination of the responses to cholera in these countries might yield some intriguing comparisons.[32] For Paris, more than for any other European capital, then, revolution had become an integral part of how members of the middle classes perceived their city.

Ever since the Great Revolution in 1789, the myth of revolution had traveled abroad and had also developed into a powerful, socially charged tradition at home. From this pivotal moment and its reenactment forty years later, in 1830, the frightened bourgeois living in

1832 internalized a set of threatening images: the masses who had taken to the streets, stormed buildings, built barricades, and beheaded the king and queen (along with many others), parading bloody, decapitated heads through the city on pikes. When lower-class Parisians once again rioted during the first cholera outbreak, many recognized familiar symbols of revolt: the crowds at the Place de Grève, the barricades, closed shops, and National Guard troops. The prevalence and repetition of these images suggest that revolutionary violence had created its own distinctive folklore.[33]

Given this powerful collective memory, this "folklore of violence," it is not surprising that Parisians compared the arrival of cholera and the resulting popular unrest with revolution rather than with some other catastrophe such as war. Because of its raw violence and unforgotten mass deaths, the Terror offered an especially compelling point of reference. "It was a reign of terror far more dreadful than the first, because the executions took place so rapidly and mysteriously," Heinrich Heine, who traveled freely in bourgeois Parisian circles, wrote to readers of the *Gazette d'Augsbourg.* "[Cholera] was a masked executioner who passed through Paris with an invisible *guillotine ambulante.*"[34] *Le Corsaire* entitled one of its editorials "The Sick Sans-Culottes,"[35] while the literary critic Alfred Nettement compared the daily mortality bulletins for cholera with the "Jacobin dictators of Paris."[36] In one of his many nostalgic flights of fancy, the aging romantic writer François-René Chateaubriand explained that "like the Terror in 1793, [cholera] promenaded in the light of day in a new world with a mocking air."[37] Another account described masked marchers who carried a guillotine through the streets of Paris, placing a black flag in the hand of Henry IV's statue "to symbolize the reign of death."[38]

As an enlightened instrument of the egalitarian death, the guillotine and the Terror it represented offered bourgeois Parisians a complex metaphor for cholera. On the one hand, it suggested (at least for a brief moment, and contrary to prevailing public opinion) that cholera, too, killed indiscriminately. On the other hand, the guillotine conjured up frightening memories of revolutionary violence linked concretely with the behavior of the lower classes, a moment also choreographed by human actors. By linking cholera to the guillotine, then, contemporaries drew on one of the more chilling and morally ambiguous images of the city's revolutionary past.

The chronological proximity of the 1830 revolution provided another convenient point of comparison with cholera, one intricately linked with bourgeois Parisians' confused understanding of their relationship to the events of 1830. Neither contemporaries nor historians have agreed on how to approach the revolution that ultimately brought the Orleanist Louis Philippe to the throne in 1830.[39] To be sure, when crowds took to the streets of Paris, threw up barricades, and demanded the overthrow of the oppressive Restoration government of Charles X, it seemed very much like a replay, albeit a faint one, of 1789. The journalists and other professionals who spoke with particular passion against a strongly pro-Catholic regime bent on undoing the "evils" of revolution and who even played a key part in selecting the future "citizen-king" ruler of France, made 1830 seem a clear victory for the Parisian bourgeoisie. At the same time, for the legitimists, the defeated supporters of the Bourbons (some of whom considered themselves bourgeois), the revolution conjured up frighteningly familiar memories from forty years before. From yet another perspective, both supporters of the July Monarchy and left-wing critics also noted that events in 1830 may have in fact changed little at the level of French society. Apart from a new king and administrative purges, they pointed out, the same elites retained power and wielded it in similar ways, thus raising the question of whether the country had in fact truly experienced a revolution at all. Within the context of such different understandings of 1830 then, bourgeois Parisians would use cholera in contradictory ways to express their dissatisfaction with the regime.

Such diverse interpretations of the 1830 revolution and the subsequent appropriation of cholera to discuss it were obviously embedded in immediate political realities.[40] While the most recent revolution had been both relatively quick and bloodless compared with its predecessor in 1789–95, the abrupt change in power had left behind fierce battles between right and left, as well as bitter divisions among the apparent victors. Both the cause and the symptoms of the chronic political instability that characterized the early years of the July Monarchy could be found in the regime's problematic relationship to the revolution that had brought it to power. Trying to ride the wave of revolutionary change while still maintaining social order, the Orleanist monarchy would never win over the right-wing "legitimists," derogatorily known as the "Carlists," the stubborn remaining supporters of the regime it had defeated.[41] At the same time, however, the king's moderate stance and the monarchy's increasing push to the center right alienated left-wing Republicans, who saw this moderation as a betrayal of the revolutionary cause. As another crisis facing a beleaguered new government, the arrival of an epidemic provided a ready metaphor for expressing political discontent.

But the links that contemporaries established between cholera and revolution also went beyond each commentator's desire to use the disease as a convenient rhetorical device. Behind the willingness to read cholera as a political indictment were the deeper social anxieties we have already encountered in Paris malade. While those who drew upon the equation may not have been fully aware of the fact, they were invoking a much deeper level of terror, which in turn gave the political satire more of a bite. In interpreting the depictions of disease and revolution, then, it is important to keep in mind how their political and social meanings reinforced one another to create a highly complex relationship between the two phenomena.

Those on both right and left saw the connection between the 1830 revolution and the 1832 epidemic as a fact, one supported by concrete evidence.[42] "We consider this disease a necessary and inevitable consequence of the events we have just experienced," editors of the right-wing Catholic newspaper *La Quotidienne* told readers, referring to the arrival of the July Monarchy.[43] Cholera's ravages on the European continent in the late 1820s and early 1830s coincided with intense political activity, a fact never lost on contemporaries. Popular wisdom at both ends of the political spectrum argued that revolutionary turmoil in Russia, Poland, Belgium, and France led to the outbreak of cholera because of the movement of troops sent to quash uprisings across the continent. Liberals and conservatives disagreed only in their explanations for the troops' presence.[44] Asking a series of rhetorical questions later in the epidemic, *La Quotidienne* went so far as to suggest that the excitement of the revolutionary upheaval in 1830 had actually predisposed Parisians to sickness two years later: "In all honesty, can we believe that all these hateful passions brought into play by the events of July had not predisposed bodies to the disease that attacked them? Moreover, can we believe that the horrible misery that has reigned for eighteen months has not in fact contributed to weakening the life organs, preparing them to host the scourge?" The editors concluded that this was indeed a real possibility.[45] M. Bellemare, a Catholic who frequently wrote of the 1830 revolution as "a revolt against the Divinity," modified *La Quotidienne*'s connection somewhat by telling the heroes of July that the revolution of 1830, like the epidemic, merely confirmed French society's ongoing and seemingly inevitable decay.[46] Or, put in Bellemare's own words, words no doubt infected by the cholera vocabulary of the day: "The materials to which the fire has been set have long been found in the entrails of the social body."[47]

One of the right's most scathing critiques of the July Revolution and its consequences appeared in a short work entitled *Paris depuis la révolution de 1830* by Jules Janin.[48] A prominent theater critic and frequent contributor to conservative papers such as *La Quotidienne, Le Messager,* and the *Journal des débats*, the bourgeois Janin made little attempt at hiding the clear links he saw between the horrors of the cholera epidemic and the failure of the July Revolution. The novella recounts the sad meeting between a disillusioned French artist and an American plantation owner, George Brown, who comes to Paris on a pilgrimage to see for himself the accomplishments of the *trois glorieuses.* The trip begins badly, for he arrives at the height of the 1832 cholera epidemic only to find that his one friend in Paris has died of the disease. The artist befriends him after realizing that the plantation owner is not a cholera patient in search of a doctor. The rest of the story focuses on a monologue by the artist who systematically whittles down the American's enthusiasm and naïveté.

The book reaches a climax when the American comes down with cholera. Clearly, George Brown's disillusionment represents that of the capital itself, as both fall sick with despair in the wake of their reappraisal of the July Revolution. Adding insult to injury, the artist invites his friends to visit the poor fellow, not to offer condolences or support but rather to see what someone who still worships the revolution could possibly look like. The thesis of the book is simple, crude, and nostalgic, summed up by the artist's concluding monologue at the American's deathbed: "And now, you see, everyone has died since July. Goethe is dead. Benjamin Constant is dead. Cuvier is dead. Bentham is dead. Scott is dead. Casimir Périer is dead. Art, poetry, political science, power, everything is dead."

Interestingly, Janin had not attacked the 1830 revolution from the standpoint of either its political or its social legacy but instead scoffed at the cultural bankruptcy of the Parisian bourgeoisie. Rather than condemn politicians, laws, or even increased agitation from the lower classes, he used an artist as his spokesman to lament the decline of elite culture. According to the artist, the July Monarchy failed to build distinctive monuments, instead relying too much on the past glory of fallen regimes. Versailles no longer hosted lavish parties, as French society had somehow become "too serious," and museums since 1830 had replaced "real art" with exhibits depicting the poor, the police, and cholera patients. By focusing on the cultural bankruptcy of the July Monarchy, Janin thus brushed past the metaphors of urban pathology so often invoked in discussions of the relationship between disease and revolution. For him, cholera represented the decline of civilization not in terms of social conflict and filth but rather in terms of a disappearing culture and a new mediocrity heralded by the rise of the masses.

Critics of the July Revolution and the regime it brought to power also used cholera cartoons to convey their views. One blamed Paris for having unleashed revolutionary ideas on the continent.[49] In figure 3, a young male traveler in tattered blue clothing embraces Marianne, the female icon of the French Revolution, dressed in red and wearing the Phrygian cap. "Ah! dear July Revolution!" the vagabond, assuming the voice of cholera, explains to Marianne, "without you I would have stayed in Northern Russia; it is you who, by agitating Poland [*en révolutionnant la Pologne*], bid me to come into this unfortunate land. . . . Thanks to you, dear July Revolution, here I am in Paris." The tricolor appears prominently at the top of the picture, with two cholera victims prostrate on the ground. In my reading, the cartoon conveys the blending of disease and revolution in several ways.[50] The flag ominously mirrors the blue, white, and red colors that emerge from the passionate embrace of cholera and Marianne at the center of the picture. Moreover, the tricolor itself contains the colors of disease and revolt, with the blue suggesting the skin color of cholera victims, and the red symbolic of blood and revolt. The flag flies over the entire scene, representing the prevalence of cholera in the heart of the contaminated July Monarchy.

A legitimist cartoon from the previous year entitled "The Devil's Indigestion" displays the July Monarchy's internal sickness even more graphically, anticipating the symptoms of cholera (see figure 4). King Louis Philippe, depicted as a devil and revolutionary (he had come to power as a rival to the French throne in 1830 and appears literally sans-culotte), hovers over a chamber pot with di-

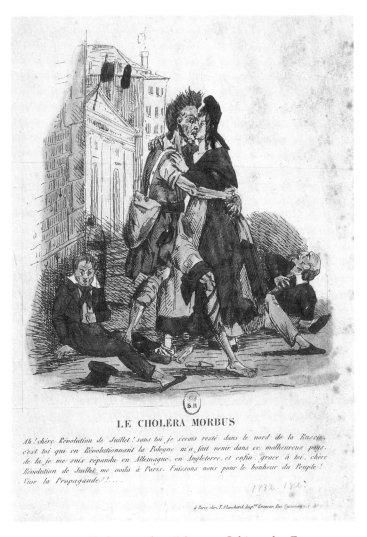

Figure 3. "Le Choléra morbus." Source: Cabinet des Estampes, no. B50536, Bibliothèque Nationale, Paris.

arrhea while vomiting out little sans-culottes bedecked with Phrygian caps. The miniature Jacobins can be seen as both symptoms and causes of the disease in the belly of the regime embodied in the king; while cholera remained a medical mystery, doctors assumed that a victim spewed out the foreign "putrid miasmas" (tiny particles that contemporary medical wisdom held to be the cause of

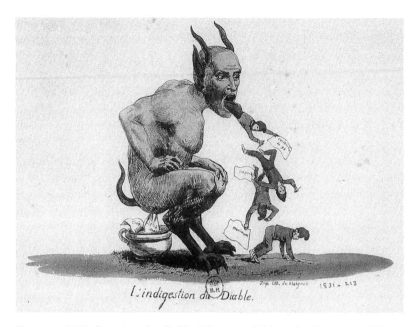

Figure 4. "L'Indigestion du diable." Source: Cabinet des Estampes, Bibliothèque Nationale, Paris. Reprinted in Patrice Bourdelais and André Dodin, *Visages du choléra* (Paris, 1987), 4.

infection) to purge the human body of unwanted elements. Cholera, like revolution, lived hidden within the (social) body until vomited forth in a stream of unwanted matter. Such a cartoon also played on equating cholera with revolution because it drew upon a particular genre of scatological caricature popular during the first Revolution.[51] Allegedly catering to the baser sensibilities of the lower classes, these playful drawings often equated the poor with excrement and vomit, the very symptoms that cholera would literally supply. The cartoon of Louis Philippe poised over the chamber pot thus invoked revolution not just through its subject matter but also by its association with a genre that depicted revolutionary excess and the transgressions of the poor.

A lesser-developed, yet significant aspect of the counterrevolutionary critique emerged in a certain nostalgia for the reign of Napoleon, a nostalgia that had a particular resonance among certain members of the bourgeoisie.[52] Because he had put an end to the chaos of the first revolution and had made a formidable impression on the popular imagination with his alleged healing of plague victims in Jaffa,[53] some saw the emperor as a model for saving France from the twin "scourges" of disease and revolt. In *Paris malade*, for example, a group of nostalgic soldiers looked back to the glory of the emperor. Napoleon "would know how to keep [cholera] outside of France," one exclaimed. "It would be [another] famous victory!"[54]

By no means did critics of the July Monarchy have a monopoly on linking disease and revolution. Those sympathetic to the *juste-milieu* tended to condemn both phenomena as evils grounded in excess. Suggesting that the exhaustion from revolutionary ferment might play a part in predisposing an individual to disease, for example, the government's preventive literature distributed to the public about cholera cautioned Parisians to avoid "excesses of any kind." This formulation included both overindulgence in food and drink and "overexcitement," as well as bathing in bath water of immoderate temperature.[55] Liberal writers pointed out that the disease would have spread less rapidly (if at all) without the uprisings in Poland and Belgium, and blamed cholera's invasion on the Russian army that was sent to oppress rebel forces. Cholera "attached itself to the caravans and the armies, . . . spilling its poisons into the war," noted one observer.[56] The concept of excess thus had a particular resonance for supporters of the July Monarchy, a regime that personified the bourgeois ethos of moderation, restraint, and balance.

A cartoon sympathetic to the July Monarchy is worth considering carefully for its critique of another kind of excess (see figure 5).[57] Entitled "Great Details about the Three Scourges of France,"[58] it offers a sophisticated blend of image and text. It consists of three horizontal sections that corresponded roughly to the three funda-mental forms of expression: image, narrative, and verse. At the top, three figures dominate: cholera flanked on the left by a Republican carrying a red flag and on the right by a Carlist seated and holding a white flag. Dressed in black and carrying palm fronds (perhaps capitalizing on the fact that the epidemic arrived at Easter in order to emphasize the July Monarchy's anticlericalism), cholera domi-nates the picture because of both its size and its shadow. The bottom portion of the improvised triptych, meanwhile, describes revolu-tionary forces brought to the surface during the 1832 epidemic. Condemning the insurgents as "anarchists of disorder," the verses praise the courage of the National Guard and credit the king with bringing calm just by virtue of his presence.

Such a cartoon must be understood as blatantly supporting the impeccable balance of the *juste-milieu*. Like the regime it defended,

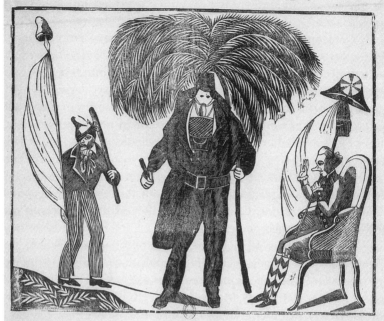

Figure 5. "Grands détails sur les trois fléaux de la France." Source: Cabinet des Estampes, no. B50357, Bibliothèque Nationale, Paris.

the lithograph stood at the middle of the political spectrum, con-demning the extremes of Carlism and Republicanism by placing them in the same visual space and under the same label of horror as cholera. Seen in this way, the idea of an extreme viewpoint was more threatening than its particulars. The extremes of the political parties, like the excesses of the lower classes and the spoiled nobil-ity, combined with the disease to constitute a threat to the moder-ation advocated by the ruling bourgeois regime.

Simultaneously attacking various aspects of Parisian society, pol-itics, and culture in the wake of the 1830 revolution, the works that juxtaposed disease and revolution in 1832 suggested an ambig-uous relationship between the city's revolutionary tradition and its bourgeoisie. The connections between cholera and guillotines, sans-culottes, Marianne, and Jacobins demonstrated how uneasy many writers and social commentators felt about a revolutionary history that had seemed to grant them increasing overt power and influ-ence. In attempting to give the disease a familiar face by linking it to a larger Parisian past, contemporaries also attacked the revolution-ary tradition as a force comparable to a mysterious modern plague. No one could control either phenomenon, and both posed a direct threat to the precarious position of a recently empowered bourgeois elite, itself brought to power by revolutionary events.

The anxiety accompanying the mixed legacy of a revolutionary past was both influenced by and would have implications for bour-geois Parisians' understanding of their relationship to both 1793 and 1830. While legitimist right-wing critics of the July Monarchy saw recent events as a continuation of the Parisian revolutionary tradi-tion, the regime's supporters seemed almost embarrassed to asso-ciate themselves with that tradition in any way, particularly in light of the Terror's raw violence, which had tainted so many interpre-tations of revolution itself. This embarrassment accounts for the predominance of right-wing imagery that depicted cholera and the revolutionary tradition. Meanwhile, those on the left were more likely to refer to 1830 as "bourgeois," a derogatory label signifying that the new regime remained quite conservative and that the so-called revolution had changed virtually nothing.[59] To further com-plicate matters, bourgeois Parisians did not necessarily share any or all of these views of 1830 and may have even changed them along with their politics.[60] Because of its diverse political meanings, then, revolution did not offer a simple metaphor for cholera, nor could images of the disease supply a clearly defined understanding of counterrevolutionary critiques.

Even when the complexity of cholera as a political symbol and its connections to the revolutionary tradition are taken into account, however, the arrival of the epidemic in 1832 forced bourgeois Parisians to confront the social implications of such a relationship. To understand why a revolutionary tradition that bourgeois Parisians viewed with such ambivalence could become so readily equated with something so new and mysterious as cholera, we must look more closely at perceptions of urban social relations as they emerged during the first weeks of the 1832 epidemic. Bolstered by initial mortality figures that indicated a far greater number of deaths among the poor, the concept of Paris malade and the city's revolutionary tradition would help give bourgeois Parisians a clearer sense of identity as they raced to establish their immunity from poverty, the poor, and—of course—cholera.

THE HAVES AND THE HAVE-NOTS

When cholera arrived in 1832, it helped integrate the image of the sick city into the revolutionary tradition by casting the lower classes in a more threatening light. Since the mysterious new disease first claimed victims from among the poor, it seemed to confirm the suspicions of many contemporaries—from medical professionals to journalists—that cholera and poverty went hand in hand. But, more important, the first epidemic also helped translate these ideas into popular discourse about urban social relations. Discussions concerning who seemed most likely to catch the disease and why, and who appeared to be exempt, as well as interpretations of these discrepancies, all revealed a process by which bourgeois Parisians established a conceptual map of the city and the epidemic that created as much distance between themselves and its perceived victims as possible. While such ideas were worked out at both an institutional and an individual level, they required little actual contact between classes. Through a series of intermediaries—namely, medical professionals, administrators, and journalists—a bourgeois sense of the epidemic reality was articulated without anyone necessarily being fully conscious of this fact. Such depictions of the disease's perceived victims often served to reinforce class differ-

ences because they were predicated upon the belief that one's superior social position played a key role in determining immunity.

Denial, however, soon clashed openly with the increasing visibility of the lower classes. The human misery so dramatically
brought to the surface by accounts such as those of doctors treating
the sick served as a growing reminder that Paris contained elements
that challenged bourgeois perceptions and values. Once the disease
began to claim victims among the wealthy, cholera—right alongside
revolution—posed a direct threat to the social immunity seemingly
enjoyed by those outside the poorer classes. As one individual in
Paris malade advised the bourgeois: "Make love, pour cool glasses of
wine, converse with your friends at court, . . . kill the time with
delicacies, but know that cholera is in your attics, that it can descend
quite suddenly and travel the three stories that separate it from your
bedrooms."[61]

The hard realities of economic life for the Parisian lower classes
during the early nineteenth century provided some genuine reasons
for bourgeois anxiety. Cholera's arrival in 1832 coincided with the
end of a period of severe economic recession that had persisted
since 1827, a fact that no doubt contributed to the increasing numbers of Parisians living in dire circumstances as well as to an ominous climate of class tensions within the capital.[62] According to one
historian's calculations, 83 percent of Parisians who died during the
early nineteenth century did not leave behind enough resources to
cover the cost of their own funerals.[63] In fact, a sizable part of the
city's more than 785,000 residents barely managed to eke out a
living on a daily basis or faced outright homelessness. During the
late Restoration and July Monarchy, for example, an estimated one
in ten Parisians was indigent—that is, inscribed on government rolls
as needing some form of public assistance. The number increases
when relying upon a broader definition, such as the percentage of
people who died in hospitals, a sign of poverty. One study has even
suggested that during economic crises half the population could be
indigent.[64] The rest crowded into crumbling tenement buildings
and residence hotels concentrated in the dark, fetid central districts
of the capital. By one estimate each inhabitant of the extremely
miserable Arcis quarter occupied only seven square meters.[65]

Set against such a dismal background, acclaimed scientific data
helped establish cholera as a disease of the "less-fortunate" classes.

During the Restoration and the July Monarchy, groups of urban investigators kept detailed accounts of exactly what they saw in the city; their hundreds of reports (sometimes several pages long) discussed individual residences, including the number of inhabitants, rooms, doors, windows, pieces of furniture, and latrines, along with descriptions of available water facilities and general impressions of the environment.[66] Formats ranged from elegantly published official reports and highly specialized articles in professional journals to hastily scrawled notes written by semiliterate doctors and appended to the minutes of neighborhood sanitation commission meetings. Recorded both as description and as numbers, these disparate pieces of information created a composite, almost three-dimensional portrait of the capital's poorer districts. As we shall see, they contributed much to popularizing statistics as an option for government policy and created a whole new way of seeing and describing the Paris environment.

Individual doctors incorporated information and assumptions from these investigations into their understanding of cholera. Discussing mortality rates in his *Histoire statistique du choléra-morbus* (1833), for example, Dr. François Marc Moreau listed the following results for the faubourg St. Denis, a district with among the highest cholera deaths:

—The wealthy class (landlords, upper-tier employees, factory owners) had 59 sick and 24 deaths; 1 death per 2.45 sick.

—The middle class (small-scale landlords, shop owners, etc.) had 135 sick and 57 deaths; 1 death per 2.35.

—The nearly indigent class or indigent class (water carriers, workers, wage laborers, etc.) had 471 sick and 218 deaths; 1 death per 2.16.[67]

During its first two weeks, the epidemic claimed nearly all of its victims from the poorer neighborhoods in the center of the city.[68] In the ninth arrondissement (the area around the Hôtel de Ville and Notre Dame, which contained the infamous rue de la Mortellerie) one in twenty-one residents succumbed to cholera, while in the fashionable first (the Tuileries and the Champs-Elysées) only one in eighty-one died.[69] Just as there had been inequality in life, such figures suggested a fundamental inequality in death as well.

With or without concrete numbers, rich and poor alike believed in the class-specificity of the new disease; such figures seemed merely to confirm a set of preconceived notions about the urban environment that cholera was so quickly coming to represent. "Cholera-morbus is doctrinaire," a theater tabloid told bourgeois readers on one of the first days of the epidemic in 1832; "it strikes and overcomes the poor classes in particular."[70] The *Journal des débats*, a prominent daily that catered to the Parisian bourgeoisie, came to similar conclusions, emphasizing the fact that "all the men stricken with this epidemic . . . come from the class of the people. They are the shoemakers, the workers who labor in textile factories. They live on the dirty and narrow streets of the Cité and around the neighborhood of Notre Dame."[71] Clearly, this disease was geographically and economically removed from the readers of such newspapers.

For the most part, writers sympathetic to the lower classes also considered cholera a disease linked to poverty. "Cholera is the personal tax of the poor," one paper sarcastically quoted a "darling of the minister's cabinet" as saying.[72] Even if satirical, the quote acknowledged the tendency to compartmentalize the disease. *Le National*, a left-wing daily quick to denounce hasty accusations against workers, reprinted the wisdom of the *Moniteur universel*, the government organ, without comment. "We repeat what we have already said, that cholera appears to prefer attacking those persons who live in unclean streets and neighborhoods, and who, because of their profession, are most exposed to poor conditions and atmospheric changes."[73] In a play sympathetic to the participants in the political disturbances during the 1832 outbreak, one character tells a worker, "All the laws are made against you; a scourge from heaven, a cholera, comes and it falls on you, while the government men tell the rich not to be afraid, that this death here isn't meant for them."[74] Even *François le fataliste*, a Republican tabloid passed among the lower classes in early April, made the point explicitly, if somewhat sarcastically:

1. —What is cholera?—For the rich it is nothing, for the poor it is the plague, it is death. . . .

2. —Why does it spare the rich?—Because they are rich.

3. —Why does it only attack the poor?—To instruct and punish them.[75]

The bitter questions and answers betrayed an implicit moral judgment, a certain fatalism that the poor had not learned some abstract, cosmic lesson, and that cholera had provided the brutal evidence of this fact. Within such a deterministic framework, poverty and cholera appeared virtually synonymous, suggesting that the lower classes suffered because of their very manner of being.

Such beliefs seemed to gain wide acceptance. Contemporary medical wisdom held that the lower classes, like the districts they inhabited, had a predisposition to disease in general, an opinion confirmed and given added vigor by the arrival of the modern plague. "It would be impossible for the commission to deny that there exists a certain kind of population, like a certain type of place, which favors the development of cholera, making the disease more intense and its effects more deadly," the official government report for the 1832 epidemic observed.[76] The public at large shared this view. The suffering classes "are unfortunately the most numerous and the most predisposed to the disease," the conservative Catholic newspaper, *La Quotidienne,* remarked. "This explains the larger number of patients taken to hospitals over those treated at home"—a reference to the fact that the better-off could afford the services of a private physician.[77] Cholera primarily attacked poorer neighborhoods, one writer believed, because "it finds bodies and souls marvelously predisposed to receiving its deadly influences."[78] Summarizing the popular idea in the crudest possible terms, one character in *Paris malade* remarked, "You'd be tempted to think that the only reason these unfortunate people exist is to wait for cholera."[79] One class's predisposition to cholera of course meant another's immunity, a fact that helped solidify a sense of bourgeois identity in opposition to the lower classes.

Accompanying the belief that the poor had a predisposition to cholera, a vocabulary soon emerged that tacitly described cholera's class-specificity. Not only did this shared medical, administrative, and journalistic discourse evoke the links between the individual and the social body, but it almost gave neighborhoods historical agency by investing them with concrete individual characteristics.[80] "We notice that it is almost always the same neighborhoods, the same streets and the same class of individual who are affected by the epidemic," *La Quotidienne* commented after printing one of its first sets of daily mortality statistics on April 3.[81] In most early accounts of the epidemic certain details provided cultural cues that enabled contemporaries to express the disease's class-specificity in a subtle, almost unconscious manner. The following report for the mayor of Lyon about the situation in Paris provides one striking example:

> [The disease] made more headway in narrow and unclean streets, where old, badly constructed buildings have narrow alleys and poorly ventilated courtyards, [and] everything [is] unclean. An impoverished population subjected to numerous hardships and neglecting all attempts at cleanliness is, in a manner of speaking, encased in this garbage.[82]

The smallest details—living situation ("homeless," "living on the ground floor, well below street level"), street and area names (rue de la Mortellerie, Ile de la Cité), arrondissement numbers (ninth, twelfth), descriptions of clothing ("dressed like a worker," "in shirt sleeves"), occupations (ragpicker, shoemaker), drinking habits ("habitual drunkard")—all served as commonly understood signifiers that immediately designated a victim's class and, consequently, likelihood of falling sick with cholera. "Such is the state of misery," noted the Lyon report, "that one doctor in a hospital affirmed that, of twenty-one patients who died in his ward, only one of them had a shirt."[83] No detail was wholly innocent.

Implicit in this lack of innocence was the belief that human agency somehow played a role in attracting the disease, especially where the poor were concerned. Frequent lamentations in the press, doctor's reports, and even the official health pamphlets condemned the vices of the lower classes.[84] François Magendie, one of the most exalted Paris physicians at the time of the 1832 epidemic, characteristically blamed "bad areas, the uncleanliness of the dwellings [and] neighborhoods, poor nutrition, fear, misery *and everything that accompanies the morals of poor, malnourished people,* for often vice accompanies misery."[85] Another doctor, who analyzed mortality figures for days of the week, argued that the highest number of cholera deaths occurred on Mondays, Tuesdays, and Wednesdays because of "excesses in which the working population indulged itself on Sundays and Mondays," a belief confirmed in the official government report.[86] The religious press in particular condemned various excesses and transgressions, ranging from intemperance and overexertion to playing dominoes and spending too many hours in gaming houses.[87]

Members of the upper classes seemed especially appalled by the apparent failure of the poor to take the disease seriously enough during the initial invasion. "Nothing is more extraordinary about the epidemic than the incredulous attitude of the working class about the existence of cholera-morbus," the *Gazette médicale de Paris* noted. Using a rather intriguing choice of a verb, it stated, "Whereas the antechambers and the salons [of the bourgeois] are infected with chlorine and camphor (medical measures recommended for warding off the disease), and whereas fear inspires preparations for taking care of the sick, the unfortunates speak of cholera as if it was something imaginary."[88] Dr. Moreau recalled that "the people seem to be braving [the epidemic] by partaking in excesses of every kind, ignoring the initial symptoms and even exacerbating them."[89] Meanwhile, aristocrats like Chateaubriand complained of drunkards seated at small wooden tables toasting the health of cholera-morbus, and told of children who "played at cholera," calling it "Nicholas Morbus" (because it came from Russia) or "Morbus the Scoundrel."[90] It seemed doubly immoral for the lower classes to bring the disease upon themselves through their vice and carelessness. By condemning the behavior of the poor in this way, better-off Parisians distanced themselves yet again from the unfortunate victims of cholera at the same time that they established an oppositional common bond with other members of the fortunate classes.

Significantly, at the beginning of the epidemic no one complained of the rich or bourgeois not taking the epidemic seriously, even though many initially wore their nonchalance as a badge of courage. Bolstered by the belief that cholera struck only the poor, many members of the upper classes were cocky, almost jovial in their first confrontations. "[My father] shrugs his shoulders when anyone talks about cholera," wrote Jacques Boucher de Crevecour de Perthes; "according to him, it doesn't exist. He eats lettuce, vegetables and generally everything the doctors forbid."[91] The Austrian cultural attaché was especially smug when describing how he first heard of the epidemic.

> It was between a cup of tea and a biscuit when they announced it:
> this didn't keep us from taking a sip of one and a bite of the other;

we weren't the least bit frightened or at least very little, and we knew that dinners, parties, shows, balls, concerts, everything would go on without interruption; the only precaution that we take, and it even has become fashionable, is to wear sachets filled with camphor, the kind which *belles dames* offer to young cavaliers, and a little cassolette with a scented lozenge made from mint and chamomile; it is in good taste to keep this little box in your waistcoat pocket and to sniff at it from time to time.[92]

Cholera, it seemed, provided a cause for celebration; it was an event that commemorated the high life of *le tout* Paris. "The best tea for protecting oneself against cholera is champagne," noted one theater journal, offering the following advice: "drink when you are thirsty, eat when you are hungry, and sleep when you get tired—voilà, the best remedy for avoiding cholera."[93] Just as the living conditions of the poor could cause cholera, so too those of the affluent could prevent it.

Like denial, the ideas of predisposition and responsibility served to isolate the lower classes (and, by implication, the threat of cholera) from "respectable" Parisians by focusing attention on aspects intrinsic to the lives of the poor. Predisposition linked disease to a world wholly foreign to the bourgeoisie, while the idea of responsibility suggested that behavior—something over which an individual had control—influenced mortality. By continually supplying a contrasting portrait of the less-fortunate districts and individuals who would be more likely to get the disease, information about cholera—be it doctors' accounts or articles in the press—thus helped create a kind of cordon sanitaire around the lower classes while establishing an opposing sense of shared identity among wealthier Parisians. The juxtaposition of statistical realities with descriptions of decrepit living conditions and debauchery seemed an unbeatable combination that suggested not only lower-class responsibility but also upper-class innocence, detachment, and—by implication—immunity.

However, an important change in the spring of 1832 soon complicated this portrait of bourgeois superiority and seeming immunity; after only three weeks mortality figures began to show increasing deaths among the wealthier classes. This development greatly altered perceptions of the epidemic among *all* Parisians. "When . . . the disease established itself . . . in all those rich neighborhoods where people flattered themselves into thinking that it would be pushed away by the beauty of the buildings, the grandeur of the streets, and the purity of the air," Dr. Métral astutely observed, "it was quite another matter, [one of] affliction and hopelessness."[94] Denial, couched in the crumbling belief that the poor were the only Parisians susceptible to the disease, now yielded to the realization that the borders between classes were in fact quite porous. At the most immediate level, members of the upper classes perceived the poor as couriers of cholera. At a deeper, perhaps even subconscious level, Paris malade and the revolutionary tradition, along with the broad definition of disease they implied, threatened to draw *all* Parisians into the terrifying underworld of the sick city.

Once the epidemic began to strike the wealthier sections of the capital, the same papers that had linked the disease to the lower classes began to condemn rich and poor alike for believing the first stories. "People who have only a vague idea of cholera's history act as if it were a disease only of the people, a disease that does not strike either the rich or powerful," warned a government report printed in the *Moniteur universel* and other papers. "This is not only erroneous but also a crazy temerity that merely provokes the indignation of the inferior classes and sustains the most absurd and dangerous prejudices." The report went so far as to list the names of wealthy people throughout Europe who had died of the disease to demonstrate that "rank and fortune have no exclusive privilege guaranteeing them [immunity] from cholera and death."[95]

Such information served a double function. On the one hand, it helped counterbalance the outrage at the beginning of the epidemic, when many protested the appearance of names and addresses of cholera victims in the press.[96] In part, these fears grew directly out of the parallels contemporaries drew between Paris malade and revolution. Even if it seemed less threatening to link cholera with the lower classes, one still had to consider how these potential revolutionaries might react to such a distinction. "Fortunately, foresightful Death cast a few rich corpses to the poor," Janin observed, because "these rich corpses have appeased the voice [of the people]."[97]

On the other hand, such information about mortality across class lines warned Parisians that socioeconomic boundaries were not sacred, thus forcing them to appreciate the true extent of their own vulnerability. "We no longer speak of anything but deaths; we do nothing but lament," the Austrian cultural attaché recorded in his diary less than three weeks after describing the fashionable sachet filled with camphor. He listed numerous wealthy acquaintances and government officials who had died, and exclaimed: "Everyone suffers or thinks they are suffering. The churches draped in black, coffins, carts for bodies, hearses on every street, women in mourning, everywhere death or its symbols—voilà the lugubrious spectacle that Paris presents."[98] Only when death had become a visible individual reality to the bourgeois could someone in deep denial accept it; not until bourgeois Parisians, with their prized sense of individuality and need for self-expression, fell sick and began describing their experiences in their memoirs, in the press, and to each other did they truly grapple with the personal implications of the disease. Lacking the basic luxury of having the time to describe their encounters, the poor meanwhile died in silence, leaving behind an impression of the disease as one that affected masses rather than individuals. Moreover, even the countless urban investigators who explored their daily lives with such close scrutiny rarely depicted the poor victims as individual human beings.[99] Thus, once cholera crossed beyond its social cordon sanitaire, it took on a new meaning, as those looking from the outside finally began to understand its terror from the inside.

A clear indication of the panic among the upper classes emerged when they resorted to the classic response to previous epidemics, flight. In the first weeks thousands of Parisians were reported to have deserted the city. "Although the cholera evidently first attacked the poorer classes, the rich still very promptly took to flight," Heine reported. "Certain parvenus should not be blamed for fleeing since they probably thought that cholera, which came such a long way from Asia, does not know that lately we have grown quite rich on the stock exchange and, mistaking us still for poor scum, will force us to bite the dust.[100] *Le Globe*, the Saint-Simonian paper, and one more likely to be critical of the wealthy, accused them of fleeing behind a cordon sanitaire formed by the mountains of Auvergne, presumably a reference to the location of summer homes.[101] Meanwhile, the socialist Louis Blanc portrayed a hectic and desperate exodus to the provinces. "When the stagecoaches were crammed full of pale travelers [a reference to those who did not need to work outdoors], people left in regular carriages and later in simple carts; . . . the rich fled, taking with them the work, the bread, and the life of the worker!"[102]

While the stories may have been exaggerated,[103] they were convincing enough to prompt a campaign urging citizens to remain in the capital. It was especially important that government officials, as leaders of the community, remain. Setting a well-publicized and popular example, King Louis Philippe and his family did not flee to one of their many summer residences. His public courage also shamed other government officials into remaining in the capital. When the wife of one official died of cholera, for instance, he thought briefly of fleeing to Switzerland with his family, but decided against it, for fear that his associates would consider him a coward.[104] Meanwhile, the *Moniteur universel* offered a lesson by describing the unfortunate ordeal of a wealthy woman who had left cholera-infested Vienna for France, only to succumb in Paris. "The fatigue brought by this moving about can encourage the disease," the article claimed, "and the moves bring about much suffering for all the transactions they impede."[105]

Although persuasive, in a sense the government's attempt to show how the disease cut across social boundaries ultimately backfired. Rather than bringing about a sense of common purpose and destiny, the outbreak of cholera created a need to reinforce boundaries, in large part because the lower classes had been made visible by the epidemic. "This epidemic brought out, from God knows where, the physiognomies of a type wholly unknown," a character in *Paris malade* observed. Describing "physiognomies of uprisings" and "physiognomies of epidemics," he invoked a wide range of sensational, mysterious images depicting a subterranean population who wore shirts made of paper and lived like rats, sleeping in narrow passages between walls.[106] Here in the shadows, cholera and revolution had fused once again as the disease came to embody a wide range of images, some of them vaguely familiar through a picturesque literature but most of them never before seen in such dramatic and immediately threatening ways.

Thus, during the cholera epidemic of 1832, upper- and middle-class Parisians became trapped within a paradox of visibility and denial. On the one hand, medical professionals and government officials helped create the idea that cholera was primarily a disease of the poor, an idea perpetuated in the pages of the press. By isolating disease within a single and largely identifiable population and by making that population highly visible through detailed description and analysis, officials presented an argument that appealed to bourgeois notions that somehow their own class remained protected. On the other hand, while it surprised few Parisians that cholera would attack the impoverished, more crowded sections of their city, the realization that the epidemic might spread across the carefully drawn boundaries between the have-nots and the haves forced them to restructure their views of urban social relations. No longer immune from cholera, bourgeois Parisians hovered dangerously close to the filth and vice of the masses that the disease now represented. In other words, the edifice of denial that they had so carefully constructed to protect themselves now led to questions about their own responsibility, as they too fell sick.

When Parisians confronted the first cholera epidemic, they faced not only a mysterious disease but also one that both illuminated and eventually helped reshape urban social relations in the capital. Arriving on the heels of the revolution in 1830 and playing into a revolutionary tradition ever-present since 1789, the 1832 crisis helped create a new view of the lower classes by concretely bringing together the two distinct threats of Paris malade and revolution for the first time. Seen another way, the terror of Paris malade epitomized by the 1832 cholera epidemic had become part and parcel of the revolutionary tradition. Within this context of the intertwining of disease and revolution, contagion threatened to bridge the gaps between classes in a number of ways. Viewed literally, contagion in the form of cholera spread from the lower to the upper classes, demonstrating that the bourgeois could not remain smug in their assumption that they were immune from the disease. In a more abstract sense, the new information emerging about the lower classes itself represented a form of contagion, for it made them visible while linking them to the general decay of the capital that affected all Parisians. Put another way, to catch cholera did not mean simply falling sick with a strange disease; rather it played into a preexisting constellation of social and cultural circumstances unique to Paris during the first part of the nineteenth century.

Thus, a number of features distinguished perceptions of cholera in 1832 from those of prerevolutionary epidemic diseases. First, in the preurban and newly industrializing era, agriculture and rural life in general had played a far greater part in defining health priorities. Post-revolutionary public health efforts focused almost exclusively on cities and the problems created by their increasing human population. As an urban phenomenon, cholera compelled bourgeois Parisians to look closely at narrow streets, dank alleys, and people they saw as desperate and rootless packed too tightly into small, fetid hovels. Moreover, it forced them to connect disease with another important and terrifying urban phenomenon, revolution.

Second, with Catholicism on the wane and the abolition of the three "estates" after 1789, bourgeois Parisians had to come to terms with a new conception of the lower classes and their relationship to cholera. Under the old regime, poverty in France had been both a widespread and a basically accepted fact of life. As we shall see, only in the 1820s did researchers and social commentators begin to work through the implications of poverty having economic rather than sacred roots, thus suggesting that an individual might escape it through his or her own efforts. Once bourgeois Parisians came to equate poverty with lack of initiative rather than with fate, it influenced their understanding of the relationship between poverty and disease. The concept of the epidemic expanded beyond the Enlightenment definition to encompass not just its environment but also its victims as part of the epidemic itself. While someone in the eighteenth century might blame the arrival of a pestilence on vagabonds, beggars, or even the wrath of God, no one had considered scapegoats an intrinsic part of the epidemic experience in quite the same way as their modern counterparts; the members of a population might catch and even carry a disease, but they never literally were disease in the sense that later victims of cholera would be.

Finally, those who shaped notions of disease and public health in the old regime had not spoken with the universalizing voice of the bourgeoisie. As we shall see, the accelerated expansion of the public sphere in the first half of the nineteenth century brought one segment of the French population—the poor—under scrutiny at the same time that it invited another—the middle classes—to observe the results. It is to this problem that we now turn.

2

Cholera's Messengers

In the months and weeks leading up to the 1832 and 1849 cholera epidemics, Parisians learned about a new disease through the words of medical professionals, government officials, and journalists. More than writers who did not publish in the press, religious leaders, or artists, these distinctly nineteenth-century representatives of bourgeois culture knowingly and unknowingly created the images of the outbreaks and determined how they would be transmitted to the public at large. Through policy choices, rhetoric, and publicizing certain kinds of information, the three distinct, yet overlapping, groups borrowed strategies used during past plagues but also invented new responses as they went along. Often seeing themselves as intermediaries rather than as creators or inventors of ideas, these men in fact were unwitting agents shaping perceptions of cholera, themselves, and the world in which they lived. As "messengers," then, they were decidedly not passive transmitters of views about cholera; rather, they possessed enough expertise and power to shape their message in the very process of conveying it.

This chapter steps back from cholera to take a close look at its storytellers within the broader context of post-Enlightenment and post-revolutionary Paris. As elite members of the middle classes, medical professionals, administrators, and journalists each brought their own bourgeois values and ideas to the discussion of the epidemics. All believed in rationality, progress, and human perfectibility, qualities that made them optimistic about the possibilities of fighting the epidemic threat at the very moment they discovered the real dangers lurking in Paris malade. They also believed that information enabled men to understand themselves and their relationship to the environment and that, accordingly, it should be collected and disseminated for the benefit of all. Finally, they shared a common perception that their values and actions were somehow universal, that in pursuing their own interests they were acting for the greatest common good. Here, objectivity and neutrality also played an important role, for they strengthened the idea that certain actions could be beyond human subjectivity and petty political interest. Put another way, cholera's messengers were products and perpetuators of the Enlightenment ideas so central to nineteenth-century bourgeois culture.

Just as the Enlightenment provided the intellectual and cultural underpinnings for their beliefs, the revolution of 1789 played a significant part in allowing members of each group to emerge as prominent social and economic actors during the first half of the nineteenth century. After doing away with the monarchy and the aristocracy, revolutionaries in 1789 sought to fill the void by performing ambitious experiments that blended politics and culture and that would influence everything from the daily life of the average citizen to the role and raison d'être of government.[1] Replacing the authority of divine right and the patronage of a court society that centered on the person of the king, the new regime relied upon Enlightenment ideals of rationality and objectivity to invent a state intended to differ as much as possible from its arbitrary predecessors. Such values would open the possibility for power to rest in the hands of experts, trained professionals who approached government service as a career more than a sinecure. The revolution thus cleared the way for professions[2] such as medicine, administration, and journalism to flourish. With training, expertise, and the new respect that accompanied "careers open to talent," professionals played important roles as creators of a distinctively modern French government and society. During the turbulent decades when the legacies of revolution—the expansion of the public sphere, the increasing strength of the middle classes, and the beginnings of mass culture—were being absorbed, these men both benefited from these changes and helped make them more far-reaching and permanent.

The following pages will show how each set of cholera's messengers contributed to the epidemic tale in different—sometimes contradictory and sometimes complementary—ways to create a portrait of life and death in the capital. Doctors had particular significance because of their growing expertise, which stemmed in part from actual experiences confronting disease and in part from the increasing professionalization of French medicine. Administrators such as police officials and civil servants also enjoyed an increasingly prominent role as policymakers, information gatherers, and recordkeepers, a trend begun by Napoleon and highlighted during the epidemic crises. Finally, perhaps more than any other group, journalists captured the spirit of the postrevolutionary age as the press came to play an increasing role in shaping public discussion and debate.

THE MEDICAL PROFESSIONALS

At the time of each cholera outbreak official almanacs listed some fourteen hundred names under the category *service de santé* for the Department of the Seine.[3] Along with *officiers de santé* (the lowliest health position established during the Revolution), interns, and medical students, these doctors, surgeons, and pharmacists made up the bulk of formally trained "medical professionals" who told the epidemic story. Through their writings in professional journals, memoirs, official reports, correspondence, published lectures, doctoral theses, and treatises, these men[4] carried on a lively and open exchange that revealed what they considered to be the essence of cholera and what measures should be taken to stop it. All had some kind of formal medical training, though its quality and nature varied, and nearly all wrote about the epidemics based on their firsthand experience.

Moreover, nearly all medical professionals were from within the ranks of the middle classes by virtue of training as well as temperament. Not only did medical students tend to come from this group, but certain factors barred individuals from the lower classes and the aristocracy from entering the profession. The expense and time commitment required by formal medical training, for example, excluded most people without some form of independent wealth. To attain the position of *officier de santé*, a candidate needed to spend six years apprenticed to a doctor, five years working in a hospital, or three years studying in a medical school before passing a series of three examinations. The more prestigious doctors (*médecins*), meanwhile, had to study at least four years at a medical school and then take the national *concours*, a six-part competitive examination that included sections in Latin. And, after 1821, just to enter the schools students needed four years of liberal arts training.[5] Should a young man be fortunate enough to complete his studies, establishing a practice usually required further financial outlays, particularly if a doctor wanted to attract the "right kind" of clientele to his practice.[6]

At the same time, the very act of practicing medicine created a barrier between even the wealthiest, most respected doctors and the nobility. With its emphasis on hands-on experience, the clinical teaching that now dominated medical training placed medicine dangerously close to the lowly realm of a skilled trade; doctors, after all, could be perceived as apprenticing themselves to learn their craft. In addition, physicians who treated the greatest nobility essentially did so as servants; the nature of their relationship (receiving fees for services, being summoned to the home of a client) suggested an underlying inequality. Thus, despite the fact that some doctors mingled freely with the Parisian elites while others lived in virtual poverty, the dual nature of their profession as a blend of theoretical learning and a trade placed them squarely within the ranks of the middle classes.

Despite these similarities, however, differences between medical professionals and other healers, conflicts among medical professionals themselves, and struggles with administration and religious officials, meant that a coherent voice about cholera would emerge only with great difficulty. Although most medical professionals essentially came from the ranks of the middle classes, they had a wide range of incomes and political views, not to mention approaches to medicine. A hierarchy persisted even after the Revolution sought to abolish it, with doctors from the Paris Faculty of Medicine occupying the top of a pyramid that sloped downward to include even those of the humblest means. As a result of this system, one of the most open professional conflicts of the 1830s and 1840s raged between doctors and health officers.[7] As a struggling elite within a struggling profession, doctors often found themselves waging constant internal battles to gain legitimacy, power, and recognition—battles not unlike those ravaging French society as a whole during the first half of the nineteenth century.

Formally trained doctors also inevitably competed with a wide variety of other healers.[8] "Irregulars" reminiscent of those from the old regime continued to be the dominant caregivers in an environment where many remained hostile to medical elites. For the average Parisian who belonged to the lower classes, the irregulars had certain distinct advantages over their formally trained counterparts, largely because educated practitioners were too expensive and socially remote. Insecure in their status, defensive doctors often tried to impress patients with their scientific knowledge, a self-fashioning—as many contemporaries realized—not always commensurate with their actual abilities.[9] Moreover, especially when all healers faced a mystery like cholera, their practices showed some striking similarities. During both epidemics, for example, advertisements offering a colorful collection of anticholera syrups, drops, baths, and vaccines appeared prominently in the back pages of popular newspapers; as proposed remedies they were not that different from the hundreds of petitions heard by the National Academy of Medicine at the same time.[10] Thus, Parisian medical professionals faced the difficult task of distinguishing themselves from the competition while winning the confidence of the city's wary population.

Much of the problem lay in the relative newness of medicine's development as a modern profession, a complex process that did not begin in earnest until after 1789.[11] The Revolution swept away the Catholic institutional structure, thereby removing—at least officially—medicine's most serious ideological opposition. Because it abolished (at least temporarily) hierarchy and outlawed the guild structure that had been the guardian of privilege, the Revolution also created a climate in which the notion of a profession could thrive. For medicine this change meant a brief dismantling of the Faculty of Medicine and the revocation of all licenses to practice healing issued during the old regime. This "clean slate" provided critics of the previous system, such as Antoine François Fourcroy and François Chaussier, with an invaluable opportunity to revamp medical education in accordance with the Enlightenment ideas of the day.[12] Among the many changes that Fourcroy and Chaussier recommended to the National Assembly in 1794 and that were gradually put into law over the next half century, two stand out as being most significant for our story. First, building on the success of earlier French medicine, the reformers placed clinical teaching at the heart of medical education. Rather than reinterpreting ancient texts as they had in the past, students would now learn through experience. They would observe patients firsthand in the wards and clinics, or, as the report succinctly put it, they were to "read little, see much, and do much."[13] Second, Fourcroy and Chaussier introduced the first Paris chair in Medical Physics and Hygiene, thus helping make the study of epidemics and ultimately of public health an integral part of formal medical training. At the very moment when the Revolution sought to abolish distinctions within the ranks of the medical profession, it implicitly encouraged the early forms of interdisciplinary work that lay at the root of public health and its eventual approach to cholera.

The Napoleonic period also made its own important imprint on subsequent medical professionalization and the fight against cholera. Beyond implementing revolutionary reforms such as those for medical education, Napoleon helped solidify a strong working relationship between medical professionals and the French state. Unlike previous rulers, the emperor consciously sought to tap the vital bourgeois energies that had been released in 1789 by bringing "experts" such as physicians, surgeons, and pharmacists into the "halls of power" where they served as administrators, consultants, and appointed officials.[14] Even if this proved a largely symbolic gesture, it helped to create a climate in which medical advice might play a prominent public role, as can be seen in the dramatic national campaign to inoculate French citizens against smallpox under the Empire.[15] The Napoleonic period also saw the creation of the Paris Health Council, which, as we shall see, played an important part in establishing an administrative body for responding to health crises such as epidemics.

Along with the planned reforms of changing medical education and drawing doctors into state service, the period of turmoil between 1789 and 1815 also had unintended consequences for how the medical profession would emerge in the time of cholera. The revolutionary and Napoleonic wars, for example, provided a modern precedent for mobilizing an organized medical corps in the face of immediate disaster.[16] Many of the doctors who would serve during the 1832 cholera epidemic trained in the Napoleonic battlefields. There they learned to treat hundreds of patients under difficult conditions, while military discipline taught them to keep detailed statistical records related to health. The urgency of wartime reinforced the importance of practical (as opposed to theoretical) knowledge, which was already associated with the clinical method; it also broadened the scope of this experience beyond the walls of the hospital or clinic to the open fields of battle. More than a change of locale, this shift helped redefine the relationship between medicine and the state. Just as the revolutionary *levée en masse* established a standing army, the large-scale mobilization of doctors for the same war effort helped create a medical corps, an idea that could be easily translated to peacetime use. Given these experiences, it is no coincidence that subsequent accounts would describe "the March and the Effects of Cholera" and that medical professionals would initially "fight" it as an outside enemy.[17]

One key group in the fight against cholera had been particularly shaped by the wartime experience, the hygienists.[18] Intellectual descendants of the Royal Society of Medicine founded by Félix Vicq d'Azyr, these men sought an explanation for disease through rigorous investigation of the environment in which it developed.[19] Though the vast majority of this quasi-official group consisting of doctors, chemists, pharmacists, and administrators had some form of medical training, the ranks of the hygienists expanded to include architects, engineers, and civil servants who participated actively at meetings with the prefect of police and in exchanges in the medical press.[20] Whether because of this hybrid membership or because most of the physicians drawn to this group tended not to come from ranks of the medical elites, the hygienists initially shared a certain outsider status with their predecessors in the Royal Society of Medicine. Unlike their old regime counterparts, however, by the 1820s they had a substantial professional following abroad,[21] not to mention the full ear of government at home; for the first half of the nineteenth century, France was the center of the Western medical world, and public health contributed heavily to this reputation.[22] Despite this prestige, the hygienists rarely drew public attention to themselves. Even their most prolific members worked quietly behind the scenes in official and unofficial capacities. But though the names of leading hygienists such as Louis René Villermé and A.J.B. Parent-Duchâtelet perhaps remained obscure to most Parisians and though the term *hygienist* was never explicitly used to describe a legitimate authority in the responses to the 1832 and 1849 epidemics,[23] this group would play a crucial role as messengers of cholera.

Because of the hygienists' diverse professional backgrounds, institutions played an especially important role in bringing them together. The Paris Health Council (Conseil de Salubrité de Paris), first established in 1802 to advise the prefect of police on unhealthy situations in the capital, gained significance only around 1820, at about the time the hygienist movement was beginning to coalesce.[24] The Council's regular meetings provided an open and lively forum where physicians, engineers, architects, and government administrators could discuss common concerns pertaining to the health of the Paris environment. As the movement gained momentum, the *Annales d'hygiène publique et de médecine légale,* founded in 1829, provided a means for reaching a broad professional audience in print. In the words of the masthead, this unofficial organ of the hygienists served as a "repertoire of all questions relating to public health, considered in their relationship to subsistence, epidemics, professions, establishments and institutions of hygiene and salubrity." Thus, articles covered subjects as diverse as the newest statistical methods, findings of recent studies about vaccinations, pregnancy, antisepsis, cesspools, sewers, slaughterhouses, and housing conditions, as well as speculation about the nature of civilization. Through the minutes, articles, and reports published in these forums, the hygienists reached out to other medical professionals, government officials, and—during the cholera epidemics—the broader public who read the articles reprinted in the popular press.

Like the majority of medical professionals, the hygienists continued to be influenced by Enlightenment ideals such as optimism, confidence in science, knowledge through observation, and the value of hands-on experience. Rather than concentrate on the internal functioning of the human body, however, they explored the vast environment of the social body through the newly evolving concept of public health. In the introduction to his *Appréciation des progrès de l'hygiène publique depuis le commencement du XIXe siècle,* which appeared in 1839, Dr. J. F. Rameaux offered what has become a widely quoted definition.

> Public health concerns itself with the man in society, and considers him as a species. Religion, government, morals and customs, institutions, relations from man to man, and from people to people—all of this is its jurisdiction. In a word, [public health] touches upon every aspect of our social existence; it does even more, for, as [P.J.G.] Cabanis would have it, it tends to perfect human nature generally.[25]

A first reading of Rameaux's definition reveals the undeniable traces of Enlightenment optimism inherent in the promise of human perfectibility, along with the placement of religion and morals within the scope of detached human analysis. But the meaning of such a definition changes when put into context. Rameaux wrote it at the height of the hygienists' influence, when they engaged in zealous quests to locate and report the increasing filth and poverty of the French capital in the name of civilization and the public good. Because the hygienists concentrated on the darkest sides of Parisian life, even Rameaux's glowing description carried their haunting "discoveries" within it. The conceptual breadth of Rameaux's description reflected the broadest possible definition of disease itself, one that encouraged contemporaries to see cholera not just in terms of the physical environment (climate, topography) but in the context of society, of the human practices and interactions embodied in Paris malade. Such an all-encompassing definition of public health helped open aspects of daily life to possible professional inquiry.

Ironically, then, public health paved the way for an unprecedented penetration into private space. The capital's revolutionary tradition, the growing fear that Paris had become a sick city, and, eventually, the threat of cholera inspired a series of both formal and informal investigations that enabled men such as the hygienists to explore private life in the name of a vaguely defined public good. They looked at everything from public squares and open-air markets to cesspools and private dwellings in order to identify unclean areas where the putrid miasmas of disease might likely arise. Complete, diverse, and scientific, this modern approach to public health was a methodology of observation and quantification applied to the increasing problems of urban and industrial life: overcrowding, waste removal, stagnant air, and tumble-down lodgings, to name but a few. By making the Paris population and its environment the object of systematic investigation, the hygienists turned Paris into a laboratory in which the population replaced the individual human body as the primary unit of analysis. Moreover, responding to fears of Paris malade, these investigations made it perfectly clear that "population" referred almost exclusively to the urban poor.

Looking back on his service during the first cholera epidemic, François Marc Moreau, a prominent physician and hygienist in the northern part of Paris, gave a revealing sense of the investigations' character in his 1833 work, *Histoire statistique du choléra-morbus dans le quartier du faubourg St.-Denis*. His material came from a careful scrutiny of registers from emergency first-aid stations and hospitals, reports of house calls, and death certificates, as well as from police documents. Calling for "facts collected without preconceptions," Moreau articulated a much-repeated view. "To trace the general history of the epidemic that has ravaged the city of Paris," he explained, "the knowledge of detailed facts is of an absolute necessity: it is necessary, in a manner of speaking, to follow this epidemic not only in each neighborhood but even in each street, in each house, to penetrate, if it is possible, into each dwelling, and to have for each and every one of these places exact and thorough documentation."[26] Here, as in all investigations of the 1820s and 1830s, detail was of greatest importance: doctors like Moreau sought to understand society by breaking it down into its smallest components. These details could then be counted and classified in order to draw preliminary conclusions from the results.

Even though hygienists belonged to different political parties and were drawn together by a genuine concern for the sheer volume of human suffering, their investigations created an image of Paris that fit in with their professional training and bourgeois background. First, the medicalized view of the population and urban space articulated by doctors such as Moreau, Villermé, and Parent-Duchâtelet probed the links between material and economic conditions on the one hand and health and "civilization" on the other. They measured humanity's progress by focusing on the characteristics of the population and its environment that related to health: births, deaths, diseases, and basic sanitary conditions.[27] Second, as representatives of bourgeois professions, the hygienists framed health and unhealth as class issues. By directing public attention to the insalubrious conditions of poor neighborhoods, they provided the legitimacy of a medical vocabulary for discussing problems of social inequality in forums outside the professional literature. Moreover, since they dwelled more upon unhealth than health, they helped to forge a sense of bourgeois identity, giving their fellow Parisians something to define themselves against through the rich and detailed descriptions of another world.[28] More abstractly, when hygienists invoked objectivity, they could not help but harness it to speak in the interests of their class, particularly since objectivity had been at the core of bourgeois thought since the eighteenth century. By writing and publishing a simple report about the Paris environment, for example, a hygienist needed to have begun with certain questions that rested on conscious or unconscious underlying assumptions about the sorts of things worth inspecting and the reasons for doing so. Moreover, the format of a written report and its dissemination also suggested the pervasiveness of bourgeois values because everything from the premise for undertaking the investigation to the level of literacy required to read it shaped how physicians, administrators, and eventually journalists would interpret the information it contained. Ideas such as order, neutrality, detail, penetration into the hidden world of the poor, and the need for readers to come to a given problem based on each individual's interpretation of the facts, all spoke directly to the sensibilities of bourgeois Parisians in the 1830s and 1840s. This approach helps explain why the hygienists had little trouble seducing the dominant French middle classes with their ideas about public health and cholera.[29] At the same time, they helped to shape this ethos by making it more solid and tangible through the backing of science. Whether fully conscious of their role or not, the hygienists both represented and influenced the interests of their class.

One of the most intriguing examples of how medical professionals served as cholera's messengers surfaces in the debates over the contagiousness of the disease. During the Restoration increasingly heated conflicts raged between the contagionists, who believed the disease to be transmitted between individuals, and the anticontagionists, who linked it to the environment. The debate, which filled medical journals and spilled into the pages of the popular press, was highly charged and complicated for three reasons. First, because no one understood how a disease such as cholera was transmitted, writers could easily muster credible evidence to support either position. Second, despite the passion and the ultimate differences between sides, the lines of battle were not always clear-cut. The actual terms of the argument changed constantly, as did people's understanding of the problem and its larger consequences. People could, for example, vehemently proclaim themselves on one side of the issue while actually appearing to espouse ideas from the other, thus creating an underlying sense of destabilization at the very moment when everyone clamored for concrete explanations. And, finally, as it surfaced in the 1820s and 1830s, the debate was less about the actual causes of a disease than about the broader implications of responding to a mysterious crisis of potentially major proportions.[30] When doctors and health officials argued over cholera's contagiousness, they opened the door to rethinking the nature of human interactions within the Paris environment and asked what role government and medicine should play in the daily lives of citizens. By tracing the contours of the complex debate among contemporaries, then, we can gain some idea of the issues at stake, not just for the medical professionals but also for anticontagionism's underlying relationship with the broader economic, political, and social concerns of bourgeois Parisians.

The contagionist approach had the force of the past on its side and seemed to make common sense. From ancient times and up until the 1820s, the dominant medical wisdom held that epidemic diseases from plague to cholera were highly contagious, brought about through contact facilitated by trade, war, migration, or simply by forces outside the given community. Accordingly, governments such as the one that faced the 1720 plague in Marseille had taken measures not unlike those used for fighting any external enemy: erecting barriers, isolating suspected invaders, and encouraging individual households to fortify themselves against the invasion by remaining indoors. Measures such as instituting cordons sanitaires and quarantine, like burning the goods associated with a victim, were tangible and familiar; they made governments and doctors who knew little about a given situation appear to be taking decisive control over it. This illusion of control helps explain why Restoration health policy so enthusiastically embraced the contagionist position in its crusade against yellow fever in 1822 and in subsequent preparations against cholera.[31]

In the first decades of the nineteenth century, practical experience, along with the frightening underworld of Paris malade so dramatically revealed in the hygienists' investigations, made many medical professionals less confident than they had been of traditional contagionist arguments. Encounters with typhoid, yellow fever, and plague during the Napoleonic wars formed the ideas of the future leaders of the public health movement, an education that convinced them of the noncontagious nature of most epidemic diseases.[32] Later, the failure of quarantine during the Spanish yellow fever epidemic further challenged the ancient hypothesis. Similarly, the unsuccessful measures taken to fight cholera in eastern Europe made the anticontagionist conclusions seem almost irrefutable.[33]

Linked to the hygienists' investigations of urban space, this "medicine of places" saw the environment as central to the outbreak of disease, a revival of an old idea that dated back as far as contagionism.[34] The strong correlations that the hygienists found among filth, poverty, disease, and death convinced them of the dangers that lay in putrid miasmas, the poisonous air that arose from repulsive matter such as stagnant water, cesspools, rotting garbage, decaying animal carcasses, and decomposing corpses. Cleaning out unsavory and foul-smelling areas, they believed, would eradicate a disease such as cholera better than quarantine.[35] Based on these observations physicians such as Nicolas Chevrin launched a serious campaign against what they perceived as massive ignorance and entrenched thinking, an effort that won an official endorsement from the recently revived Royal Academy of Medicine in 1828. Thus began a steady campaign to win over government officials and residents of the capital. For reasons that will become apparent, the July Monarchy rapidly adopted the anticontagionist position, and in the spring of 1832 the official government organ, the *Moniteur universel*, published numerous reports by doctors supporting the view that the city's filthy, dark, overcrowded conditions were responsible for the outbreak of cholera.[36] By 1849 the view had gained enough support among the medical community and lay press so that few treatises or memoirs mentioned the debate at all.

Based on what we now know about cholera, both contagionism and anticontagionism made correct and incorrect assumptions about how the disease worked. Over the course of the century, the discoveries of John Snow, Robert Koch, and others would produce the greatly reformed view of contagion now known as the "germ theory," a kind of contingent contagionism in which bacteria or other microorganisms serve as transmitting agents that bring about the spread of infectious diseases. Thus, contagionists rightly argued that humans helped transmit cholera and that it did not spontaneously generate from decaying piles of putrefying matter, while anticontagionists correctly insisted that the cleanliness of the environment was an important factor.

Perhaps because both sides could cite concrete evidence to support their claims, the issue of contagion remained far from resolved at the time of the 1832 cholera epidemic. Even the most influential medical leaders at the time of the first outbreak found it difficult to commit to one side or the other in the face of conflicting evidence.

François Broussais, the immensely popular and respected theorist of "physiological medicine," for example, expressed the confusion that many of his contemporaries felt in 1832. On the one hand, he pointed out, one never found isolated cases of cholera. "When this disease breaks out in a house," he wrote in a published study of the first epidemic, "it almost always affects several people." On the other hand, evidence suggested that not everyone in the infected houses always fell sick, notably doctors or other health officials who came to tend victims. "Looking at all these facts," he concluded, "I do not know if I should admit to calling it an infection. As for contagion, this is not admissible if one understands contagion to mean something like [what happens] in the case of smallpox." In the final analysis, Broussais's monograph supported anticontagionism.[37]

The confusion of Broussais and others arose partly from semantics. Because most doctors had a clear idea of what cholera was not rather than of what it actually was, it proved difficult to arrive at a satisfactory definition of contagion. "In their writings not all doctors have given the same meaning to the word contagion," one physician noted, complaining that they had "often argued over words, without much use to science."[38] Even by the time of the second epidemic, when the debate had apparently been resolved in favor of anticontagionism, some doctors still called for a more nuanced interpretation of the problem. "Cholera is only *contagious under given circumstances*," three doctors from the National Academy of Medicine concluded in 1849.[39] Given the imprecise and constantly changing definitions, the lines between contagion and anticontagion could never be clear-cut, and thus the debate continued to be a source of controversy and anxiety among medical professionals in spite of some attempts to present a unified front.

It is not easy to explain why medical professionals, government officials, and, eventually, opinion in the press came to embrace anticontagionism by the mid-1830s.[40] In order to overcome the inertia and common-sense appeal of contagionism, anticontagionists had to make powerful claims of their own, claims that appealed to the new logic of the post-revolutionary era. At the same time, the victory of anticontagionism would help recast these concerns by infusing them with the increasing respectability of scientific authority.

Economically, anticontagionism provided a doctrine virtually tailor-made for the Parisian bourgeoisie, a fact that goes a long way toward explaining its content as well as its success.[41] Few contemporaries masked their beliefs that quarantine and border protection made poor business sense, particularly when (at least in theory and in public discourse) laissez-faire economics had come to capture the imagination of the dominant middle classes who benefited most from the July Monarchy's coming to power. The restriction of trade and travel resulting from a cordon sanitaire posed a direct threat to the livelihood of merchants, some of the regime's most ardent supporters. "Until now these precautions have not served any function except to hinder commercial relations between peoples," Dr. F. Foy, a prominent hygienist, explained.[42] One scholar even suggests that anticontagionism's inherent ability to alienate people from a holistic, hands-on approach to understanding their own health paralleled the alienation of labor from the process of work.[43] The idea of anticontagionism thus emerged out of the same conceptual fabric as capitalism, making it inherently appealing to many bourgeois Parisians.

Politically, anticontagionism promised novelty and an opportunity to challenge long-held assumptions. Some proponents pitched the struggle as a scientific correlate to post-revolutionary change; just as the Restoration government had advocated returning to the past by bringing back the monarchy and the Church, so too staid medical professionalism could be seen as threatening to scientific innovation.[44] Many medical professionals, for example, presented themselves as noble crusaders for reform, as men who would provide a healthy undoing of the status quo. Though not exactly at the forefront of radicalism once the July Monarchy came to power, many hygienists and medical doctors tended to emerge on the left of the political spectrum,[45] and anticontagionism initially had a certain rebellious appeal for members of the middle classes. Once it had become an accepted doctrine, however, anticontagionism took on the role of helping maintain the status quo so cherished by defenders of the July Monarchy. It allowed city officials to penetrate more easily than they had in the past into the lives of less-fortunate French citizens through investigation and increasing regulation of everything from buildings to diet. Moreover, the miasmatic theory of disease helped provide the scientific justification for the concept of Paris malade because disease could now be defined as an internal enemy, one intrinsic to the Paris environment.

Implicit in the environmental conception of disease that surfaced in the post-revolutionary era were deeper anxieties about poverty and the lower classes who might once again take to the streets as they had after 1789. By placing the blame for cholera on the putrid miasmas that emanated from piles of garbage, anticontagionism shifted the burden from the individual to the environment, from the internal world of the victim to the external world in which that victim lived. Moreover, anticontagionism further compounded the class-specificity of the disease by influencing how hygienists would try to answer the question of where cholera came from and by determining how they would ask the question in the first place. Or, put another way, because the hygienists never studied the dank alleyways, open cesspools, and piles of rotting refuse in the city's wealthier neighborhoods, their notion of putrid miasmas remained confined to the world of the poor. At the same time, by focusing attention on the environment, anticontagionism shifted responsibility to an abstract collective entity, a "them" as opposed to an "I" or even an "us." The growing prominence of the individual over the course of the nineteenth century initially reinforced a bourgeois, class-based notion of the "I" that tended to ignore members of the lower classes. As indicated by the middle-class outcry against printing the names of individual victims, cholera was not to be seen as the disease of an individual.[46]

Culturally, anticontagionism helped provide a medical justification and means for establishing the kind of order that the Parisian middle classes so desperately sought after the turbulence of the early nineteenth century.[47] It granted investigators permission to seek out dirt, to study it, quantify it, and finally to present it in neatly packaged reports that could be safely shelved in a library or government office. Moreover, the victory of anticontagionism pointed to the growing credibility of medical professionals as major guardians of French order and stability; fifty years earlier, the Royal Society of Medicine probably did not have the political power to defy an enduring conception of disease, let alone the cultural clout to triumph over the common sense and tradition that had dictated such a definition for generations. And, finally, like the concept of public health, the debate over contagionism revealed how and to what extent many problems in French society and culture were being conceptualized in medical terms. It is noteworthy, for example, that as industrial capitalism grew in influence, especially after 1830, medical metaphors ("the social body") continued to dominate economic ones ("the social machine").

To look ahead, the medical professionals and, most notably, the hygienists provided the city government and popular press with the key assumptions and methods for telling the epidemic story and refashioning it as they went along. As members of the Parisian middle classes, they developed their ideas within the ethos of this group, while also reaching out and teaching their fellow citizens to see the city and cholera in a particular way. By linking the disease to the putrid miasmas of the Paris environment and by introducing detailed investigations to study it, they would have a profound impact on the city's response to the immediate crisis as well as on the ultimate relationship between medicine and government.

THE ADMINISTRATORS

Cholera was perhaps the French capital's first truly bureaucratic disease; its second set of messengers could be found toiling in the capital's growing warren of administrative offices, where they compiled and collated statistical data, submitted reports, and issued circulars. This group consisted of trained administrators, office workers in the prefecture of police, and sometimes even medical doctors. As collectors and recorders of information, they left behind some of the richest quantitative documentation about epidemic deaths as well as qualitative descriptions of life in different parts of the capital. Concerned more with order and social stability than with curing individual patients, these bureaucrats waged their battle against cholera as intermediaries among medical professionals, the state, and the Paris population. Through their reports and decrees, which appeared in newspapers and on posters throughout the city, they helped shape residents' perceptions of cholera by telling them what actions they should take to prevent the disease and how to recognize its symptoms, as well as where they should turn for help. But while the web of information gathering and dissemination appeared more far-reaching than during earlier epidemics, it was by no means monolithic; even as officials called for "rigorous exactitude" in gathering facts about Parisian life, the crisis of cholera exacerbated inconsistency, confusion, and conflict.

The history of cholera's bureaucrats must be viewed within the larger context of a changing role for the post-revolutionary bourgeois state.[48] During the old regime the French government functioned through a relatively arbitrary distribution and exercise of power centered around the king and the nobility of the royal court. Someone interested in a government position frequently purchased it, inherited it, or received it as a favor. Because government offices were increasingly lucrative for a financially strapped regime, it became more and more difficult to change the system. Under such circumstances, even the most zealous administrators might just as easily receive their posts by chance as by design, while the less enthusiastic had little incentive for devoting any attention at all to their duties. During the eighteenth century, men such as Turgot, Malesherbes, Necker, and Maurepas attempted some rationalization of the French bureaucratic structure with the creation of institutions such as the Ecole des Ponts et Chaussées in 1747.[49] Moreover, we have already seen how the Royal Society of Medicine provided an important precedent for a medical administration by establishing a system of "correspondents" in communities throughout France who provided regular reports to the Society. The Revolution would abolish the Society as a royal entity, at the same time that it cleared the way for government bureaucratic reform more generally. When the National Assembly outlawed the sale of offices in 1789, for example, it opened the way for the development of a government apparatus explicitly based upon merit rather than upon patronage or purchase. Moreover, after 1792 the new state began to perform the recordkeeping functions that had traditionally been the responsibility of church officials.

With its roots in revolution, the administrative apparatus that would use bureaucracy to fight cholera gradually came into being over the early decades of the nineteenth century. By introducing the first blueprint for a French secular bureaucracy, Napoleon set the stage for broad reforms in what would later be called "the golden age of administration."[50] His public commitment to establishing a meritocracy and his desire to bring order after the chaos of revolution, as well as his translation of military discipline into civilian life, all influenced the creation of an administrative base from which a rational, uniform system might emerge. His reforms, however, concentrated primarily on organizing an upper strata of loyal bureaucrats without consciously aiming to create a homogenous, complete, regularized administrative structure down to the most fundamental level of daily tasks.[51] After Napoleon, the European peace that prevailed during the Restoration and the July Monarchy provided an opportunity for the development of a state apparatus not intrinsically tied to war abroad. Moreover, international relations generated enough stability for officials to turn their attention to developing the guiding principles for the routine running of a bureaucracy. Freed from the demands of mobilization against enemies abroad, officials could devote attention to internal crises such as Paris malade and epidemics.

By the time of cholera, a culture of bureaucracy had taken root in the capital, which contributed to the expectation that the disease could be fought administratively.[52] Works such as *L'Art d'obtenir des places* (1816), *La Bureaucratie* (1825), *Moeurs administratives* (1825), and *Moeurs administratives dessinées d'après nature* (1828) offered both witty and pragmatic advice about how to climb the unwieldy administrative ladder to success. Moreover, the first administrative law course in 1819, along with the growing use of preprinted forms to record routine information during the July Monarchy, reflected and perpetuated the accepted reliance on bureaucracy. Also, within the administration, 250,000 functionaries[53] had access to a growing variety of periodicals specifically devoted to their profession. The prevalence of bureaucratic culture could be found too in numerous spoofs that appeared during the July Monarchy.[54]

The bureaucratic culture reflected the ambitions and goals of the newly liberated bourgeoisie.[55] The growing number of administrative positions generated by an expanding bureaucracy provided employment opportunities for upwardly mobile middle-class Parisians eager to keep themselves above the ranks of artisans and workers. Reflecting the new prestige of government employment, the average wage of administrators was nearly twice that of workers.[56] Moreover, like medical professionals, bureaucrats were perceived as occupying a prominent middle ground between manual and intellectual labor. "In a word," *La Doctrine de la Tribune des employés* asserted in 1849, "the functionary [*employé*[57]] is the laborer of the pen. Worker by virtue of his manual labor, man of letters by thought, he encompasses both the artisan and the artist; he is the natural link between the material and liberal professions."[58] Finally,

the promise of professional advancement fit in with the broad notions of progress coming to dominate bourgeois thinking in the
post-revolutionary decades. While bureaucracy represented the essence of stasis for anyone who had to deal with it, it functioned in
large part by inviting its employees to rise within its ranks to increase their economic and social status.[59]

The modern bureaucracy also reflected the bourgeois ideal that
rationality, universality, neutrality, and objectivity should super-
sede political interests.[60] Napoleon understood, for example, that
he could run a more effective administration by drawing upon talent rather than blind political loyalty and argued for recruiting his
personnel accordingly.[61] Moreover, as the prescriptive literature of
the 1840s explained, the ideal bureaucrat should be trained to op-
erate freely within a variety of institutional structures independent
of politics. He should rely upon "his intelligence, his accumulated
knowledge, [and] his time," which he placed at the disposal of "a
public or private administration, a commercial or industrial enterprise."[62] Obviously, however, politics did play a role, particularly as
administrators and party leaders came to understand power as part
and parcel of an expanding state in times of crisis such as the cholera epidemics.

More than any other branch of the city administration, the Paris
municipal police exemplified the complex political nature of the
bureaucracy that would play such a key role in shaping responses to
both epidemics.[63] The connections between police and administration stretched back well into the old regime, and persist in the
current French term *police*, which refers to both law-enforcement
officers and policy. Building upon this traditional relationship, Napoleon made the police the linchpin of his administration, an arrangement that would carry over into the Restoration and July Monarchy.[64] In a city racked with fears of continuing revolution, crime,
poverty, vice, and disease—in Paris malade—the police occupied an
especially important position that extended well beyond appre-
hending criminals and spying on political adversaries of the regime
in power. Despite the many problems that tarnished their reputation as an efficient force on the streets of Paris,[65] the police in fact
played a much more important role behind the scenes as they managed and staffed the capital's most powerful administrative apparatus. One official estimated that the police signed an average of two

thousand papers a day and explained that "the [police] bureaus are the true centers of power."[66] In his *Etudes administratives*, published in 1859, the former prefect of police Alexandre Vivien explained how the bureaucrats "prepare, deliberate, organize; they are the thought and the intelligence," while because of their direct contact with Parisians, the "active officers" served as "the eyes [and] the arms of the administration."[67]

During the cholera epidemics the police performed a variety of functions that made them the most important executors of government policy and the most visible symbols of its authority. When ragpickers destroyed garbage carts and angry crowds attacked individuals whom they accused of trying to poison them during the early days of the 1832 epidemic, for example, the police both made arrests and produced reams of paperwork to chronicle the events. Police also helped to transport patients to emergency first-aid stations, to maintain order in the cramped quarters, and to supervise the removal of bodies. Beyond keeping physical order, the police also performed many of the key administrative tasks that would make the cholera outbreaks appear so closely managed. For example, under the leadership of Henri Gisquet, the prefect from 1831 to 1836, each neighborhood *commissaire* was required to submit a daily report about the political and social climate of the neighborhood for which he was responsible, which included mortality figures as well as the names of people who entered first-aid stations. The prefecture of police also supervised the organization and coordination of emergency medical services in all neighborhoods and issued the time cards that physicians filed with the government when they performed their services. Finally, the police also verified that a particular medical professional deserved an honorary medal after each epidemic.[68]

The municipal police enjoyed such prominence during both cholera outbreaks in large part because of Paris's unique administrative role as both the country's largest city and the capital of a centralizing state.[69] As in the past, the city administration—rather than the national government—had primary responsibility for combating the epidemic disease and for financing the battle. But since the Revolution, when Paris had formed its own distinctive, rebellious "Commune," officials had been wary of endowing a single person with the necessary power to run the city. As a consequence, the prefect of police, the prefect of the Seine, and the mayors of each of the city's twelve arrondissements shared authority. Writing some years after his service as prefect of police, Vivien explained the differences between his responsibilities and those of the prefect of the Seine. Whereas the prefect of the Seine was entrusted with "the most brilliant tasks" (arts, beautification, and so forth), the prefect of police was left to handle "the most difficult jurisdictions, [that is,] every stern measure [such as] the running of prisons, making arrests, etc."[70] The prefect of police, then, had tremendous power within the city's administrative structure, power that reached well beyond law enforcement.

One of the most revealing examples of the Paris administration in action is found in the establishment of a public health bureaucracy to deal with both epidemics. Inspired by news of cholera from eastern Europe, the prefecture of police issued a series of circulars and decrees in the late summer of 1831 that described the formation of one central and forty-eight neighborhood health commissions. Noting the failure of previous health measures to provide adequate and accurate information about the urban environment and acknowledging "the dangers of a disease that has ravaged northern Europe," most of the decrees were quite explicit: they sought to create a regular, efficient, detailed, and complete bureaucratic apparatus for gathering information concerning matters of public health.[71] "It is necessary . . . to divide up the tasks so that they can be executed with greater regularity, by bringing together and classifying the results," one report proclaimed. "In a word, there needs to be a central point where all observations, all the councils can come together, where the administration can weigh all the information relevant to taking its actions."[72]

Such commissions seemed ideally suited for carrying out the kind of detailed investigations of the urban environment called for by the new methodology of public health. For example, the best way to ensure "an active, efficient surveillance," the initial police circular of August 20, 1831, announced, was to create a health commission (*commission de salubrité*) for each part of the capital. Charged with investigating and notifying authorities of unclean areas where cholera might likely emerge, each district commission (*commission d'arrondissement*) was to be made up of six "pillars of the community" (*citoyens notables*), among them, two doctors and one pharmacist (all appointed by the prefecture of police), three notables (designated by the prefecture of the Seine), as well as the mayor of the arrondissement, who would serve as president. At the neighborhood level, the *commission du quartier* was to consist of similarly appointed persons who, accompanied by a policeman and an inspector, would visit "all the buildings in their neighborhood, seeking out causes of insalubrity, advising residents of the danger, and enjoining them as much as possible to find a remedy."[73] Clearly, the commissions were to leave no stone unturned, as subsequent circulars encouraged them to visit everything from the hidden spaces occupied by ragpickers, merchants, or artisans to various public institutions frequented principally by the poor.[74] In the words of the *Journal des commissions sanitaires*, the goal of the commissions was to "enlighten both authorities and inhabitants of the capital about all the measures that, because of the grave epidemic manifest in Europe, have become of such lively interest in Paris and all of France." The editors appealed to "the patriotism and enlightenment" of anyone who might be connected with the epidemic to refer any relevant documents directly to the journal so that they might be disseminated to the public.[75]

Because the commissions represented a new assertion of government authority, their credibility became a central concern of the administration. Accordingly, they were to include members whose "social position would make their example influential."[76] All members were to be chosen from among "enlightened men" and must have "indispensable knowledge in order to comprehend fully the causes of insalubrity and the means of remedying it." To make these investigations, the city government relied especially heavily on medical professionals, who would provide valuable scientific resources because of their training, as well as legitimacy because of their social standing. Ideally, the commissions were also to have influence over "the somewhat more enlightened segments of the population, [such as] foremen or even intelligent workers."[77] For the state, then, the commissions were intended to present a credible means of maintaining order by creating an organization for battling the epidemic.

Many approached the establishment of a centralized bureaucratic structure with some reservations, however. On the one hand, the prefecture of police was to serve as the central hub of a clearly

defined bureaucracy, one fully integrated with the Conseil de Salubrité from 1802. If the commissions failed to provide sufficiently
detailed information regarding their investigations of Parisian
neighborhoods, the prefect was to encourage uniformity and thor-
oughness by enclosing a blank table listing specific categories to be
completed by each member.[78] On the other hand, the decrees that
set up the sanitary commissions clearly created an apparatus that
emphasized local autonomy and initiative. Thus, although the decrees frequently stressed cooperation between individual members
and among the various commissions, they also invited each unit to
maintain "an essentially municipal character."[79]

By encouraging local autonomy and seeking officials of well-
established social standing, the administration created a situation
of continued—and perhaps inevitable—friction between the prefecture of police and the commission members. Despite the prefecture's constant assurances to the contrary, members often complained that they had little power other than to offer suggestions.
"Their principal, I would say even their only, means of accomplish-
ing anything was through persuasion," noted one doctor looking
back on his service in the Luxembourg quarter.[80] Writing in his
memoirs, another physician, Dr. F. L. Poumiès de la Siboutie, displayed similar frustration. He observed that although the city
seemed eager to send in investigation teams, officials displayed
considerably less enthusiasm about following up on his group's
suggestions. "According to its custom, the Administration put these
documents into boxes," he recalled. "Some effort was made [to do
something with the documents], and then that was it."[81] Thus, the
first months of the *commissions sanitaires* were marked by friction,
ambiguity, and disorganization, in spite of the carefully articulated
measures for forging a working alliance between the bureaucracy
and the medical profession.

Since the commissions established in conjunction with the first
epidemic had been disbanded shortly after the departure of cholera,
new ones had to be established in 1849. Though they had comparable responsibilities, the tone of the documents indicated that the
government no longer seemed as concerned with creating a new
image or discovering methodologies for exploring problems in the
urban environment. Now, the commissions had become a permanent part of a larger bureaucratic structure much more broadly

focused on problems of public health. The law of December 18, 1848, established a permanent Conseil d'Hygiène Publique et de Salubrité (Council of Public Health and Salubrity), which had much the same bureaucratic organization and many of the same responsibilities as the 1832 *commissions de salubrité*.[82] Although the decree offered fewer detailed guidelines than the comparable measures in 1832, the post-1848 discussions of health commissions present a picture of much greater bureaucratic coordination and centralization. And now, under the authority of the Ministry of Agriculture and Commerce, the commissions took on a more national and permanent character. Paris lost its position of autonomy, sharing administrative power on an equal basis with provincial prefectures. Moreover, the regularly established intervals for meetings, as well as their desired contents and the established channels for reporting them, gave the commissions a permanent place within the French bureaucratic structure for the first time.

Cholera's administrative messengers thus provided a structure for collecting and disseminating information about the epidemic reality and thereby created perceptions of it. Their efforts suggested officials' underlying assumption that through an objective, rational deployment of human resources the bureaucracy might yield valuable responses to an epidemic crisis. While innovations ranging from the use of preprinted forms to the establishment of a rigorous bureaucracy helped to create a particular image of the epidemic reality, the view of the epidemics that ultimately emerged was the product of failed experiments as much as of preplanning and design. At the same time, the work of bodies such as the *commissions sanitaires* revealed points of collaboration and conflict between administrators and the medical professionals, whose duties and jurisdictions frequently overlapped. Doctors worked within the system, for example, at the same time that they challenged it. Relying on many of the documents produced by this bureaucracy, the press would in turn create and disseminate its own picture of cholera.

THE JOURNALISTS

After the initial excitement at the beginning of the 1832 epidemic, an entertainment daily, *L'Entracte*, printed a modern parable that demonstrated the central yet problematic place the press occupied for the public.[83] Entitled "A Correspondence," the article consisted of a fictitious exchange of letters between a writer and Cholera-morbus, "a man all in black and having an evil look." Cholera opened the exchange by informing the writer that he should be ready at high noon, when the disease's servant would come for him. The intended victim casually wrote back that he would gladly oblige but that noon was too early because he had an important article to finish that day. Upon learning that the writer was in fact a journalist, Cholera gave him a reprieve, saying that, had he known the writer's occupation, he would never have bothered "a person whom I cherish as much as he respects me." Cholera politely thanked the journalist for his help in claiming more victims and promised the writer somewhat perversely: "I'll never forget you as long as I live." After receiving such a warm letter, the journalist asked Cholera's permission to publish it, which the disease gladly granted, saying that he would "refuse nothing to kindly journalists." The article ended with the writer's suggestion that, given the affection Cholera had for journalists, their occupation offered the best immunity against catching the disease.

Humorous and sarcastic, the epistolary exchange reveals an ambivalent attitude toward the press and its prominent role in conveying information through the printed word. Such a mixed view stemmed in part from journalists' unsavory reputation as unscrupulous, money-grubbing men of limited political and personal integrity. Caught between personal ambition, duty to employers, and an expanding public sphere that touted the ideal of rational debate, journalists personified the dilemmas of the public citizen in post-revolutionary France. Crudely put, public expectations rarely mixed well with one's private interests, and thus journalists of the July Monarchy found themselves in an awkward and precarious position.[84]

Journalists' individual identity crises translated into those of a newspaper itself. For example, publishing "A Correspondence" suggests *L'Entracte's* own fundamental confusion about its role in educating the public about the dangers of the press. On the one hand, the cooperative, almost conspiratorial, relationship between Cholera and the journalist revealed a certain animosity toward and resentment of the glib mainstream press. The fear inspired by sensationalist newspaper articles, the piece suggested, constituted a danger as formidable as the epidemic itself. Because current medical wisdom held that fear predisposed one to catching the disease, it lent a certain legitimacy to the modern parable's implicit argument that the press spread cholera by spreading news of it. On the other hand, the content of the correspondence as well as its inclusion in the paper clearly demonstrated the power of the press, a power that might just as easily be used against the epidemic. If journalists took their responsibilities seriously, they wielded influence that could help fight the fear that had given the disease free reign.

Despite comparatively low circulation figures, the press played an important role in the creation and transmission of politics and culture during both cholera epidemics.[85] The most frequently cited and widely circulating political papers, such as the *Journal des débats*, *Le Constitutionnel*, and *Le Courrier français*, had subscription rates of six to eleven or twelve thousand copies during the 1830s and 1840s. Even the wildly popular *Le Siècle* and *La Presse* hovered around twenty thousand, while comparable British papers routinely boasted circulation figures over fifty thousand.[86] With the average subscription in the 1830s costing about one-tenth of a worker's wages and with little street vending to speak of until 1848 (most dailies had to be purchased through expensive up-front quarterly or annual subscriptions), newspapers remained a luxury for a majority of Parisians until the end of the century.[87] Nonetheless, the number of "active readers" in France climbed from 53 percent of men and 40 percent of women in 1831 to 68 percent of men and 52 percent of women in 1851.[88]

But subscription or even literacy figures provide only a crude picture of a paper's potential influence. As the prefect of police pointed out in 1831, "One issue of *Le Constitutionnel* [a paper with greater appeal among the less-literate Parisians, who tended toward the left] sometimes has a hundred readers, while one issue of *La Quotidienne* [a royalist Catholic paper] has but one or at the most a family."[89] Many papers were indeed passed from hand to hand. For the modest fee of ten centimes, curious Parisians could also read newspapers in small lending libraries or in the local café, or they could listen as another read them out loud.[90] Finally, as we shall see, by influencing the exercise of government power, newspapers would also have an important impact even on Parisians who did not read them.

Perhaps more than doctors and administrators, who had been among the messengers of past epidemics, journalists emerged as the quintessential storytellers of the first "modern plague." By the time of the cholera outbreaks, new definitions of politics and the public combined with changes in technology and reading habits to shape a newspaper press that would have been unrecognizable to anyone half a century earlier. Although stories like "A Correspondence" suggested that many remained wary of this new press, nearly everyone accepted the fact that the newspaper had become a fundamental part of Parisian political and cultural life. "Today journalism is an established power," a popular booklet entitled *Physiologie de la presse* informed readers in 1841. "Everything is done on behalf of newspapers, and nothing can be done without them." The anonymous work went on to explain how journalism was "the most powerful and virtuous of the four branches of government."[91] Even foreigners remarked on the central place of the press in Paris. In a report to his ruler about French customs in the mid-1840s, for example, a Moroccan scholar reserved a special section for describing Parisian newspaper culture. "All in all," he concluded after extolling the virtues of a frequent and available commodity, "the gazette is of such importance that [a bourgeois Parisian] would do without food or drink sooner than do without the newspaper."[92] By the time of cholera the Parisian press enjoyed enough power to provoke comment, yet not so much power that it was taken for granted.

The relationship between journalism and cholera must be seen within the larger question of how the Parisian newspaper developed into a powerful bourgeois institution over a relatively short period of time. Between 1770 and 1850 the political and cultural history of the Parisian press followed two parallel, yet sometimes interrelated stories. On the one hand, the development of a vital opposition press propelled by revolution, debates over censorship, and conflicts over party politics contributed to a standard political narrative of a newly important institution seeking power. On the other hand, the form and content of the French press were intricately bound up with the Parisian bourgeoisie's economic and cultural ascendancy during the late eighteenth and early nineteenth centuries; entrepreneurs invested in newspapers as an economic venture, at the same time that "vernacular print capitalism" was beginning to play a greater role than other more immediate ties in creating a sense of shared identity among bourgeois Parisians.[93] The confluence of the political and cultural narratives enabled the Parisian press to be both oppositional and a guardian of a new status quo, a fact that helps explain the inherent, yet logical contradiction in "A Correspondence."

Because factors such as government regulations, high costs, limited production capacity, and widespread illiteracy prevented a wide and regular newspaper culture from developing in the capital prior to 1789, the history of the modern press in fact begins with the Revolution.[94] Supporters and critics alike saw the newspaper as an integral part of the revolutionary process, an idea that would contribute significantly to attitudes toward the press during the cholera epidemics. By toppling a repressive regime and an entire social class of aristocrats, the Revolution had unleashed the press and a torrent of new political ideas. Along with providing important narrative accounts of revolutionary events, the more than 130 dailies that began circulating for the first time in 1789 helped generate a new, vastly larger audience eager to read them.[95] Even if the majority of these papers were only sporadic and short-lived, they provided a forum for the many new experimental ideas spreading throughout the capital. One no longer needed to be present at Assembly meetings or other events to know what happened or to express an opinion on the subject. Moreover, newspapers' immediacy, initial availability through street hawkers, and relative low cost enabled journalists to proclaim themselves de facto representatives of the Third Estate, at least until wary government officials could agree upon a satisfactory means of regulating them.[96] During the early excitement of 1789 the newspaper thus both described the events and became a fundamental part of the revolutionary process by doing so.

From its revolutionary outset, the modern newspaper had particularly strong bonds with bourgeois culture, bonds that would influence the character of the press as a messenger of cholera. Most of the Revolution's journalists came from obscure families of the middle class, while a subscription or the entrance fees to a reading room constituted luxuries not readily available to anyone below the ranks of the middle classes.[97] At the same time, by abolishing censorship and state-regulated monopolies, the revolution of 1789 set the stage for the commercialization of the press, which would make the newspaper trade attractive to bourgeois investors.[98] Running a paper required someone with the precarious modern blend of financial stability and a willingness to take risks, qualities most likely found in a bourgeois; few others had either the capital or the willingness to purchase the basic materials such as printing presses, ink, paper, or the labor to produce and distribute a newspaper. Because the press had been so instrumental in releasing the fury of a new public in 1789, subsequent regimes further compounded the newspaper's bourgeois character by requiring significant amounts of caution money designed to be beyond the means of the threatening lower classes.[99] Although these facts do not mean that all revolutionary papers carried bourgeois ideas or catered merely to bourgeois readers, they do shed some light on why the newspaper so easily developed into a bourgeois institution in subsequent decades.

If, as a representative of the Third Estate, the press had brought the bourgeoisie into politics, as a "Fourth Estate" it completely recreated the terrain on which the battles would be fought by the time of the first cholera epidemic. Of course, the newspaper provided a tidy means for supporters and opponents of 1789 to continue fighting through much of the nineteenth century. By replacing the barricade with the printed page and by spilling ink instead of blood, the ideological conflicts of revolution and counterrevolution could be played out over and over again in every attack on a ruler or his policies. The critic Alfred Nettement, who deplored the commercialization of the press during the July Monarchy, explained in 1845 that "a newspaper [had originally been] supported financially by those whose political views it expressed; it was a flag."[100] To be sure, the fifty years after the Revolution were the heyday of Parisian newspapers' close public identification with a single political opinion of a given editor or publisher, a fact that created a political landscape deceptively easy to map.[101] The discussions of the relationship between cholera and revolution outlined in the previous chapter emerged within this context. More abstractly, the postrevolutionary press helped perpetuate the idea that public knowledge through the printed word was central to exercising power. In the bourgeois ideal, every reasonable man should be literate and educated in order to make the rational choices required in a democracy. As relatively cheap, disposable commodities that could be quickly produced and distributed to individuals, newspapers provided the potential for universal access to such information. By creating and fulfilling popular demand for information, newspapers made themselves indispensable avenues of political as well as economic and cultural power. At the same time, the press helped crystallize the concept of a "public opinion" in the form of an audience that could be appealed to and used.

Because of its increasing and novel power, the newspaper itself became a political object different from, yet tied to, its content. Expressed in the concept "freedom of the press," this deeper politics emerged as a contest between journalists trying to maintain their revolutionary rights and government officials seeking to restrict the newspaper's potentially inflammatory impact upon the newly liberated masses. More than an argument over who should control thought, the debates raised fundamental questions regarding the nature of authority and the origin and transmission of ideas, as well as about how truth should be determined.[102] In some sense, journalists who had fought for revolution in the streets or in the pages of their newspapers helped keep Enlightenment thought and the revolutionary tradition alive by shifting their battles to the censor's office and the courtroom. Perhaps for this reason, many bourgeois, long after they had distanced themselves from so many other aspects of the revolutionary tradition, still defended the press, the institution that had become quintessentially theirs in the wake of 1789. When championing hard-won freedom of the press in subsequent generations, for example, they defended a liberal desire to allow ideas to circulate freely like currency and merchandise. But their calls for a free press also served as a rhetorical shorthand for guaranteeing members of the bourgeoisie a permanent voice in politics.

The agitation for freedom of the press culminated in the 1830 revolution, which both contemporaries and historians have specifically linked to bourgeois journalists.[103] Charles X's increasing defensiveness led to his infamous July Ordinances, part of a poorly planned coup d'état in which, among other things, he attacked newspapers as "instruments of sedition and disorder."[104] The legislative proclamation quickly led to a public spectacle that galvanized bourgeois Parisians to support the press and its revolution, at least initially. Journalists fought on the barricades,[105] reported the events, and called Parisians to arms by drawing attention to the threatening nature of the king's assault. And not only did they play a key role in toppling Charles X, but these men were also instrumental in goading a reluctant Louis Philippe into assuming the crown as the "citizen-king, a myth they created for him.[106] Finally, by making the news itself news, the journalists of 1830 had crystallized the self-consciousness of the press as a political, social, and cultural force, a fact that would later shape how writers presented their relationship to the epidemic reality.

As a regime that came to power only reluctantly and one that found itself with enemies on both ends of the political spectrum, the July Monarchy had an ambivalent relationship to the press similar to the sentiment expressed in "A Correspondence." On the one hand, Louis Philippe tried to take advantage of the revolutionary momentum by supporting both the journalists and the bourgeois crusade for freedom of the press that had brought him to power. To this end, he revoked all censorship laws and even encouraged the publication and distribution of papers throughout the capital. On the other hand, the regime had to defend itself against vicious attacks on the monarch from both the left- and right-wing press at a time when events such as the 1832 cholera epidemic convinced authorities that life in the capital could easily dissolve into disorder. Louis Philippe so much loathed how the French press ridiculed him that he reportedly read only *The Times* of London, and, after a brief honeymoon of only a few months, his regime clamped down heavily on "political and moral offenders."[107] Strong attacks came in the wake of the disturbances that accompanied General Lamarque's funeral several weeks after the initial invasion of cholera in June 1832, while even more stringent controls went into effect in September 1835.[108]

The period after 1848 marked a clear end to the role of the mainstream press as a revolutionary force and the beginning of its growing role as the guardian of the bourgeois status quo. During the early weeks of the Second Republic the provisional government lifted a stamp tax and briefly did away with the requirement of caution money. Moreover, by introducing universal male suffrage, the new regime increased the number of potential readers and contributors to a political press.[109] When the climate turned sour after the bloody June insurrection, however, the anxious provisional government once again clamped down on the press, with a particularly chilling effect on the smaller radical newspapers. Meanwhile, the campaign and election of Louis Napoleon Bonaparte as president of the Republic, in December 1848, revealed that politicians were coming to rely upon the modern newspaper as a potent political force. By the time of the second cholera epidemic, contemporaries had become conscious enough of the press as a vital influence that they complained of its silence.[110]

Innovations in technology and in the content of papers also reflected and helped forge a strong relationship between bourgeois culture and the modern French press.[111] Technologically, new production processes and equipment made the newspaper widely available.[112] At the same time, industrial capitalism created a climate open to experimentation, in which entrepreneurs such as Emile de Girardin contributed to altering the relationship between politics and the modern press. In some sense, Girardin's life paralleled the evolution of the French bourgeoisie he would ultimately seduce; to make up for the fact that he was the illegitimate son of a noble general, he perpetually sought recognition through ambition, speculation, and financial prowess.[113] The lives of other mid-nineteenth-century journalists displayed a similar pattern: a young man of elite education arrives in Paris without friends or money and eventually manages to find his way by taking risks and selling his political soul.[114]

The eventual success of Girardin and others during the mid-1830s stemmed from cutting subscription rates of their popular papers, such as *La Presse* and *Le Siècle,* in half and making up the lost revenue by luring businesses to place ads based on the vastly larger audience attracted by the low rates.[115] In addition, serialized novels, known as feuilletons-romans, drew in thousands of mostly middle-class readers eager to follow daily accounts of vice and crime in exotic places. In works such as *Les Mystères de Paris* and *Le Juif errant*, writers like Sue conjured up images of Paris malade that bore some striking similarities to the explorations of the hygienists. Perhaps more than the reduced subscription costs, this innovation drew an increased segment of the Paris population into the world of mass-distribution print. During the July Monarchy critics of the genre such as Nettement saw feuilletons-romans as the logical outcome of an ongoing process that ended in the depoliticization of the French press by the mid-1840s.[116]

Despite the beliefs of Nettement and others that the modern newspaper had succumbed to the apolitical lure of fashion and entertainment, however, the modern press was in fact helping to expand the definition of politics beyond the traditional concerns of party debates and foreign policy. The stories that middle-class Parisians eagerly followed in the feuilletons-romans provided them with a new conceptual framework for understanding Paris malade in the most vivid terms. Moreover, as some larger papers abandoned politics for lighter fare, the emergence of a new genre of smaller, specialized newspapers began politicizing the problems of feeding and housing the city's growing numbers of poor. The rise of socialism and a powerful Catholic religious revival during the second half of the July Monarchy helped create the audience for a rapidly proliferating number of small newspapers such as *L'Atelier* (1840), *La Ruche populaire* (1839), *La Revue du progrès* (1840), *L'Ami du peuple* (1845), *La Réforme* (1843), and *La Bonne Foi* (1849), most of which began as established alternatives to large circulation dailies such as the *Journal des débats*, *Le Constitutionnel*, and *Le Courrier français*.[117] An acknowledged part of the Parisian journalistic and political landscape, such papers were both a symptom and a cause of shifting sensibilities toward the poor that would have an important impact on responses to cholera in 1849. Even if many of these papers had probably been started by bourgeois, their very existence was an explicit acknowledgment that the concerns of lower-class Parisians had become politically significant. At the same time, they indicated that the press was now perceived as a valuable tool for winning over a broader public.

The evolution of the government organ, the *Moniteur universel*, the most important paper during both epidemics, offers another important and wholly overlooked example of how the avenues of politics were being broadened with the advent of a more widely disseminated daily press.[118] Founded at the very beginning of the 1789 revolution, the *Moniteur* was one of the first "information newspapers" in France, which meant that it tried to supply detailed news items with a minimum of commentary. In one of the earliest attempts to create objective rather than interpretive news, the *Moniteur* based its content on the "exactitude of facts, clarity in style, [and] scrupulous fidelity to the transcriptions of debates."[119] Originally, this had been an economic ploy on the part of its founder, editor, and publisher, the book-trade magnate Charles-Joseph Panckoucke, to find an uncrowded niche in the chaotic, yet lucrative publishing scene during the spring of 1789. Under Panckoucke, the *Moniteur* provided readers with verbatim accounts of National Assembly proceedings, along with the full texts of laws, treaties, and administrative circulars. To market his paper's objectivity in a dramatic manner, Panckoucke departed from the standard format of Parisian dailies by borrowing a large folio size from late eighteenth-century British newspapers. The combination of seemingly dispassionate information conveyed on such a large scale no doubt contributed to initial impressions of the *Moniteur* as an unparalleled voice of authority. Moreover, Panckoucke and subsequent editors quickly learned that this format had enduring economic advantages; as governments began clamping down on press freedoms during the waning years of the Revolution and the Empire, the *Moniteur* survived each change in regime by making itself both inoffensive and indispensable.[120]

For readers, meanwhile, even if they did not all actually receive and read it, the *Moniteur* assumed a central role as a representative of state authority, particularly in a time of crisis such as during the cholera epidemics. According to comments made almost in passing, many readers fundamentally accepted the paper's dry objectivity as part and parcel of the abstract government power it had come to represent. "Inflexible as destiny, it has registered the acts of each successive government with the same cold blood for the past forty years," the *Physiologie de la presse* noted in 1841. "The *Moniteur* is not a paper devoted to discussion, it is a stake on which ministries post their official announcements."[121] Even if he meant it somewhat disparagingly, Hugo also acknowledged the *Moniteur*'s universalizing, objective power when he characterized it as the post-revolutionary equivalent of the *Encyclopédie*.[122] The paper thus enjoyed considerable influence because of its official stature. During both epidemics, for example, nearly every paper in the capital reprinted substantial portions of its pronouncements, minutes from meetings of the *commissions sanitaires*, and police circulars without comment. Thus, many Parisians learned either directly or indirectly from the pages of the *Moniteur* how they should recognize the first symptoms of cholera, which sections of the city seemed most affected, and the size of charity subscriptions.

As was the case with doctors' reports, bureaucratic circulars, and other faithful, "authentic" recorders of official policy, the *Moniteur* also produced a highly subjective bourgeois objectivity. Drawing upon the Enlightenment ideal that reasonable men should interpret facts for themselves based on careful reading and study, the *Moniteur* presupposed a certain shared, preexisting knowledge as well as the leisure time to read and interpret the information it supplied. Like the paper's dry recounting of commerce and trade figures, its verbatim accounts of laws and parliamentary debates spoke most directly to the small group of bourgeois men immediately engaged in these activities. Moreover, the paper's choice of news items for its *partie non-officielle* and their position in even the most bland column layout, not to mention the paper's very existence as a government organ, all created a particular slant on current events, whether or not editors were fully conscious of all implications and possibilities. Like medical professionals and police officials, the journalists who provided information for the *Moniteur* did so anonymously, relying on a replication of detailed facts to present highly subjective interpretations through an allegedly objective stance. The *Moniteur universel* was, in effect, the quintessential bourgeois journalistic institution precisely because it claimed to be universal, objective, and neutral.

Most Parisians had only indirect exposure to the *Moniteur*, however, a contact mediated largely through a variety of more explicitly subjective papers that also experimented with new journalistic techniques.[123] The *Journal des débats, Le Courrier français, Le Constitutionnel, Le Bonhomme Richard, Le National,* and *La Quotidienne* were among the thirty or so papers published in the capital during the July Monarchy.[124] By the time of the cholera epidemics, most Parisian dailies averaged four to six large-format pages. Except for papers such as *Le Charivari* or *La Caricature,* whose raison d'être was the illustration, no Parisian paper in the 1830s and 1840s tried to be either devious or fetching. With no headlines, cartoons, or other graphics to set off a story, and with the few blatant advertisements relegated to the final page,[125] the papers relied exclusively on the quality of the printed text to attract readers. By drawing upon the *Moniteur*'s authenticity, these papers sought to heighten their own credibility while offering alternative views of party politics within the capital. As newspapers created largely by and for a middle-class readership, they perpetuated bourgeois ideas and values both in their content and by virtue of their very existence.

Alongside the daily newspapers, a proliferation of professional journals further attested to the expanding cultural power of the press and its relationship to the Parisian bourgeoisie during both epidemics. Beginning in the 1820s, for example, as many as seventy new periodicals dealing with medicine and public health were circulating in the French capital.[126] While some clearly addressed a lay audience hungry for medical remedies, the majority seemed to speak directly to members of the profession and no doubt played an important part in creating at least a superficial sense of identity among doctors.[127] In addition to the *Annales d'hygiène publique et de médecine légale* (1829), journals such as the *Gazette des hôpitaux civils et militaires* (1828), the *Gazette médicale de Paris* (1830), and the *Gazette de santé* (1833), to name but a few, appeared in Paris, with subscribers probably numbering below a thousand.[128] Significantly, the medical periodicals outnumbered their counterparts in jurisprudence and beaux-arts by nearly four to one.[129] Seeing themselves as men of the world, many Parisian doctors offered contributions not just in medicine but in literature and politics, particularly since medicine had not yet developed the precise scientific vocabulary that would soon distance it from the lay public. Moreover, as we have seen, medical professionals' methodology of observing and recording exactly what they saw further solidified a relationship between medical power and print. Perhaps the most important paper for the medical profession as a whole was *L'Union médicale,* founded in 1846, a year after the watershed congress in which doctors had formally committed themselves to establishing a profession. The paper departed from previous journals by supplementing traditional medical information and instruction with a conscious program of representing the interests of doctors, pharmacists, and veterinarians as a profession.[130]

During both cholera epidemics medical equivalents to the *Moniteur* appeared, a telling indication of the cultural power of the press and the medicalization of French society more generally. Along with the *Moniteur*, popular papers mined these journals for cholera news with the stamp of medical authority. During the first outbreak, for example, the *Journal des commissions sanitaires établies dans le département de la Seine* provided statistics on mortality and recovery, résumés of case reports by famous doctors, and brief descriptions of the latest books on cholera, as well as an open forum for medical professionals to air their views. At the same time, the *Gazette médicale de Paris* started a small spin-off journal that appeared three times a week to accommodate all the latest news about the epidemic.[131] By 1849, *L'Union médicale* had gained enough stature to serve as the oracle for cholera news, a fact that, as we shall see, generated some controversy. By creating such a specific forum for discussing cholera, these papers underscored the importance of the epidemic as an event worthy of ongoing public attention in print. But, at the same time, they provided a voice of authority that legitimated accounts in less-specialized papers.

As "A Correspondence" indicated, the modern press occupied a powerful, yet ambivalent place within the Parisian popular imagination. Both a subversive force and a potential defender of the bourgeois status quo, the modern press was by no means a monolithic entity in complete economic, political, or social agreement. Duels among editors and conflicts between government censors and journalists, as well as competition for readers, all suggested attempts to stake out a highly contested terrain that no single group could define, let alone possess. Moreover, the press itself was extremely divided among political factions. Put another way, at the time of both cholera epidemics, the press did not have a fixed purpose or identity, even if contemporaries tried to locate one by creating fictitious exchanges between such unlikely conspirators as Cholera and journalists.

Taken together, cholera's messengers would shape an image of the epidemic reality based on their backgrounds as bourgeois Parisians. Products of Enlightenment and Revolution, these members of recently empowered professions led a struggle against the disease based on such values as confidence in science, human rationality, reason, hands-on experience, objectivity, and neutrality, as well as a belief in universalizing truths. At the same time, however, the hard realities of Parisian life brought to the surface by cholera forced them to refine these conceptual tools. The understanding of cholera as a disease grounded in class differences, for example, did not readily fit with the notions of equality and universality that were so central to Enlightenment thought. Moreover, the suffering and human misery brought to the surface in Paris malade baldly contradicted ideas of progress and human perfectibility.

More concretely, cholera's messengers were united by their shared role of transmitting information within the context of post-Enlightenment and postrevolutionary Paris. To further its goals, each group both benefited from and contributed to the creation of a "commerce of information," perhaps the most important weapon at their disposal when so little could be done about cholera. Especially in a society where access to information was so limited, their control over it gave them unprecedented power and leverage. Through medical reports, mortality figures, advice for cures, and accounts of these activities, cholera's messengers managed to create a specific image of the epidemics precisely because they collected and interpreted information about them. At the same time, the quest for such information would enable each of the three groups to penetrate into areas and lives that had previously been hidden from view and to shed light on this darkness for other potential observers. In this sense, bourgeois culture was in fact about creating transparency; the very idea that information should be accumulated and made public was one of the fundamental tenets of bourgeois liberal thought. Or, as Foucault argued through much of his work, the universalizing power of bourgeois culture lay in the discovery and exploitation of the idea of equating knowledge and power; this equation explains the pivotal role played by cholera's messengers.

But while medical professionals, administrators, and journalists shared a common bourgeois identity and values grounded in the legacy of the Enlightenment and Revolution, their power was in fact uneven and incomplete; they did not constitute a monolithic, seamless web of repressive state power. Limited by inconsistent or insufficient information, inefficiency, confusion, as well as by their own doubts and fears, these men struggled to fight cholera as best they could. Moreover, as we shall see in the following chapters, the three groups not only suffered from internal conflicts but also vied with one another as they grappled with an epidemic mystery and its many unforeseen consequences.

3

Inventing Perceptions
of Disease and Government

To gain an understanding of the complex interactions among medical professionals, administrators, and journalists, I now turn to three areas where their authority intersected during both epidemics. Through the creation and distribution of health instructions, the establishment of emergency first-aid stations, and the collection and dissemination of daily mortality figures, cholera's messengers forged a working relationship with one another at the same time that they created perceptions of each outbreak and their own attempts to fight it. Moreover, this newly evolving relationship among the medical profession, bureaucracy, and the press was a key component in the consolidation of bourgeois authority in the mid-nineteenth century. Not only did most medical professionals and government officials come from the "rising bourgeoisie," but—as revealed by the content and tone of their writings—they wrote with members of that class firmly in mind.

The official responses to cholera, however, should not be viewed as part of a conscious scheme of bourgeois hegemony aimed at brutal oppression of the poor. Rather, reactions to the epidemics must be explored for what they reveal about a bourgeois class in the process of redefining its bases of power and legitimacy at a time when its supremacy was by no means assured. When the disease first threatened Paris in 1832, the administration had not yet developed a coherent set of responses, let alone an efficient bureaucratic public health apparatus. Despite the limited experience during the yellow fever threat of the early 1820s, government officials had a narrow understanding of strategies they could use in the impending crisis, while their raison d'être had not yet been clearly articulated or established. Moreover, even considering the relatively highly developed character of the centralized French administration and the country's leading world role in both medicine and public health, a collaboration between medical professionals and the administration was not a foregone conclusion in 1832, nor was it obvious what form such a possible collaboration might take. And, finally, without strong precedents of active government intervention in areas of health, cholera's messengers needed to respond to a crisis constantly being reshaped by shifting expectations linked to the disease as well as to the revolutionary tradition and Paris malade. By 1849, the rhetoric, expectations, and justifications for the steps taken by cholera's messengers revealed a new confidence and a less open sense of class antagonism than had been the case in 1832.

This chapter is organized conceptually around the health instructions, the emergency first-aid stations, and the presentation of daily mortality figures. By contrasting 1832 and 1849 within each section, we can focus on the nature and content of each type of response and see how cholera's messengers interacted under different trying situations.

THE *INSTRUCTIONS POPULAIRES*

Published and widely distributed at the height of both epidemics, the *instructions populaires*, or popular instructions, became one of the most important conduits of information between the government and its citizens. Upon first glance, these pamphlets provide concrete, welcome facts for fighting a mysterious epidemic and seem to have been written for members of less-fortunate classes, as suggested by the title *popular* instructions. However, a careful look at the content, layout, and rhetorical structure of the documents reveals the ways in which administration officials attempted to use doctors' advice to shape bourgeois impressions of both government actions and the nature of the disease itself. Moreover, by looking at the underlying assumptions behind the *instructions* in 1832 and 1849, we can gain fresh insight into how bourgeois authority and culture became dominant within the supposedly objective realm of medical advice.

As early as mid-November 1831, the Department of the Seine published its first set of popular instructions under the auspices of the prefecture of police, and when the epidemic reached the capital six months later, the administration had forty thousand copies printed.[1] Amidst mortality statistics and detailed information about emergency first-aid stations, the *Moniteur* suggested that the arrival of the pamphlets was a sign that officials had matters well in hand.[2] Based on observations made by medical teams that had investigated cholera in eastern Europe, the fourteen-page printed booklet was signed by members of the Central Board of Health, appointed by the prefect of police.

Politically, the popular instructions helped promote the power of bourgeois government by underscoring the legitimacy of the newly arrived July Monarchy and Paris administration. At a certain level, the widely publicized document revealed a desire to establish the government's credibility independent of medical authority at a time when both the state and the medical profession were struggling to establish authority and legitimacy. The prefect of police, Gisquet, stated the goal explicitly enough. Describing the pamphlet in his memoirs, he boasted that it went into "the minutest details, so that each person could ward off cholera, or [at least] follow the best curative regimen *without even having to resort to the help of medical wisdom.*"[3] With frequent references to cures being "administered" rather than "provided" or "given" by doctors, moreover, the rhetoric of the document itself suggested that the administration had placed its stamp upon medical ideas. In one classic example the *instruction* wrapped up its discussion of acceptable home remedies by advising, "Even though these different means should be put into use as soon as possible, they must be administered with order and without too much haste."[4]

Because of the credibility of the Paris medical profession, however, officials usually found it more useful to profit from medical authority rather than to bypass it. In the instructions, the administration even placed itself in the lofty position of distinguishing acceptable from unacceptable medical wisdom. Urging the public to follow "the *rigorous* observation [of these] rules for preservation," the pamphlet warned Parisians not to be taken in by the "alleged preservation and curative means whose properties greedy charlatans push in newspapers and announce on posters plastered on the walls of the capital." The administration wished to establish itself as the principal judge of legitimate knowledge and thus assured Parisians, "If authorities were fortunate enough to know such a [successful] method, they would not fail to publicize and recommend it."[5] At the same time, officials faithfully reflected the current wisdom of the Paris medical establishment, which remained deeply skeptical of therapeutics in general.[6] The administration's desire to prevent unqualified remedies from entering the marketplace also contributed to the credibility of the mainstream medical profession at a time when it was struggling to establish itself as the sole arbiter of power by eclipsing alternative practitioners. In this way, government authority played a key role in validating some doctors' prestige at the same time that it exploited the struggle to assert its own power.

To be sure, the *instruction* shared certain characteristics with such "charlatans," who pushed anything from miracle diets to special anticholera syrups and drops in the back pages of popular newspapers.[7] The government's trump card, however, was its credibility, its promise to offer the public knowledge based on reasoned, thorough medical observation, description, and experience. Appropriating authority from the medical profession at a time when no one understood the cause of, progress of, or cure for cholera, officials participated in the creation of a new means of interacting with the inhabitants of the capital that placed primary emphasis on the new bourgeois regime as a source of power.

The instructions also contributed to the dominance of bourgeois culture more subtly by promoting the values of that class in widely distributed print. Most important, the pamphlet spoke directly to the individual lay reader. Striking a delicate balance between detail and plain language, the *instruction* appealed to the rational, self-interested, confident citizen who could read and think for himself. While some kind of *instruction* had been a standard official response to plagues in previous centuries, such documents had been written principally for town elders, justices, and other civil servants in order to offer advice on how best to govern the population during the crisis.[8] The *instruction populaire* issued during the first cholera epidemic represented a dramatic departure; the pamphlet adopted a common-sense approach in which it called upon individual citizens to take an unprecedented amount of responsibility for both their own health and the well-being of society. Moreover, the instructions thrived because of the proliferation of print culture, which made them readily available to an increasingly literate public. With forty thousand copies allegedly circulating in the capital in addition to the versions reprinted in newspapers, the instructions were among the most widely disseminated documents in the capital at the time.

Thus, the pamphlets were a potentially influential way of disseminating and forming bourgeois attitudes toward cholera.

By appealing to the individual as the principal unit in society, the *instruction* also provided a medical correlate to laissez-faire, in which each individual contributed to the greater good by working in his or her self-interest. In this case, however, the "invisible hand" was that of a marionette because officials used the appeals to self-help to further the seemingly contradictory end of orchestrating public behavior. Discussing everything from the specifics of how dwellings should be cleaned and aired to the details of clothing, diet, and moral conduct, the official pamphlet offered preventive measures as well as concrete steps to take should one come down with the disease. Diet occupied a particularly important place, in part because it was an area over which the (bourgeois) individual had greatest control. Acknowledging the fact that each individual had foods that could be digested only with difficulty, for example, the remarkably detailed *instruction* suggested that "each person should study his stomach." In general, however, fatty, salted meats, charcuterie, heavy pastries, aqueous vegetables such as cucumbers or beets, and large quantities of fruit were all to be avoided, as were excessive eating and drinking of any kind. This attention to the details of diet made disease prevention a strictly individual matter.

Appeals to the individual lay reader created a special role for detail because, as the doctors writing the *instruction* no doubt understood, minute facts helped evoke the texture of personal experience. Thus, the *instruction* spoke to each reader through its impressive mastery of detail at the same time that it had to train Parisians to understand the value and meaning of the details themselves. In other words, not everyone could "study his stomach," unless, as the pamphlet instructed, "each person [became] familiar with the first signs which indicate that an individual will be, or already is, stricken with cholera." The *instruction* provided ample details as a guide. I quote the following passage at some length to give an idea of the quality of knowledge presented to the average reader. Note the breathless, almost romanticized portrait, which lends both specificity and urgency to the description:

Sudden weariness or a sudden feeling of fatigue in all limbs; a feeling of heaviness in the head, as when one is exposed to carbon va-

pors; dizziness, staggering, mild deafness, pallor of a leaden hue, a blu-
ish color on the face, with a *peculiar* alteration of the features; there
is something odd about the expression, the eyes lose their bright-
ness, their brilliance; a loss of appetite; thirst, and a desire to sat-
isfy it with cold drinks; feelings of oppression, anxiety in the chest
and [feelings of] heat and burning in the pit of the stomach; passing twinges of pain in the ribs (that is to say below the areas that begin at the hallow of the stomach in calculating from top to bottom); rumblings in the intestines (gurgling), accompanied above all
by colic followed by a loosening of the bowels in the base of the stomach; sometimes this loosening seems to reduce the pain; the skin becomes cold and dry; sometimes it becomes covered in cold sweat.
Some patients experience shivers along the spinal column of the back,
along with a sensation as if someone blew cold air on their hair.[9]

While waiting for a doctor, the patient was to be covered with wool
blankets (heated if possible), and those attending were to rub the
body ("with vigor and for a *long time*") with a dry brush or a coarse
cloth soaked in a mixture of *eau de vie*, strong vinegar, mustard flour,
camphor, pepper, and garlic. Vaporized baths could also be useful,
and so the pamphlet provided a suitable recipe.[10]

The exhaustive use of detail in the instructions both enhanced
officials' credibility and reveal their sense of awe as they faced
cholera in 1832. The ability to narrate new details grounded in expertise provided administrators with a reasonably easy means of
managing the epidemic in such a way that they appeared to be more
in control of the situation than they actually were. The sheer volume
of details, combined with the prefecture's self-declared monopoly
on legitimate knowledge and the canonization of the instructions in
bold print, gave the measures an undeniable authenticity. At bottom, however, the details also revealed a struggle to attain much-
needed knowledge. Reading the pamphlet from 1832, one is left
with the feeling of going on a voyage of discovery in which certain
key points obviously remained an unsolved medical mystery. Here
the act of description itself was not enough; even if this ability to
describe the disease and possible remedies gave the administration
the credibility to treat it, the growing numbers of random deaths
that soon threatened the most respectable neighborhoods called
government authority more and more into question.

Perhaps because the pamphlets had been conceived and written
by medical professionals and distributed through a government

bureaucracy and the popular press, the story told by the details spoke with particular clarity to bourgeois Parisians and reflected the values of their class. Frequently, for example, the *instruction* made a point of stressing moderation and restraint. "Sobriety [meaning *moderation* in both food and drink] cannot be recommended enough," officials cautioned, because "there are many examples which prove that cholera comes on after excesses at table." According to the principles of the *juste milieu*, excesses of any kind, such as fear, indulgences of the flesh, or even bath water of immoderate temperature could all be potential sources of cholera.[11] Such advice was based on a modified version of the ancient system of medical knowledge known as "the doctrine of the non-naturals." Coming from the works of Hippocrates and Galen, the orderly system was predicated upon the idea of *balance* among elements both inside (humors) and outside (air, water, food) the body. The key to good health was to achieve a state of equilibrium, which would keep a disease such as cholera at bay. In its late eighteenth-century reinterpretation, the doctrine championed rationality and self-help in order to attain the precious balance among the elements that constituted "health," a set of ideas that had a remarkable affinity with bourgeois values.[12]

Moreover, in some places the pamphlet called upon Parisians to live like good bourgeois in order to be spared the ravages of cholera. No one who truly thought about it, for example, could expect the poor to avoid fatty meats, move to other rooms during the day, have curtains around their beds, or have the plumbing and latrines that the instructions recommended they keep so clean.[13] A larger number of passages in the pamphlet, however, targeted the lower classes by name or by custom, a fact that ultimately reinforced widespread belief in the class-specificity of the disease. Again, keep in mind the rich details of daily life:

> Unnecessary domestic animals should be taken away. Refrain from raising pigs, rabbits, chickens, and giving food to pigeons, etc., in areas reserved for humans, [especially] in small, stuffy courtyards.
>
> Residents should all keep an eye on one another in this regard [*devraient à cet égard se surveiller mutuellement*], particularly in populous neighborhoods; they should, moreover, each take their part in contributing to the cleanliness of the streets, especially when the streets are narrow. This is in everyone's interest.[14]

Many people, especially those in the less-fortunate classes, have the very bad habit of sleeping and, upon waking, of placing their bare feet on the cold floor. Some even walk like this. This practice cannot be condemned enough, especially when cholera rages.[15]

Such naive outrage betrayed how little the pamphlet's authors assumed middle-class Parisians understood about the lives of their less-fortunate neighbors. Not all paupers walked in bare feet out of spite; far too many did so out of necessity, as revealed by the countless investigations of urban space in the 1820s, some of them conducted by the very medical professionals responsible for the *instructions*. This stylized portrait of (unhealthy) lower-class life provided a revealing contrast with that of the (healthy) bourgeois.

Similar contrasts served to warn bourgeois Parisians against *behaving* like the poor. Among the lower classes the excessive consumption of alcohol constituted a particular danger, though by no means did officials advocate complete temperance in the manner of their American counterparts.[16] Even while the *instruction* claimed that "common practices, especially among the working class," of drinking *eau de vie* on an empty stomach could prove deadly during a cholera epidemic, it made no attempt to stop the custom.[17] Instead, the pamphlet suggested people restrict their consumption of wine to that of superior quality. In effect, "drinking" became a synonym, a code word, for "poverty" and its supposed direct links to cholera. By implication, one needed only to avoid the habits of the poor in order to maintain a safe distance from the disease.

Significantly, the pamphlet used two somewhat incompatible rhetorical strategies to encourage Parisians to fight the epidemic. As we have seen, one placed emphasis on the individual. The other, by contrast, focused on the *environment* in which that individual lived, not just in terms of immediate surroundings but also in terms of Paris malade. Seen in this way, cholera was an intrinsic part of the world in which the poor lived. If the lower classes would pay greater attention to the cleanliness of their dwellings and their bodies, the document seemed to argue, they would stand a much reduced chance of falling sick. From the perspective of the middle classes, such passages were quite reassuring; by tacitly linking the disease with the filth and vices of the poor, the upper strata of Parisian society spared themselves both responsibility for the epidemic and anxiety over catching the disease.

Individual and environmental approaches to cholera could coexist in part because the idea of the individual, like that of the environment, had a different meaning depending upon the class being described. From the perspective of bourgeois writers, social commentators, and—to some extent—even doctors, few concrete individuals existed amidst the massive numbers of poor who filled the Paris streets in the same way that they might in a respectable parlor. To be sure, the bourgeois Parisian who survived was many times more likely than a struggling worker to have the luxury of recording his or her personal experience in a memoir that was preserved for posterity. Even if some from the lower classes were literate, they probably lacked the supplies (paper and pen), the free time, and the sense of destiny that propelled so many bourgeois to record their encounters with cholera. Inequalities in treatment further enhanced this discrepancy because more affluent Parisians could afford to send for doctors and were thus treated in the privacy of their own homes. Under these circumstances, even the most harried doctor would feel compelled by the victim's family (his paying clients) to record the situation of the individual death in detail. The poor, meanwhile, either went to the overburdened, make-shift emergency first-aid stations scattered throughout the capital or died without treatment. In either case, they more likely became casualty figures than part of a disclosing narrative that made them into individual human beings. The fact that neither firsthand experience nor written evidence allowed most bourgeois Parisians to know members of the lower classes as individuals made it easier for them to imagine the group, like the disease, as part of Paris malade.

The two rhetorical approaches to cholera also reflected the *instruction*'s ambivalence about the larger scientific debate over contagion. (See Chapter 2.) To some extent, the links between the disease and the environment of the lower classes reflected the anticontagionist position, though the *instruction* of 1832 was careful to avoid overtly taking sides in the controversy. In fact, the word *contagion* did not appear anywhere in the brochure. This was a conspicuous and deliberate omission; not only did the contagionist debate dominate much of the medical discourse at the time, but also *la contagion* had become a careless synonym for cholera in many official and unofficial accounts of the epidemic. Preferring words such as *la maladie, le mal*, or simply *le choléra*, the *instruction*, through rhetoric, removed contagion from public debate as well as from the private individual's unconscious association.

Written by prominent medical professionals who had been appointed by the prefect of police, the brochure sometimes seemed to walk a fine line between both sides of the debate, which indicated that it still remained far from settled. At one point, for example, the *instruction* encouraged contagionist measures such as isolation of infected individuals, noting that it would be "useful, whenever possible, to place the patient in a room separate from those occupied by the other members of the family." Moreover, in an interesting nineteenth-century reinterpretation of measures taken against the plague (which called for burning the victim's clothing and linens), the *instruction* replaced fire with water by calling for items to be thrown into a vat of hot, soapy disinfectant.[18] The use of water and soap as cleansing agents echoed measures being taken on the city streets, the standard response to any infection in the early nineteenth century.[19]

Clearly, however, the *instruction* indirectly endorsed the anticontagionist view, which linked the causes of cholera to the "putrid miasmas" of the unsanitary Parisian environment. "Cleanliness is always very necessary for [good] health,"—few statements could be as direct.[20] Elsewhere noting that those who breathed "pure air" ran a much lower risk of contracting the disease, the *instruction* asked inhabitants of the capital to "air things out in the morning and again during the day by opening doors and windows as often and as long as possible. It would also be good to place a large pottery container filled with chlorinated water in each occupied room. [A long footnote provides an exact recipe.] Finally, the circulation of air can be further encouraged by building a large, blazing fire for a few minutes in the fireplace."[21] In addition, "dung, excrement, debris from animals and vegetables require special attention. To avoid the accumulation of these materials, they should be cleared out as often as possible."[22] The *instruction* thus called for throwing dwellings wide open to the outside world rather than closing them in on themselves, as suggested by the contagionist legacy of the plague. Filth and stagnant air—not infected individuals—characterized what anticontagionists tellingly labeled "homes [*foyers*] of infection."

The popular instructions that circulated at the height of the 1832 cholera epidemic suggest ways of trying to understand how and why bourgeois values came to dominate French culture in the early nineteenth century. By implying the administration's monopoly on legitimate preventive measures, by bringing the individual into the process, as well as by creating the very image of the disease itself as a product of the environment and as essentially class-specific, the forty thousand pamphlets distributed throughout the capital played a significant part in shaping popular attitudes toward the government, disease, and urban social relations. Moreover, the long descriptions and rigorous detail made the 1832 pamphlets part of a process in which officials discovered cholera by writing as much about it as they possibly could. More than being the final word about the disease, then, the early instructions served as a revealing introduction.

During the second epidemic, the instructions played a far less obvious role in creating perceptions of disease and government. In 1849 the prefecture of police published a similar *instruction;* it contained most of the same information as its predecessor, but its prominence and detail had diminished considerably.[23] Printed in January and issued the following April, the official *instruction* began with an immediate disclaimer, typical of the official literature at the time:

> Since the invasion of cholera in Paris, the progress [of the epidemic] observed day by day with care has fortunately rendered all special health measures unnecessary. There is every reason to hope that there will be no need to resort to these special measures.

Moreover, information from abroad was "of the type that would reassure the population." All across Europe, the eleven-page pamphlet told readers, this second outbreak seemed to be affecting "a far less considerable number of inhabitants" than in 1832. The lower incidence of disease, officials argued, could be explained by a weaker epidemic. Moreover, they also cited "ameliorations introduced in hygienic conditions [in the areas] where the majority of the population of Europe lives today," without mentioning specific improvements.[24] Even so, the prefecture noted, printing such "hygienic advice appropriate to present circumstances" was a useful preventive measure.[25]

While certain phrases, the general organization, and the content of the new *instruction* revealed that the 1832 pamphlet had served as a blueprint, the documents from each epidemic displayed significant differences. The layout of the pamphlet in 1849 reflected a new philosophy of simplicity and confidence; whereas dense printing and long paragraphs had characterized the first version of the booklet, the second was spacious, often presenting information in a single, direct sentence. Contrast the following with the earlier descriptions of aqueous vegetables, bad wines, and fatty meats:

> Peace of mind is always one of the conditions most favorable for health, even more so during an epidemic.
> Moderate, wholesome, regular eating habits [that are] adequately substantial are among the precepts of hygiene that are important to observe.
> Every disruption in daily habits [*les habitudes de la vie*], every change in eating habits that seem healthy [*dont on se trouve bien*], is a disturbing change.[26]

Such simple, crisp language suggested that measures for fighting the disease did not need to be explained as thoroughly to a population that now had come to understand the language and its implications quite fully.

In 1849 the *instruction* paid token homage to medical wisdom with a few scattered references, but the real message was that the administration's pronouncements regarding cholera were legitimate in and of themselves. Unlike the first epidemic, during which officials depended on medical professionals to provide information and treatment as well as the stamp of legitimacy, the second outbreak saw the administration undefensively asserting its independent power and authority. By the time of the second epidemic, the administration had clearly triumphed over the medical professionals by absorbing their anticontagionist ideas without relinquishing political power. When the *Moniteur* published the measures in April 1849, for example, it no longer felt compelled to introduce them as representing the latest findings of prestigious doctors.[27]

Moreover, the 1849 pamphlet did not implicitly address members of the middle classes, as its counterpart had done during the first epidemic. Instead, it spoke openly to the entire population of Paris, confronting the issue of class more boldly. Having dropped the tacit charges against the filth and immoral behavior of "the less fortunate classes," the booklet abandoned the biased vocabulary of class-specificity. "If the disease can attack all individuals irrespective of their social position," the *instruction* told readers in its only reference to the issue, "everyone can also take the precautions that we generally consider the most appropriate measures for avoiding being stricken."[28] The layout, format, rhetoric, and even the direct language of the 1849 pamphlet said that all classes—not just members of the bourgeoisie—confronted the epidemic in the same way. No longer could anyone hope for implicit immunity.

At the same time, the pamphlet was more explicit regarding the issue of contagion. Almost more than in 1832, the imprint of the hygienists could be felt throughout the *instruction* in 1849. "Cholera is not contagious," it boldly (and erroneously) proclaimed; "one can now lavish attention upon those stricken with this disease without fear."[29] As in 1832, the pamphlet recommended that garbage be kept to a minimum and dwellings be frequently aired out, all to guard against the putrid miasmas presumed to cause cholera.[30] Even at the most fundamental level of nomenclature, the document bore the unmistakable stamp of the hygienists. In 1832, for example, the section dealing with precautionary measures had been entitled "Behavior to Observe to Preserve Oneself from Cholera," while the 1849 equivalent had become "Hygienic Precautions to Take during the Epidemic." The word *hygienic* was a conspicuous choice, for it replaced the subjective category of behavior with the seemingly more objective one of a scientific fact.

THE *BUREAUX DE SECOURS*

Along with the *instructions populaires,* the emergency first-aid stations scattered throughout the capital served as one of the most prominent images in the press of the Paris administration's fight against cholera. And, as with the instructions, the stations made a much bigger impression in 1832 than in 1849. "A red lantern placed at the entrance marked these asylums of mercy," wrote one contemporary, describing them with a mixture of anxiety and awe, "and night or day you could see horses ready to dash anywhere where the Contagion brought death."[31] Called *bureaux de secours,* the stations sent out doctors to make house calls or offered temporary care until a consenting patient could be transported to a hospital. Like the hospitals, they provided care especially for members of the lower classes, who could not afford the services of a private physician. Moreover, the stations acted as conduits of information for authorities monitoring the progress of the epidemic in every neighborhood of the capital.

Like the *instructions populaires,* the first-aid stations were a key link between the government and bourgeois perceptions of it. "The medical stations were morally, politically, and medically advantageous," a report about the situation in Paris explained to the mayor of Lyon after the first epidemic. "They help dissipate fears that there is not enough aid; they bring together the population and the Administration, and all useful remedies can be found in them."[32] The 1832 system of *bureaux de secours* not only tested the government's resources and responses but also provided an opportunity to establish a new kind of authority based on a tenuous combination of administrative skill and medical wisdom. Here in the front lines of epidemiological battle, where the administration and medical professionals worked most closely together, emerged many of the acute tensions that hampered the flawless collaboration between medicine and the state.

Initially, the system was part of a compromise that, while never explicitly stated, had its roots in the controversy over contagion. Fearing the contagiousness of the disease, several administrators had argued in favor of isolating cholera patients in special hospitals to be located on the outskirts of the city. Such a solution, however, meant that it would be difficult, if not impossible, to transport victims quickly enough, and thus officials concluded that each hospital should designate specific wards for cholera patients, a system that would be supplemented by a network of emergency first-aid stations. Influenced by the anticontagionists, the administration had foregone a kind of therapeutic quarantine in favor of placing treatment facilities within the capital. The compromise, however, was but one part of an ongoing struggle between the administration and medical professionals, a struggle that played itself out in the planning, publicizing, and functioning of the *bureaux de secours.*

On November 19, four months before the arrival of the 1832 epidemic, officials presented a detailed plan for implementing a system of emergency first-aid stations.[33] Prepared by a special subcommittee of the prefect of police's Commission Sanitaire, the two-part report covered nearly everything concerning a station's organization and functioning. The first section described how each two-room office should be furnished, listing items down to the number of chairs, blankets, bottles, pans, goblets, and candles, as well as specific quantities of medication. The second part of the report provided detailed guidelines on personnel, including how doctors, pharmacists, assistants, and medical students should be selected for service, the number of hours they should work (they were required to sign timecards), and the types of records they should keep about each patient they treated. Under the supervision of the prefecture of police, the local *commissions sanitaires* in each arrondissement informed medical professionals from their districts when and where they were required to serve their four-hour shifts.[34]

The elaborate plans for the *bureaux,* and especially the fact that they appeared prominently in the *Moniteur* and subsequently in other major newspapers once the epidemic had arrived, are among the most striking features of the 1832 outbreak. Given the lack of scientific knowledge about cholera, such measures "prepared with great care" (as the introduction told readers) contributed to the image of a government taking the initiative during a crisis. As with the *instructions populaires,* the publicized descriptions promoted the government's credibility at a pivotal moment of uncertainty during the early 1830s. Moreover, the detailed presentation of the *bureaux de secours* in the press followed the hygienists' belief that presenting intricate facts was the most advanced method for combating the epidemic. It seemed that providing detail—a specific and new conception of knowledge—was the key method for both presenting and preventing the crisis of cholera. And, even more, providing such detail was a way of making scientific ideas public.

Born of an impressive plan, the *bureaux* often worked better in theory than in practice, especially when the epidemic hit Paris with full force in the first two weeks of April 1832. M. Boulay de la Meurthe, the chief doctor of a *bureau* in the Luxembourg quarter, painted a characteristic and especially vivid portrait in his daily log. On April 6 in his hasty, abbreviated handwriting, he complained of extreme fatigue and overwork resulting from attempts to treat "an alarming number" of cholera victims. The following day his tiny two-room station received as many as forty patients an hour, a number so large that he was unable to take the time to file the required reports with the prefect of police. On April 12, "The night was very hard, and the doctors didn't have a single moment's rest."[35] Lecturing at the Collège de France, the influential physiologist François Magendie confirmed this chaotic picture, denouncing panic-stricken, lazy, or opportunistic aides. "More than once when I arrived at an inopportune moment," he lamented, "I had the misfortune of seeing all my nurses gathered around a pot [of food], without being the least bit disturbed by the cries of the dying."[36]

More numerous than general complaints of overwork, however, were doctors' specific criticisms of the administration. Frequently, they lambasted officials who ignored their requests for supplies and vehicles to transport victims.[37] Boulay found the prefecture of police especially parsimonious when it came to providing sustenance for his staff. "It's urgent that they change the wine," he threatened for a third time on April 13; "otherwise it will itself become a cause of cholera in our first-aid station." Blaming an order from Gisquet that severely cut back deliveries for no apparent reason, he called the move "*vile* because of its stinginess, and atrocious because it risks the lives of the people in the medical service."[38] The *Gazette des hôpitaux civils et militaires,* a paper often critical of administration policy, denounced "M. Gisquet's sad circular" as demonstrating how little gratitude the prefect had for medical professionals.[39]

Deeper tensions between medical professionals and Gisquet emerged when the prefect of police announced that he would be adding an accountant to the permanent staff of each *bureau*. These men were to work under his direct orders, balancing books, paying medical students and aides, ordering medications and supplies, as well as guarding against any "abuses that might take place."[40] Boulay welcomed the innovation sarcastically, asserting that he was "pleased, because I'll no longer have to deal with my most intolerable chore, accounting." But he quickly dissolved into anger. "For heaven's sake, now we're even being invaded by offices, boxes, and bureaucrats. Our service functions as the pinnacle of economy and rapidity. A useless middleman [*un agent inutile*] will only make things work with more difficulty and expense."[41] He concluded with an urgent plea for the mayor of his arrondissement to consider the consequences carefully. But apparently his call went unheeded, for a few days later, on April 18, a postscript in his log noted in small, defeated handwriting the arrival of "M. Capron, our accountant." Perhaps in an act of passive resistance, Boulay promptly dispatched the unfortunate Capron to distant parts of the neighborhood to collect pharmacists' receipts.[42] But, even so, the administration had openly challenged medical authority and had won.

For its part, the city administration unknowingly juggled financial and bureaucratic efficiency, on the one hand, and a growing (if still quite abstract) sense of its own potential power on the other. The National Assembly had voted only a limited emergency credit of two million francs to pay for the capital's relief services, a sum that legislators of the liberal July Monarchy believed would be supplemented by municipal funds and by "inexhaustible individual charitable sources."[43] The city administration thus faced the immediate problem of fighting cholera with extremely limited financial resources. Officials sent out constant pleas to the mayors and members of the *commissions sanitaires* of each arrondissement to encourage economical, regular, and orderly services in medical stations throughout the city.[44] To encourage efficiency, the prefecture of police eventually provided preprinted forms to facilitate record-keeping and the gathering of statistics. Moreover, in another effort to save money, the city immediately disbanded most of the *bureaux de secours* once the number of victims began to decline markedly in mid-May. Even after a second wave of cholera hit the capital in the middle of July, officials seemed reluctant to reopen any of the stations for fear that they would be too costly. Evidently, the government's frugality was of a nondiscriminating nature. This characteristic became apparent after the epidemic, once officials had decided to award medals to outstanding medical professionals for their services. One recipient wrote that he was originally promised a gold medal but that the administration allegedly "for reasons of cupidity" reduced it to silver and ultimately to bronze "for the same reason, and because cholera had vanished entirely."[45]

In the face of financial constraints, the administration clearly demonstrated a desire to establish credibility and to assert its power over the medical profession just as the doctors were beginning to organize and claim their own authority. As in the *commissions sanitaires* and the *instructions populaires,* the prefect relied heavily on the authority of doctors as medical experts to lend the *bureaux de secours* a sense of legitimacy, but the administration, not the medical profession, dominated official responses to the crisis of cholera. By publicizing the elaborate system of first-aid stations through posters and highly detailed descriptions in the press, the prefecture of police provided valuable information and contributed to its own image of taking active steps to keep the situation under control. Not only did the prefecture of police preside over the opening and closing of the *bureaux* in each of the city's forty-eight neighborhoods, but it also dictated the exact details of their functioning, first through the guidelines of the November 19 report and later by introducing a nonmedical authority, the accountant, into each medical station itself.

—⟡—

Despite important advances made by the French medical profession during the 1830s and 1840s, a close examination of the new guidelines for the *bureaux de secours* during the second epidemic reveals that the administration now had even more of an upper hand. At first glance the lists of personnel and furniture remained essentially unchanged, even down to the order of their appearance in the booklets.[46] But while the new system borrowed quite heavily from its predecessor, a close inspection reveals changes suggesting that the relationship between medical professionals and administration officials had become more amicable. Tensions between bureaucrats and doctors persisted, but now the documents contained no hints of the struggle for power apparent during the first epidemic. Rather, the administration clearly asserted itself as the commanding authority in the battle against cholera. And, unlike its strategy in 1832, the city's reliance on medical professionals to lend credibility to the enterprise was slight. With continuity among the lower ranks of bureaucrats and little increase in the Parisian public's respect for doctors since the first epidemic, reliance on administrative measures offered a logical possible avenue for fighting cholera.

From the outset, city officials asserted their power in both plans and preparations for the implementation of the system of *bureaux de secours*. Although no scientific breakthroughs had suggested new medications for curing cholera, the city made changes regarding those to be kept in each station. A few new items appeared, such as seltzer water and mixtures for chloride, a liquid used for cleansing, but, more interesting, the quantity of most medications required on the premises had been cut in half. Given the extent of complaints against the prefecture for failing to provide enough supplies in 1832, the reduction was a significant act that reflected a new kind of administrative initiative; rather than relying solely upon past medical experience, officials now interpreted the gravity of the situation and prescribed a modified solution of their own. Further evidence of the government's tightened grip in 1849 was the introduction of an "agent of the administration" into each of the *bureaux*. Presumably a formal replacement for the accountants during the first epidemic, the new officers performed a much wider range of services, from balancing books and keeping track of medications to collecting doctors' timecards and recording vital information about the patients treated. Whereas in 1832 doctors had complained that the presence of such an outside authority interfered with their work in treating cholera patients, the new agents met with no documented resistance in 1849, a sign that administrative involvement had become an accepted part of the medical stations' functioning.

Despite the fact that the administration seemed so much in control, officials acted slowly in putting the system into effect. Though the epidemic was declared on March 18, newspapers did not mention the report about instituting neighborhood *conseils de salubrité* and a system of *bureaux de secours* until nearly two months later, on May 13. And as with the *instructions populaires,* the press downplayed the epidemic by offering almost no detail.[47] Moreover, in many cases the stations themselves did not open until well after the rapidly rising number of deaths could no longer be ignored. As late as June 5, for example, an anxious prefect of police had written to the mayor of the fourth arrondissement for help in securing new facilities.[48] On June 7, over three months after the epidemic has been declared, the Conseil de Salubrité of the first arrondissement began meeting on a regular basis.[49]

In an attempt to assert its newly achieved professional status, which had begun to crystallize during a major conference in 1845,[50] the medical community condemned the administration for its delays in establishing the *bureaux de secours.* "We have learned that medical aid is being organized through each neighborhood mayor's office [*mairie*]," *L'Union médicale* noted on June 9. "It is certainly late, but this really is not the time to offer recriminations."[51] Looking back, E. A. Duchesne, who served on the sanitary commission of the eleventh arrondissement, rhetorically asked, "Did the government take all the measures necessary to lessen the likely ravages of this new epidemic?" And he answered, "I do not think so."[52]

To defend itself, the administration pointed to the rest of Europe, where the epidemic seemed less severe than in 1832, a judgment it made independent of the medical profession. Moreover, regardless of the second invasion's actual severity, the city administration's preparation for implementing the *bureaux de secours* had already demonstrated further independence from the medical community. During the first outbreak the government had relied heavily on doctors for both information and for establishing credibility based on links to science and knowledge. Having gained practical experience and legitimacy as the leading crusader against cholera in 1832, the government no longer needed medical professionals, except to provide treatment. By delaying the opening of the *bureaux* in spite of prevailing medical opinion, by introducing an "agent of the administration" without resistance from the medical community, by limiting the quantity of medications without doctors' advice, and by controlling the response to the epidemic itself by learning to use the press, administrative power had clearly triumphed over medical authority. More important, cholera had been transformed from a predominantly medical problem to one that could now be treated with administrative actions.

THE *BULLETINS DU CHOLÉRA*

"In the mornings people opened the newspaper with trembling hands," one Parisian recalled in his memoirs about the first epidemic. "They weren't looking through them for political news anymore. . . . What they really wanted were the casualty figures."[53] Appearing prominently in most major newspapers, the *bulletins du choléra* had a significance all their own, one unmatched by any other official representation of the outbreak. Printed as tables, the figures stood in stark contrast to the rest of a densely printed newspaper page. In a very real sense, they represented the early nineteenth-century equivalent of a photograph for a population quite literally learning to see information in new ways.[54]

The bulletins served as a key link between the medical and administrative investigations of Paris on the one hand and the largely upper- and middle-class readership of the popular press on the other. Not only did the daily mortality figures provide the public with a running account of the epidemic's progress, they also were among the few concrete pieces of information available at a time when cholera remained an unsolved medical mystery. As miniature, daily versions of the earlier, more comprehensive statistical inquiries, the bulletins helped make the hygienists' ideas—faith in quantification, the desire for objectivity, and the need to present information publicly—a part of the popular imagination when Parisians thirsted for any cholera news they could find.

Conditions seemed especially ripe for placing the daily bulletins at the center of government policy and public consciousness in 1832. The ideas of the hygienists helped to propel statistical description to the forefront of scientific knowledge, while this enthusiasm for figures had greatly improved techniques for their collection and dissemination.[55] Moreover, as literacy, newspaper circulation, and newspaper availability increased, and as the Parisian middle classes were brought more directly into the political process, the press became an increasingly valuable tool for promoting the image of an administration fully in control of the crisis. Thus the power of statistical description and particularly the *bulletins du choléra* resulted from the convergence of two previously distinctive developments that were forced together for the first time during the cholera outbreak. On the one hand, the hygienists had helped make medical knowledge a legitimate concern of government, while on the other the growing need to engage the public—redefined to encompass a greater segment of the population—had forged a new role for the press and its representation of the epidemic.

The *bulletins du choléra* were such a novel innovation for presenting an ongoing epidemic reality to the public that Parisian papers initially engaged in a lively and heated debate on the subject. *Le Corsaire,* an entertainment daily that often poked fun at the government, observed that the "sad lists of mortality don't diminish the scourge, they only serve to heighten fears," and consequently it never published them.[56] The Saint-Simonian newspaper, *Le Globe,* hesitated to present the bulletins, explaining, "Not everyone is strong enough to endure this daily enumeration of pain and suffering that strikes their neighbors."[57] One haughty theater tabloid ridiculed the obsession with statistics in general, condemning publications that competed for readers by offering "the prettiest, the longest, the most complete lists of the dead and dying."[58] This paper, like others that refused to print the figures, was apparently convinced that the information would serve only to frighten the public.

More often, however, papers took up the cry for "rigorous exactitude," accusing the government of willfully misleading Parisians with grossly reduced figures. *Le National,* a left-wing daily fervently opposed to government policy, automatically assumed that published mortality figures were only half the real number.[59] Another popular newspaper went so far as to express concern that Paris did not have "a central place where papers could obtain information [that was] rigorously exact."[60] *Le Bonhomme Richard* waited a couple of weeks before passing judgment, announcing that the civil register contained a much larger number of cholera deaths than did the *Moniteur,* a commonly held assumption, suggesting that the official figures lacked credibility.[61]

The avid quest for Truth must be viewed in the context of how difficult it was to secure and report information about deaths. While post-Napoleonic France was renowned for its highly centralized bureaucratic apparatus, the cumbersome system was by no means prepared to collect and record the avalanche of information that inevitably accompanied a cholera epidemic. Even in normal times reporting a death was a major bureaucratic chore. To record a death in Paris and thus ensure that it would be counted with the mortality figures, one needed a doctor's confirmation, a witness to certify it, a member of the mayor's office to collect the announcement, and a notary to register it.[62] On the average it took approximately three days after a death for the information to make its way into daily newspapers. The daily bulletins, then, required an efficient, uniform, and coordinated strategy among neighborhood hospitals, first-aid stations, and those who reported house calls. In reality, however, the quality and quantity of information varied considerably among arrondissements and even among individual medical stations, especially during the busiest periods of the epidemic.[63]

Though the complexity of reporting a death made it seem a nearly impossible task, the press campaigned aggressively to present the truth to readers. Accuracy, or "exactitude," was of the utmost importance for medical and administrative purposes and for presenting the epidemic to the public at large. "Our readers are grateful to us for telling them the entire truth, regardless of how sad this truth [is]," the *Journal des débats* boasted during its earliest coverage of the epidemic. "Better to know [the truth] such as it is than to allow the public to be misled by the thousands of exaggerated stories that circulate about this fatal event."[64] In writing of the early mortality figures, one popular newspaper warned its readers: "This information is exact; but we are far from presenting it as the complete portrait [*tableau complet*] of cholera cases observed during the day." Citing the fact that "no regular service [for collecting data] has yet been established," the editors pointed out that "many observations have gone ignored, just as many that have been given lack authenticity." For the following day the paper promised a table that would provide the most up-to-date information on the epidemic.[65] Even the *Moniteur* apologized to its readers for failing to include figures it had yet to receive from the suburbs.[66]

Such disclaimers implied that editors believed an epidemic Truth could be placed within readers' grasp simply by presenting enough facts about cholera. In 1832 the truth constituted a reality that was within humans' capacity to record, if not to understand. Accordingly, it had to be discovered and could be presented to the public concretely through the *bulletins du choléra*, even at a time when no one really understood the disease. By picking up a daily paper such as the *Moniteur* or the *Journal des débats*, one could potentially come close to touching Truth both figuratively and literally because ideally the paper contained the known facts that would illuminate this truth.

Because truth conveyed through daily statistics had rarely been an ongoing part of public discourse, officials did not initially grasp how to appropriate the bulletins' social and political power in 1832. Relying largely on trial and error, authorities experimented with how best to present and use them. On March 31, for example, the *Moniteur* took the lead by publishing the first *bulletin du choléra*, which listed reported cases as well as actual deaths (see figure 6). In keeping with the government's naive desire to present everything known about the epidemic, the bulletin also contained the names, occupations, and addresses of the victims.

PARTIE NON OFFICIELLE.

INTÉRIEUR.

Paris, le 30 mars.

IIᵉ BULLETIN SANITAIRE DE LA VILLE DE PARIS.

État des personnes atteintes du Choléra depuis le 22 mars jusqu'au 30 mars à minuit.

9ᵉ *Arrondissement.* — Lecomte, 40 ans, rue Saint-Paul, 5.

8ᵉ — Martin, 65 ans, forgeron, rue des Lombards, 21, mort.

12ᵉ — Démoui, 67 ans, journalier, place Maubert, 10, mort.

9ᵉ — Inconnu, portier, rue Bautreillis, 13.

9ᵉ — Inconnu, trouvé par un garde municipal sur le boulevard Beaumarchais.

7ᵉ — Legris, 32 ans, ouvrier en acier, rue de la Verrerie, 5.

11ᵉ — Barry (veuve), rue des Francs-Bourgeois, 4.

10ᵉ — Mauguin, 44 ans, couvreur, rue de la Vierge, 1, morte.

9ᵉ — Lemaire (veuve), 64 ans, rue des Nonaindières, 5.

9ᵉ — Salomon, 11 ans, rue de la Mortellerie, 124.

9ᵉ — Catin, tailleur de pierres, rue de la Mortellerie, 135.

9ᵉ — Puault, taillandier, rue de la Mortellerie, 136.

12ᵉ — Clidière, 56 ans, indigent, rue du Chardonnet, 8.

9ᵉ — Anqueville, 30 ans, cocher de fiacre, rue Bautreillis, 15, mort.

9ᵉ — Inconnue (femme), portière, rue Bautreillis, 13, morte.

6ᵉ — Petit, 6 ans et demi, faubourg du Temple, 35, mort.

7ᵉ — Carmuat, 72 ans, balayeur, rue de la Tixeranderie, 71, mort.

7ᵉ — Gaudrau (femme), 35 ans, rue Saint-Antoine, 55, morte.

6ᵉ — David, rue du Cimetière-St.-Nicolas, 12, mort.

12ᵉ — Cambillard, boulanger, rue Galande, 47, mort.

12ᵉ — Godet, 64 ans, peintre en bâtimens, rue Traversine, 28.

12ᵉ — Mandar (femme), 64 ans, journalière, rue du Chardonnet, 15.

12ᵉ — Mazou de Saint-Michel, 71 ans, chiffonnier, rue des Boulangers, 15.

6ᵉ — Duret, palfrenier, rue de l'Orillon, 8, mort.

4ᵉ — Caboche, 25 ans, couvreur, Appori-Paris, 36.

10ᵉ — Chérel, 45 ans, journalier, avenue de la Bourdonnais, 85.

11ᵉ — Ledoux, 29 ans, domestique, rue Galade, 12.

10ᵉ — André, 68 ans, marinier, rue de la Boucherie, Grua-Caillou.

9ᵉ — Morel, 54 ans, scieur de long, rue de la Mortellerie, 86.

10ᵉ — Richard (veuve), 73 ans, fileuse, avenue de Breteuil, 13.

10ᵉ — Foucquety, 29 ans, fumiste, rue Sainte-Marguerite, 9.

9ᵉ — Leunilcieux (femme), 52 ans, journalière, rue aux Fèves, 19, morte.

9ᵉ — Marjud, 70 ans, charpentier, rue des Marmouzets, 24, mort.

7ᵉ — Florence, 73 ans, journalier, passage Sainte-Croix-de-la-Bretonnerie, 26.

9ᵉ — Bourgeut, 58 ans, maçon, rue de la Mortellerie, 28, mort.

9ᵉ — Montpellier, 37 ans, cordonnier, rue des Marmouzets, 38, mort.

11ᵉ — Barrochat, 70 ans, terrassier, rue Saint-Jacques, 52, mort.

12ᵉ — Langlois, 69 ans, cordonnier, montagne Sainte-Geneviève, 24.

9ᵉ — Cauiel, 39 ans, cordonnier, Marché aux Fleurs, mort.

11ᵉ — Vidault, 41 ans, distillateur, rue de la Parcheminerie, 5, mort.

9ᵉ — Bricqville, 41 ans, maçon, rue des Marmouzets, 27, mort.

9ᵉ — Raphanel, 29 ans, marchand de cirage, rue aux Fèves, 16.

11ᵉ — Pedretié, 21 ans, vitrier, rue de la Parcheminerie, 5, mort.

7ᵉ — Nugues (femme), 34 ans, dentellière, rue Grenier-Saint-Lazare, 14.

7ᵉ — Chervaz, 19 ans, commissionnaire, rue des Blancs-Manteaux, 38, mort.

9ᵉ — Laferté, 60 ans, tailleur, rue Bautreillis, 13, mort.

7ᵉ — Dupont, 48 ans, vannier, rue de la Vannerie, 6. Decreuville (veuve).

9ᵉ — Huot (femme), 60 ans, marchande, rue de la Mortellerie, 34.

9ᵉ — Bador, 48 ans, journalier, rue de la Licorne, 12.

7ᵉ — Thoru (Mathieu), 45 ans, maçon, rue de la Coutellerie, 23.

12ᵉ — Marcot, portier, rue Saint-Julien, 10.

12ᵉ — Delavalle, 70 ans, reutier, rue des Carmes, 23.

12ᵉ — Mauceau (femme), 55 ans, garde-malade, place Maubert, 39.

Sautier.

Ve Billet.

Hubert.

10ᵉ — Chambaud, 14 ans, avenue de S-ger, 7.

10ᵉ — Baisse, 18 ans, ouvrier en tabac, rue de la Bucherie, 12.

9ᵉ — Ve Lemoine, 64 ans, blanchisseuse, rue Malart, 15, morte.

10ᵉ — Thirion (femme), 59 ans, couturière, avenue de Lowendal, 21.

10ᵉ — Legrand (femme), 67 ans, avenue Lamotte-Piquet, 8, morte.

Dufeu, lancier, mort.

9ᵉ — Beau (Frédéric), 35 ans, chartier, rue de Jouy, 5, mort.

178 personnes atteintes du choléra au 30 mars, à minuit, dont 118 du sexe masculin, 60 du sexe féminin.

60 décès déjà connus, dont 41 hommes et 19 femmes.

Il reste 118 malades, dont 77 hommes et 41 femmes.

Le ministre de la guerre vient d'ordonner que les mesures suivantes fussent appliquées sans délai à la garnison de Paris :

« 1°. Chaque homme sera pourvu d'une ceinture en flanelle et de chaussettes en laine. Les conseils d'administration y pourvoiront au moyen de 5 fr. par homme qui leur seront alloués.

« 2°. A compter de ce jour, il sera fait, dans les magasins, une distribution d'une ration de riz et de vin à chaque homme.

(Ces deux articles ne concernent, pour le moment, que la garnison de Paris.)

Figure 6. Early cholera bulletin in 1832. Source: *Moniteur universel*, 31 March 1832.

Although the *Moniteur* printed the data as the most up-to-date information about the epidemic, the public did not always read it that way. The early exposés immediately caused a public outcry; because cholera struck the poor neighborhoods of the capital with the greatest intensity at the beginning of the outbreak, names from the lower classes dominated the lists. Using recognizable imagery in the form of street names, arrondissement numbers, occupations, and even family names, the initial cholera statistics seemed to present the disease and its victims as problems that could be kept at a comfortable psychological distance from the bourgeoisie by linking them to the alien world of the poor. The opposition press implicitly questioned the administration's objectivity when it attacked the government's insensitivity toward and prejudice against the poor.[67] Writing some years later, the socialist Louis Blanc claimed that printing the names had been a deliberate policy of class hegemony "either to dissipate the fears of the fortunate or to flatter their pride."[68]

It is doubtful that such rosters reassured the upper classes as the opposition suggested. Readers of the *Moniteur* (most likely to be bourgeois Parisians) immediately voiced their strong disapproval. After only three days, complaints to authorities and editors forced the paper to replace the names and occupations of victims with simple summary statistics. "The identity of a few names gave rise to terrible misunderstandings, causing considerable discomfort to families living in the suburbs," the *Moniteur* explained to readers on the day the paper shifted to using figures alone.[69] The public outcry against the lists demonstrated the extent to which both the disease and the information about it were already invested with vast social and cultural meaning. In effect the black ink of the modern press had replaced the ancient tradition of marking the houses of plague victims with a large white "X." Middle-class readers, it seemed, objected to the transformation of the epidemic into something related to individuals, even if these individuals happened to be poor; it was one thing to see cholera in the larger context of Paris malade, and quite another to see it linked to concrete human beings.

Although the daily figures promised a kind of anonymity and objectivity, they in fact helped readers and government officials discover the subjectivity of numbers, as revealed by the changing formats of the bulletins. Although the administration stopped disclosing details about individual victims, the prefect of police still provided daily mortality figures, which appeared in most newspapers until late August. The press made several attempts before settling upon a more palatable form for presenting the data to readers. On April 3, for example, the *Moniteur* opted for detail. It printed two tables, one for deaths and one for new cases, each table broken down by arrondissement or indication of residence in the suburbs, sex, and military status. The day's totals and the cumulative total for the epidemic punctuated each daily report. The following day a new category appeared, "homeless persons," a distinction that could be either reassuring (because it linked cholera safely with "the other") or frightening (because of the threat from wanderers) to the comfortably housed readers of the popular press (see figure 7).

When the hysteria surrounding the cholera outbreak reached a climax around April 5, the mortality figures occupied an even more prominent yet complex place in telling the epidemic story. The bulletins reported a dramatic rise in deaths, with nearly eight hundred victims a day in the first week of April.[70] In this context of chaos, the *Moniteur* experimented with highly stylized tables that used figures divided by thick ink lines, a format more commonly found in the hygienists' published inquiries than in a daily newspaper. Linked to the credibility of the hygienists, the tables suggested legitimacy and accuracy, which might give added veracity to the numbers contained in them. As the epidemic began to stabilize, the bulletins became simpler and more formal, stressing new kinds of information. After the initial flush of enthusiasm for figures as deaths climbed into the hundreds per day, the newspaper later conveyed only the most basic points and no longer attempted to impress the public with sheer detail. A regular, repeated, familiar format appeared to comply with expectations officials had created when making the information available in the first place. Every couple of weeks the paper printed elaborate summaries of the data it had acquired about cumulative mortality figures.[71] The epidemic and the bulletins' narration of it had become almost routine, yet not routine enough to eliminate the daily figures completely.

Once the bulletins had become a part of daily life, spoofs appeared in the popular press, a further indication of the hold that a veritable culture of statistics had on the public imagination. *Le Corsaire* printed parodies of the *bulletins du choléra* on several occasions. In the first instance, the paper compared cholera mortality with

*Bulletin officiel du 1er avril quatre heures du soir,
au 2 avril quatre heures du soir.*

NOMBRE DES PERSONNES ATTEINTES.

1er arrondt.	4 hommes	3 femmes.	
2e. ――	2	1	
3e. ――	1	1	
4e. ――	5	7	
5e. ――	3	4	
6e. ――	12	8	
7e. ――	18	14	
8e. ――	13	9	
9e. ――	13	11	
10e. ――	22	9	
11e. ――	19	5	
12 . ――	21	12	
Militaires..........	6	»	
Personnes sans asile.	19	10	
Total de la journée..	158	94	252
Total des jours précédens....................			483
Total général...............			735

DÉCÈS.

1er arrondt.	4 hommes	» femmes.		
2e. ――	2	»		
3e. ――	1	»		
4e. ――	3	2		
5e. ――	2	1		
6e. ――	8	3		
7e. ――	8	6		
8e. ――	4	2		
9e. ――	8	5		
10e. ――	12	4		
11e. ――	3	2		
12e. ――	3	4		
Militaires	2	»		
Personnes sans asile.	9	2		
Banlieue...........	»	»	4	
Militaires	»	»	2	
Total de la journée..	69	31		100
Total des jours précédens				167
Total général...............				267

Figure 7. Routine cholera bulletin in 1832. Source: *Moniteur universel,* 3 April 1832.

figures from the revolution of 1830 as well as with numbers of what it called "unexpected mortality" from the insurrection of June 5 and 6, 1832.[72] Six days later the parody was more explicit, this time offering information on criminal cases prosecuted in connection with the insurrection. "It is assured that the newspapers on sale are about to have daily bulletins of trial judgments," the paper joked. "These will be calculated like those for cholera." A "model" followed, which included categories such as numbers of judgments, lengths of sentences, and condemnations. Like the bulletins, the parody provided figures for the day and the day before as well as numbers from the previous year. Just in case the comparison proved too subtle, the mock bulletin closed by condemning state intervention, likening prison terms to the cholera measures that seemed to bring the government into every aspect of daily life. "One will be considered on the road to recovery [only] when one is under police surveillance," the paper proclaimed.[73] Such mockery not only demonstrated the extent to which disease and social unrest were fused in the minds of contemporaries but also showed how deeply the mortality figures themselves had permeated popular consciousness. The spoofs worked only because the majority of readers had internalized the cultural import of the *bulletins du choléra,* for no cultural code could have been so consciously manipulated or broken without a widespread understanding of the rules that shaped it.

Sensing the potential of the information presented in the *bulletins du choléra,* authorities sought other ways of achieving a measured balance between enlightening and alarming the public. Frequently, the *Moniteur* tried to dilute unpleasant statistical realities with what one contemporary described as "reassuring formulas, altered with remarkable talent, genuine language of nourishment for lulling the screaming baby to sleep." If mortality increased, he explained, "it was a good sign, the epidemic would not last. If the number decreased, it meant that the troubles were coming to an end. If [the number of deaths] picked up again, it was a last effort before the calm."[74] This double narrative sometimes resulted in an absurd discrepancy between rising mortality figures and the soothing mood of optimism that the paper sought to foster in its prose. On April 10, for example, the *Moniteur*'s front-page sanitary bulletin joyfully proclaimed that doctors were "almost unanimous [in supporting] the fact of the very noticeable decrease in the power of the disease." The accompanying mortality figures offered a blatant contradiction, however, since they faithfully recorded the previous day's total deaths at 861—the highest number for the entire epidemic.[75]

Such an awkward compromise between numbers and narrative make it clear that in 1832 contemporaries had not yet fully comprehended the meaning implicit in the daily information. On the one hand, officials seemed almost naively committed to furthering hygienists' ideals by objectively presenting an epidemic truth based on observation and quantifiable knowledge. As the culture of statistics would have it, describing the disease in numerical terms made it seem less baffling because when quantified it could somehow be conquered. Part of the bulletins' greatest appeal lay in their apparent innocence, their closeness to a possible truth so lauded by the hygienists, the respected thinkers of the day. Thus, by printing everything it knew about the epidemic, the government hoped to heighten its credibility.

On the other hand, the addition of a paragraph to offer a subjective interpretation of this truth suggested that both the administration and the press were arriving at a new understanding of their own position in the nexus between power and knowledge. As officials and journalists experimented with how to use the *bulletins du choléra* in 1832, the figures seem to have lost their original allure of offering neutrality and objectivity. The experiments also introduced a new balance between a traditional narrative description that used words as facts and a seemingly neutral rhetoric of statistics that relied upon numbers. The apparent impartiality and objectivity of numbers helped redefine the meaning of both "detail" and "fact." By controlling the collection and presentation of mortality figures while redefining the use and meaning of this information, officials could create the image of both the epidemic and their prefectures' attempts to fight it. In other words, not only did officials try to use their information about the outbreak to maintain control over it and the anxious population, but they also redefined what that information was; knowledge—and particularly its dissemination—became power.

As with the *instructions populaires* and the *bureaux de secours*, by 1849 officials seemed less inclined to promote the bulletins as symbols of science, progress, and a government in control of a crisis. In fact, the relative silence of the Parisian press was perhaps the most striking feature of the 1849 outbreak. Three days after the declaration of an epidemic in mid-March, the *Moniteur* first mentioned cholera in a small news item buried in the back pages. Beginning with a brief statement describing a few victims who had died in civil hospitals, the article was accompanied by a small table of mortality figures that lacked the detail of the information published in 1832.[76] Although cholera continued to claim victims in the capital throughout April and May, the *Moniteur* limited its reports on the subject to a short column entitled "Cholera News." Appearing approximately every three or four days, the feature often contained mortality figures without explanation or comment. On the rare occasions when tables replaced the numbers printed in the text, they had a simpler format than their counterparts in 1832, with fewer comparisons and statistical breakdowns by location, sex, or age. Nongovernment organs did the same. *Le Courrier français,* a popular paper that had filled its pages with news of cholera in 1832, relegated much of its coverage of the epidemic to the *faits divers* section in the back pages. Nestled among accounts of bizarre murders and sensational robberies, and stories of people who set fire to themselves or others, the information about cholera had clearly lost its privileged place.[77] Other papers, such as *Le National*, the *Journal des débats,* and *Le Constitutionnel*, followed a similar policy of only occasionally reprinting figures verbatim from medical journals. Only when the number of deaths began to rise noticeably in early June did the figures receive any prominent attention in the papers (see figure 8). But, even so, as with the popular instructions and emergency first-aid stations, it seemed clear that the administration no longer relied on statistics to perpetuate its image of being in control.

The medical press, linked to the newly emerging sense of solidarity among doctors, protested this silence most vociferously. Because of their distance from any one political party, medical journals had largely been spared the wrath of political censorship. However, the emboldened editors found themselves engaged in a turf war that forced them to defend their position vis-à-vis the administration. On March 13, when it became obvious that cholera had claimed several victims in the northern suburb of St.-Denis and would soon reach the capital, the most prominent medical journal at the time, *L'Union médicale,* noted, "For more than eight days this sad

---

MINISTÈRE DE L'AGRICULTURE ET DU COMMERCE.

BULLETIN DU CHOLÉRA.

Paris. — Journée du 10 juin 1849.

Décès à domicile..........................	477
Décès dans les hôpitaux et hospices civils........	163
Décès dans les hôpitaux militaires.............	32
Total....	672

Mouvement des hôpitaux et hospices civils.

Existant le matin..........................	1,705
Admis pendant la journée....................	335
Total.....................	2,040
Sortis.................................. 47 ⎱ Décédés............................. 163 ⎰	210
Restant le soir.............................	1,830

Mouvement des hôpitaux militaires.

Existant le matin..........................	485
Admis pendant la journee....................	88
Total...................	573
Sortis. .... 36 ⎱ Décédés.......................... 32 ⎰	68
Restant le soir.............................	505

Le chiffre des décès à domicile signalés pour la journée du 11 juin s'élève à 211, mais toutes les déclarations n'étaient pas encore connues.

Dans les hôpitaux le chiffre des décès est de 181.

Figure 8. Cholera bulletin from the height of the 1849 epidemic. *Moniteur universel*, 11 June 1849.

fact has been known, and no official communication has yet been addressed either to the Academies [of Science and Medicine] or in professional journals. We can do nothing but criticize this silence."[78] By mid-May, after more than three thousand Parisians with cholera symptoms had entered hospitals, the editors attacked the National

Academy of Medicine for remaining silent, demanding, "What has it got to hide?"[79] At about the same time, the *Gazette médicale de Paris* lamented the fact that its "colleagues of the press" had failed to register a united complaint about the silence from the administration and the National Academy of Medicine.[80] Shortly after the epidemic had peaked, toward the end of June, the *Gazette des hôpitaux* joined other medical journals in issuing a plea to the government to keep statistics as accurately as possible.[81]

Individual doctors argued for publishing statistics on both pragmatic and moral grounds. Many of them, such as the editors of *L'Union médicale*, believed that regular information would quell what they considered the exaggerated fears of Parisians. Condemning the administration, the respected medical journal announced that "this hesitancy [to provide information] is vexing; it produces precisely the misfortune that it wants to avoid."[82] Editors of the *Gazette des hôpitaux* saw the problem in terms of the government's need to maintain a certain public image. "What kind of confidence can the people have in the administration that is charged with giving them assistance," the editors wondered, "when they see this administration hiding the truth to achieve a goal that they cannot always understand?"[83]

Perhaps Paul Caffe, director of a clinic at the Hôtel Dieu and a veteran of the first epidemic, understood the government's role in the culture of statistics best of all. Arguing that continuous and clearly presented mortality figures had spared London considerable panic in 1832, and conveniently forgetting the social unrest that contributed to even greater malaise in Paris at that time, he noted that "officially produced truth is the only way of responding to exaggerations in every sense: far from causing panic, truth always calms; [it] reassures the frightened and destroys calculations that are sometimes knowingly false."[84]

Caffe's observation was both to the point and uncannily modern. Like his contemporaries, he feared the consequences of withholding information. But he also clearly saw "truth" where others saw Truth, while understanding the government's active role in *producing* it through statistical description. This idea of "producing truth" marked an important contrast with the quest for objectivity and rigorous exactitude that had preoccupied officials during the first epidemic. In 1849 the administration seemed much more self-aware;

not only did officials realize the power implicit in the bulletins, but they were also more savvy about just how this information could be both created and presented. The administration's use of statistics had subtly shifted from a mere rendering of truth to the production of it.

To be sure, since 1832 the meaning of the figures had changed in such a way that many contemporaries now considered it the administration's *duty* to publish them and the public's *right* to read them. "Publicizing statistics is an obligation that the municipal administration must religiously perform at very frequent intervals," wrote Caffe in a remarkably articulate and candid appraisal of the problem. "Everyone has the right to be informed of what is taking place in the city, above all at the moment when each one plays his part in the public interest."[85] Officials, it seemed, had violated a contract that they had unknowingly signed when they first promised the most detailed and up-to-date figures about cholera in 1832. Moreover, because the number of papers and their circulations had increased over the course of the 1830s and 1840s, the public in 1849 expected that the press could and would provide an open forum for presenting the information at the same time that more papers began taking the initiative in presenting data not necessarily drawn from the pages of the *Moniteur*.[86]

By 1849 standards of rigorous exactitude no longer dominated statistical description. Not only was less information available to the public, but papers also did not always print the most detailed or accurate figures. Having no common source, the political papers' casualty reports varied wildly between understatement and gross exaggeration. *L'Union médicale,* for example, accused the *Moniteur* of publishing a figure that was "far below" its own.[87] The popular *Journal du peuple,* meanwhile, offered figures that differed markedly from those in other papers, perhaps partly because of frequent mistakes in addition.[88] Seen from another perspective, Truth itself had been brought into the bourgeois free market of selling copy.

More prone to gross exaggeration, the opposition press finally prompted government officials to address the problem of statistics directly. On June 8, with the number of cases rising steadily, all major newspapers carried a statement from the administration:

> In the interest of public calm, we will not hesitate to publish figures that are probably considerable but which are far from being as ter-

rifying as those spread everywhere by fear and exaggeration. People have gone as far as to say that 1200 persons have died in the city the day of June 5. We can affirm that nothing is more false: they have more than doubled the true number.[89]

This official statement represented much more than a simple desire to maintain "public calm," for ultimately it symbolized a fundamental change in the meaning of statistics and the role of the press, as well as attitudes toward government and urban social relations. Whereas in 1832 the administration had to convince the public of both the validity and the importance of the *bulletins du choléra,* by 1849 the government's role in collecting and presenting the data had gained acceptance to the point that it had become a *duty* to provide them. Officials feared that if they failed to provide information, there might be dire consequences, ranging from an uncontrolled epidemic to social unrest. In other words, the lack of statistical information during the second epidemic did not reflect a decline in such data's social or political potency; rather the cries of outrage in response to the government's silence indicated that the figures were now potent for different reasons. By successfully promoting mortality figures as symbols of science and knowledge, officials had created an enduring set of expectations and, eventually, a new social meaning for the mortality figures; no longer the discourse of distant experts, the numbers became central to telling the daily story to the middle-class citizens of Paris.

As revealed by the popular instructions, emergency first-aid stations, and mortality figures, cholera's messengers interacted in both complementary and contradictory ways to create different epidemic realities in 1832 and 1849. The medical professionals helped lay the groundwork for seeing the disease as an aspect of the Parisian environment, a fact that influenced the nature of the measures used to fight the outbreaks. Appropriating the hygienists' use of detail, objectivity, and rigorous exactitude, for example, officials established responses that relied more heavily on administration than upon medicine. Thus, although contemporaries perceived cholera as a danger to the *health* of the Paris population, the *instructions, bureaux,* and *bulletins* were as much monuments to bureaucratic as to scientific breakthroughs.

The emerging newspaper press, meanwhile, helped popularize these medical and administrative views by creating a forum in which they could be presented to a middle-class Parisian public. Through detail and plain language that described precautions, places to receive help, and information management, officials established an image of themselves and their valiant efforts to remain in control of a crisis. More than a naive attempt to assume mastery over the disease by assuming mastery over the epidemic story, the detailed descriptions that appeared in the press helped meet a set of post-revolutionary bourgeois expectations that the government had a responsibility to keep the citizens of the capital informed. Regardless of the explanation, however, such official efforts were unprecedented in French history; prior to the advent of a widely circulating press, no earlier regime had either the inclination or the ability to fashion itself with so much awareness.

The discussion of the measures used to fight cholera also illuminates a new and more complex relationship among cholera's messengers. As we have seen, collaboration emerged in a reciprocal exchange of methodology, information, and talent among individuals who had rarely worked together before. The anticontagionist slant of the popular instructions, the functioning of neighborhood first-aid stations, and the attempts to present the truth about the epidemic through publicized statistical data all relied on a considerable amount of coordination just to achieve a modicum of success. In spite of this common ground, however, the problematic relationship between the administration and medical professionals surfaced as each group sought to stake its claims, while journalists had particular axes to grind with each regime.

These shifting alliances and tensions provide insight into the different responses to cholera in 1832 and 1849. During the first epidemic, the administration and medical professionals had engaged in an open battle over authority. As a new regime struggling to maintain power and establish a sense of legitimacy, the July Monarchy needed to depend on the medical profession's growing authority. This dependence created visible tensions, such as the mixed messages about medical advice in the *instructions populaires* or the conflict over the accountant in the *bureaux de secours*. By 1849 the administration had established its position as the primary fighter against cholera, having absorbed the social and cultural prestige of the medical community. The sheer volume of information conveyed about the first epidemic, then, can be seen as a defensive strategy, one no longer required by a more fully consolidated Parisian bourgeoisie in 1849. Having established the internal complexity of this secular authority, we can now turn to a discussion of how cholera's messengers struggled to define themselves against yet another competing source of authority, that of the Catholic Church.

4

Catholicism and Cholera

Responses to cholera cannot be fully understood in a secular context.[1] Although medical professionals and administrators had created a powerful alliance by the time of the 1849 outbreak, the Catholic Church also played a significant part in shaping the complex dynamics of authority and urban social relations in the Paris environment. During both epidemics the Church participated in collecting and distributing charity, taking care of the city's many cholera orphans, running hospitals, and supervising the burial of bodies. Moreover, it offered its own alternative interpretations of the causes of the crisis and possible remedies. Such involvement often placed French Church officials in direct conflict not only with administrators and politicians who feared their power but also with doctors and scientists seeking a plausible explanation for the arrival of the mysterious epidemic.

Pronouncements from the Church hierarchy provided bourgeois Parisians such as medical professionals, administrators, and journalists with further opportunities for articulating a sense of identity. In debates over everything from explanations for cholera to the nature of charitable relief, these representatives of secular authority repeatedly found themselves forced to defend Enlightenment ideals that placed them in open conflict with the Catholic Church. For a class that approached the world as something that could be manipulated by human actors, that was optimistic about human potential, that viewed poverty as an individual's own fault, and that believed that a credible way of making money was to lend it, the belief in divine power and original sin, and the inherent honor of charitable giving advocated by Catholicism rang false indeed. Partly cultural, partly political, and partly intellectual, bourgeois animosity toward religious authority also surfaced in daily life, particularly in urban areas. For example, bourgeois Parisians tended to possess few religious objects compared with their counterparts in either the nobility or the working classes. Moreover, they usually displayed an "occasional orthodoxy," attending church only for major holidays or for rites of passage such as marriages and baptisms.[2]

This attitude toward religion did not mean, of course, that no bourgeois wanted to give to charity or was religious, or that the pious all approached their faith in the same way. Rather, the arrival of a new modern plague challenged many beliefs within a cultural and political context that helped make the rhetorical lines of battle appear with particular clarity. By giving bourgeois Parisians something to define themselves against, religious pronouncements concerning cholera revealed part of the process by which they forged a new sense of identity at the time of both outbreaks.

But given the complex relationships between religious and secular beliefs and institutions, neither world view had either the political legitimacy or the cultural clout to provide a coherent bourgeois response to cholera. Even the most cursory history of the Catholic Church in France suggests an ambiguous role for an institution that had experienced dramatic fluctuations in its authority and popularity since the eighteenth century.[3] Attacked by the Enlightenment philosophes, the Church met a major defeat in the revolution of 1789 and in subsequent de-Christianization efforts. The new, zealously secular government not only took over the vast Church landholdings and monetary wealth but also beheaded many clerics and exiled others. Catholic authority gradually returned in the years after the Directory and the signing of the Concordat, ultimately regaining prominence with the conservative Restoration government of the Bourbons in the 1820s. But once the revolution of 1830 toppled the Bourbon ruler Charles X, the institution suffered another important setback under the unsympathetic regime of the bourgeois citizen-king Louis Philippe. Just a year before the arrival of cholera, for example, the government had stood by as an angry group of men and women sacked the St.-Germain-l'Auxerrois church in the center of Paris. During the July Monarchy the rigid anticlericalism began to soften as the regime gained more confidence and turned its attention toward political enemies on the left. By 1849, two loosely connected religious revivals helped change the social and cultural landscape: an institutional reinvigoration of the Catholic Church and a grass-roots rediscovery of certain Christian values. Together, these movements once again altered the significance of and role played by religious authority.[4]

Although the Enlightenment and the French Revolution mounted successful intellectual and institutional attacks against religion, secular authorities faced numerous significant obstacles that restricted their ability to dominate Parisian life in the 1830s. Religious piety remained a complex personal issue for bourgeois Parisians, and it would take generations for secular ideas to gain a firm hold over individuals of all classes.[5] Moreover, as we have already seen, the place of even the most firmly established purveyors of secular authority was by no means secure. The inability of formally trained doctors to combat the epidemic threatened to tarnish the international reputation of the Paris medical school, while charlatans dominated the bulk of the profession well into the middle of the century. For their part, the city administration and the government of the July Monarchy also had to cope with problems of overcrowding and poverty exacerbated by the arrival of cholera.

Such instability helps explain the mood of antagonism between religious and secular officials that seemed to prevail during the 1832 outbreak. Evidence of friction between religious and secular authority emerged in many areas, from explanations regarding cholera's arrival to recommendations for ensuring its speedy departure. On one side, secular authorities emphasized the epidemic as something to be understood and explained physically: through rigorous investigation and statistical description, cleaning out run-down dwellings and neighborhoods, as well as by changing an individual's diet and dress. On the other side, the Church addressed the crisis of cholera as a spiritual matter, a symbol of the moral decay of both the individual and society. According to this view, the outbreak symbolized the wrath of God for the ongoing sins of 1789 and could be remedied only through a conscious program of spiritual renewal,— that is, a return to the faith. Because of their complex histories and their failure to provide an explanation or cure for cholera, religious and secular authorities all stood on unstable footing in 1832.

But in the uncertain world of cholera, where religion provided fewer answers while science asked more and more baffling questions, new interpretations and responses would soon emerge, often in a piecemeal synthesis of the secular and the sacred. During both epidemics officials grappled to find ways of putting a good face on their inability to stem the tide of ugly deaths. Since no one could offer an explanation or cure for cholera, the solicitation and distribution of alms occupied an especially important place in the ongoing struggle between secular and religious officials. As one of the only concrete options for fighting the epidemic disaster, charity gave a powerful voice of authority to whomever could claim to run it In other words, whoever controlled charity controlled the story being told about humanity's ability to combat the mysterious forces of nature.

To explore the relationship between religious and secular authority during both cholera epidemics, then, this chapter examines the debates over charitable relief and what they reveal about an important change in attitudes toward disease and the urban poor by 1849. Before exploring the new climate of the second epidemic, however, it is necessary to take a careful look at the situation in 1832.

NEITHER TEA NOR PRAYER

At first glance, one is struck by a prominent conflict between religious and secular authority during the 1832 epidemic. A definite bitterness and anxiety can be seen most clearly in the writings of men such as Chateaubriand, who mourned the fall of the Catholic Church in France. "If this scourge had fallen upon us during a religious century," the conservative romantic writer declared, "if it had found a place within the poetry of the popular imagination, it would have left a striking picture."[6] Waxing nostalgic, the aging aristocrat asked his readers to imagine a Paris with black flags flying at the top of Notre Dame, occasional cannon fire to alert unsuspecting travelers to avoid the city, churches filled with crowds of lamenters, processions of priests carrying candles from house to house and reading the last sacraments, the constant ringing of church bells, monks wielding crucifixes and calling the city to repent, saints' relics paraded through the streets, veiled women asking for God's forgiveness. More than casting a wistful glance toward the pageantry of past plagues, Chateaubriand's fantasy mourned the eclipse of Church authority by such unglamorous measures as first-aid stations and public health placards that encouraged Parisians to drink tea and clean their houses and streets regularly.

Beginning in the late 1820s, and especially since the revolution of 1830, a belief existed among conservatives like Chateaubriand that France, and Paris in particular, lacked a religious spirit. "Religious beliefs no longer have a magnetic pull for the Parisian who has ceased being moved by the earthly prods of hope and fear in regards to the afterlife," one writer commented.[7] A newspaper complained that Paris contained "a whole race of men who has never heard of God,"[8] while others typically described the French capital as "the crazy and impious city that believes in nothing and makes fun of everything."[9] Such appraisals received added weight from the fact that when making its French debut the disease seemed to jump unexpectedly into Paris without following the almost predictable march that had enabled contemporaries to map its progress elsewhere in Europe. One archbishop in the provinces explained the epidemic's apparent preference for the capital by noting, "Is it not [in Paris] more than anywhere else [where] His holy name has been insulted and profaned, where crosses have been torn down [and] thrown to the ground, [where] temples have been desecrated [and] pillaged?"[10] For many clerics, Paris—more than any other place in France or even the world—represented the very essence of impiety, and thus few acted surprised by the epidemic's arrival in 1832. To a devout Catholic, the triumph of religious fate over scientific predictability seemed both inevitable and natural, especially when it could be viewed as a sign of the capital's obvious disrespect for religion.

Perhaps no work made the connection between impiety and cholera more forcefully than M. Bellemare's *Le Fléau de Dieu* (The Scourge of God).[11] Little is known about Bellemare, apart from his modest contribution to the theological implications of cholera, which was written, published, and widely reviewed at the height of the 1832 outbreak. "Cholera-morbus is a scourge from Heaven more destined to enlighten than to punish [humanity]," he proclaimed, promising in a manner strikingly reminiscent of the description of the plagues in Exodus that the epidemic would last "just as long as is necessary to accomplish its task."[12] Although he made the distinction between enlightenment and punishment, his boundaries in fact appeared somewhat tenuous, as he outlined God's plans to educate both "the people" and "the men in power." His message was clear: cholera had been sent by God in order to put an end to the infidelity, corruption, and perversion that had come to dominate life in the French capital.

Bellemare found evidence to support his assertions by pointing to medicine's failure to find an alternative explanation, a condemnation that ultimately became a critique of the entire scientific enterprise. "In our lifetime human science has reached its highest degree of perfection," he sarcastically explained; "nature no longer holds impenetrable secrets: everything has been discovered, nothing escapes investigation anymore." But even after a month of research and scientific experiments, he complained, "not one solution, not a trace of light has come to our aid." According to Bellemare, doctors did not suffer from an insufficient number of subjects because, thanks to cholera, "thousands of corpses have been liberated for autopsies." And the city itself had become the victim of both the epidemic and the scientific enterprise, for Paris was "nothing more than a [surgical] amphitheater where at all hours of the day [and night] one can examine the entrails of victims."

For a pious man such as Bellemare, science had violated the sanctity of the human body in its quest for knowledge. It had, as his choice of vocabulary suggested, reduced humans to anonymous objects represented by their physical characteristics and not their spiritual being; they had become *objects* of investigation, cadavers, and even disembodied entrails, while Paris itself remained little more than an enormous laboratory of dissection. And not only had science profaned the human body, but the violation had yielded nothing.

Bellemare's work enjoyed much favorable attention in the mainstream Catholic press.[13] Shunning the most up-to-date scientific wisdom to make his argument, Bellemare had created a compelling, viable religious explanation for the arrival and subsequent course of the epidemic. His message that irreligion had been responsible for bringing cholera into the capital struck a powerful chord. At a time when medicine and government authorities seemed incapable of providing answers to the crisis, Bellemare had developed and published a bold alternative view of the epidemic and its inevitable consequences. Unlike the scientific hypotheses and secular rhetoric that had dominated the newspapers and posters plastered on walls throughout the epidemic, Bellemare's interpretation was more fully compatible with Catholic doctrine.

In addition to the fears of medical intervention and profanation of the human body voiced by writers such as Bellemare, Catholics found what they believed to be the increasing secularization of French society especially frightening. Not only had Parisians apparently lost the faith, but they also sought help from a competing authority once cholera arrived in the spring of 1832. "Society finds itself abandoned to the wisdom of doctors," *L'Ami de la religion* told readers at the height of the epidemic, "treating truth as if it has a body but not a soul." The editorial found it reprehensible that France remained the only country in the world where the need for expiations and public prayers never occurred to the administration during a time of crisis. "What is to be said of a government and of a people that in the face of death only know to seek help in pharmacies?" the editors wondered, perhaps unconsciously drawing upon the biblical story of Asa's premature death for having sought the help of doctors instead of the Lord.[14] A character in Roch's play, *Paris malade*, put it most eloquently: "hospitals are fuller than churches, doctors more consulted than priests, [and] newspapers of liberalism more widely read than psalms of penitence."[15] In the battle for cultural authority, many Catholics feared that medicine had become the unquestioned victor, a fact that greatly troubled the Catholic press.

Bourbon Catholics held particular contempt for the Orleanist government. From the beginning, religious authorities condemned the administration of the July Monarchy for its lack of a spiritual base. "The government shows no sign of [acknowledging] the religion professed by thirty-three million French people," Chateaubriand lamented; "it neither prays nor cries at the altars of the people." In England, "land of liberty" (and Protestants!), he explained, officials called for prayers and fasts, while in France theaters remained open even on Easter Sunday.[16] Moreover, many believed, secular authority could never fulfill humanity's most basic needs. "One senses quite clearly that earthly power does not suffice for reaching the heart and spirit regarding questions of life and death," a Catholic daily told readers in the early days of the epidemic, "and that religious prayers . . . have a different eloquence, a different resonance, a different result from administrative circulars."[17] It was as if the soul had somehow departed from the responses to cholera, leaving behind a body of cold, bureaucratic material measures, a frightening vision of modernity. *L'Ami de la religion* put it eloquently when it used a premodern military metaphor that played on older ideas about humankind's place in the universe: "Unfortunately, when it comes to knowing where to place their confidence, [the men of the administration] only have one arrow in their quiver; they always come back to hygiene, blankets and socks. As for those who have more faith in help from above than from medicine, [the government] has nothing to offer in this respect."[18] Secular authorities could offer physical remedies, religious writers believed, but material goods could do little to stem the preexisting spiritual crisis made visible by the arrival of cholera. To those who saw the epidemic as a religious rather than a hygienic crisis, secular authority appeared inflexible and inappropriate, but, above all, irreligious.

Church fears of government anticlericalism had some basis in reality.[19] The administration of the July Monarchy followed a policy decidedly hostile to Catholic authority. After his ascension to power in July 1830, King Louis Philippe sought to check the influence of the Church, in part because it had been one of the main sources of support for the rival branch of the Bourbons. Just weeks after the revolution, the government amended and the king issued a revision of the 1814 constitutional charter, which had set the tone for a post-revolutionary monarchy after the fall of Napoleon. While the 1814 version had restored the principle of divine right, the new charter explicitly stated that Catholicism was no longer the official state religion, but rather, according to article 6, "the religion professed by the majority of the French." Moreover, because all religions were to have equal recognition, the civil government was to have the final say in religious matters because of its "neutrality." And, unlike its predecessor, the July Monarchy refused to extend privileges such as landholdings and tax breaks to Catholic religious orders at the same time that it slashed the state budget for religious expenditures.[20] A small, yet revealing detail confirmed that Louis Philippe had made his point; shortly after he came to power, the influential Catholic newspaper *L'Ami de la religion et du roi* dropped the word *king* from its name to become simply *L'Ami de la religion.*

The July Monarchy's official stance against the Church no doubt influenced the regime's approach to cholera. The administration repeatedly shunned religious prayers by devoting all its energy to promoting hygienic measures such as cleaning and airing out dwellings, washing public squares with chlorine, and encouraging citizens to take warm baths while drinking tea of moderate temperature. The government also made a conscious effort to eclipse religious authority by drawing attention to areas where it now dominated traditionally ecclesiastical functions. Members of the royal family made frequent and well-publicized visits to local hospitals offering consolation to victims, while most newspapers published lists of individuals who had contributed money to government relief efforts. Such actions were unquestionably secular, with the pro-government newspapers making little or no mention of the Church and its active participation in collecting and distributing aid. A study of medals awarded to Parisians for their help in the 1832 epidemic revealed that of the 336 medals given to individuals in the first, sixth, tenth, and eleventh arrondissements, only five went to the clergy.[21] Because Church officials did participate in numerous relief efforts, the government clearly found it either unnecessary or threatening to acknowledge these actions. Such reticence was but one indication of the animosity the bourgeois state held toward the Church.

Moreover, a lively anticlericalism permeated articles in the secular press. "Are certain priests praying for us or for cholera-morbus?" the theater tabloid *Le Corsaire* wondered at the height of the urban disorder that accompanied the early days of the outbreak.[22] The republican *National*, meanwhile, printed a letter from an intern in the Hôpital de la Pitié who was disgusted by the fact that a priest threatened a cholera patient (an English Protestant) on her deathbed with "all the torments of hell if she did not change her religion." The writer condemned what he called "such misplaced, absurd zeal" and concluded that "true religious freedom could not exist in hospitals until a priest . . . would only be admitted upon the spontaneous and formal demand of a patient."[23] After the epidemic, Roch fictionalized the incident in his epic play, *Paris malade,* an indication that it had become an important part of cholera folklore.[24]

Publicly then, the rhetorical battle lines had been drawn between the religious and secular responses to cholera. Attacks in Catholic papers such as *L'Ami de la religion* and *La Quotidienne*, as well as the writings of men such as Chateaubriand and Bellemare, seemed to suggest that a return to a world dominated by religion had a certain appeal. Heated articles in the secular press, meanwhile, revealed that neither the bourgeois July Monarchy nor the medical profession felt secure in their apparent victory over tradition. At a certain level, this battle was political, with the cholera epidemic providing yet one more occasion to offer commentary about the change in regime after 1830. Here the embittered pro-Catholic, right-wing Bourbon legitimists, composed largely of aristocrats like Chateaubriand, fought the upstart July Monarchy, the regime of the Orleanist "citizen king" who wore a suit and carried an umbrella to symbolize his sympathies with the liberal middle classes. Children of Enlightenment values, many bourgeois Parisians saw the institution of the Church as the outmoded champion of a class and way of life that threatened their livelihood. Louis Philippe relied on these bankers, entrepreneurs, and professionals for support, and in many ways the regime's responses to cholera reflected the expectations of that class.

At another level, the religious and secular rhetorical stances represented a deep concern with the effects of the epidemic and human powerlessness to stop it. The magnitude of cholera's devastation in 1832 helped to create a battle with the peculiar quality of having both sides on the defensive, a fact that explains some of the rhetoric's vehemence. Because cholera remained an enigma, the conflict was displaced to larger issues. At stake was the increasing prevalence of a bourgeois anticlerical world view that might determine cultural priorities. The epidemic's arrival in the turbulent decades after the French Revolution made obvious a vacuum that religious and secular authority alike sought to fill.

At the very beginning of the 1832 epidemic, the prefect of police, Gisquet, wrote a letter to Msgr. Quélen, the archbishop of Paris, promising him that neither the eminent religious figure nor his entourage would encounter any difficulties when they visited patients in hospitals throughout the capital.[25] The following day, the head of the Bureau Sanitaire in the prefecture of police wrote to confirm Gisquet's message and also took the opportunity to ask the archbishop to pray for him, for his "young, Christian family," and for the duties he must carry out as the head of the Bureau Sanitaire. "Blessed am I if [my responsibilities at work] could be acceptable to God," he concluded; "he alone *is able* to give me the strength to carry them all out with the zeal and charity of a Christian."[26]

Such a story indicates that even in a climate of animosity between Church and state, religious and secular worlds intersected in many

ways. Clearly, government officials wary of Church authority understood that the archbishop's traditional sphere of influence lay in
the hospital and blessing the sick, and that it was probably in the
administration's interest to accommodate itself accordingly. The
king himself quietly attended mass on a regular basis, even as he
publicly chipped away at certain Church privileges.[27] Moreover,
while executing his administrative duties, a bureaucrat could easily
have deep-rooted religious beliefs, just as members of the clergy
could look to hygienic measures as useful models of efficiency. In
fact, subtle conceptual and rhetorical overlaps between religious
and secular wisdom could be found everywhere, in Church and
medical documents alike. Not literal equations, these links show a
kind of intimacy that contemporaries perceived either consciously
or unconsciously between two worlds that intersected in new ways
at the time of the 1832 epidemic.

In its April 17 issue, for example, France's most prominent Catholic daily, *La Quotidienne*, carried an advertisement for the official
scientific journal of the epidemic, the *Gazette médicale de Paris*, right
next to one for a book entitled *Afflictions et repentir*, a collection of
recommended prayers for warding off the disease.[28] *Le Corsaire*
seemed especially taken with the parallels between religious and
secular wisdom. In one issue, for example, it complained that the
previous day's Bourbon (and, by implication, Catholic) newspaper
had carried two contradictory articles about cholera. "In the first
one," the openly agnostic editors explained, "they write that this
disease is a scourge sent by God himself, that all of human science
will try in vain to get rid of it, while in the other they assure us that
simply by popping sugar every day we will never get sick. What
logic!"[29] Even Catholics, the editors seemed to argue, were learning
to accept secular advice, and they should admit the fact openly.

Telling overlaps between religious and secular ideas could also
be found in the use of language. For example, one of the most
popular synonyms for cholera was *fléau* (scourge), a term also long
associated with a kind of religious transgression but appropriated
by both religious writers and medical doctors.[30] "[The French gov-
ernment] thinks that even if science cannot stop this terrible
scourge," one doctor explained, "at least it will be able to reduce the
epidemic's violence."[31] Even the official medical report for the epidemic slipped into using the religious word in its discussion of

cholera and urban social unrest when it noted that "political commotions, generally short-lived, do not evoke the same terror as the presence of a terrible scourge."[32] In the hands of secular authorities (perhaps themselves products of a Catholic upbringing, as in the case of the young bureaucrat above), the religious word *scourge* had become a careless synonym for more neutral terms such as *cholera, the epidemic,* and *the crisis.*

Sometimes humor served as a vehicle for pointing out the coexistence of religious and secular wisdom. Six days after Easter, *Le Corsaire* printed the following pithy comment: "Tea is such a fine prevention against cholera that Odry proposes singing a *Te Deum* in its honor! It would be the apotheosis of tea."[33] At first glance, the statement offered a simple, witty play on words in French. As one of the preventive measures most commonly recommended by doctors in printed health instructions, tea (*thé*) was pronounced the same way as the "Te" in *Te Deum.* But, on another level, the paper's seemingly irreverent quip, like the odd juxtaposition of the advertisement for the *Gazette médicale de Paris* with the advertisement for the book *Afflictions et repentir,* brought together religion and medicine within a context that questioned the authority and capability of both. If tea were as effective as officials claimed, the statement in *Le Corsaire* implied, no one would need to resort to prayer. Or, conversely, if prayers provided an adequate solution, there would be no use in advertising medical wisdom. Underlying such casual wit was a basic realization that cholera remained a mystery and that, given this fact, both religion and medicine shared equal access to failure or to truth.

Even the official Church pronouncements on the disease revealed a complex and ambiguous attitude toward secular authority. Once the epidemic had claimed its first victims in late March, Archbishop Quélen issued a mandate that outlined measures to be taken by Church authorities. Calling for public prayers and extra masses, the three-page document also listed specific songs to be sung on each day of the week and ordered parish priests to sing a *Te Deum* every few hours. One of the most striking features of the epidemic's first religious document, however, was the deference it showed to scientific authority. Acknowledging "doctors' almost unanimous advice" that raw vegetables and restricted eating could predispose one to cholera, the archbishop lifted the fasting rules imposed because of

Lent.[34] A second mandate issued three weeks later admitted a general feeling of human powerlessness and called on a combination of religious and secular measures to defeat the epidemic. The letter urged local priests to set up associations for men and women to offer help to cholera victims. But, in advocating the formation of these organizations, the archbishop made sure to distinguish them as supplements rather than replacements for state-supported relief. "Far from hindering parish or civil administration efforts to provide aid," the letter stated, "these associations are on the contrary auxiliaries and reserves for supplying what might not otherwise be provided."[35] In making such a distinction, the archbishop's letter clearly yielded to government authority, a pragmatic as well as a symbolic endorsement in the years after 1830.

Even more intriguing was the archbishop's call for supplementary prayers after the epidemic had settled in the capital for several weeks. The first in a list of several ordinances issued on April 18 stated:

> A Quarantine of prayers will be said in all of the diocese to ask God to end the scourge that devastates the city of Paris and the suburbs. This Quarantine will begin on Easter, April 22, and will end on May 31, the day of Ascension.[36]

Here, the important word is *quarantine,* which has a double meaning in French, just as it does in English. On the one hand, it denoted a quantity of around forty, a number having special significance for Western religion: the forty days and forty nights of Noah's ark, the forty days that Jesus fasted in the desert, the forty years during which the Israelites wandered in the wilderness, and so on. More specifically, "the holy quarantine" indicated the forty days of Lent and referred to a specific set of prayers to be read in the spring. But quarantine also had its modern, secular meaning, referring to a practice that as early as the twelfth century isolated individuals suspected of bearing an infectious disease for a period of forty days. Although the linguistic history lacks precision, it seems probable that this concept ultimately associated with the secular world of public health had its genesis in a religious practice.[37] Thus, when the Church invoked "quarantine" in the spring of 1832, it underscored the importance of a religious idea, that of ritual purification. But it did so in a context which inadvertently assigned that idea a prominent secular meaning; quarantine had been one of the first measures considered by the administration before the triumph of anticontagionist ideas had linked the disease more to decaying refuse than to human contact. Thus, an ancient religious concept of purity and segregation had been the root of quarantine, one of secular officials' most often-used responses to the invasion of epidemic disease.

Beyond rhetoric in documents, religion and medicine intersected in the healers themselves. Because of historical congruencies between religion and medicine as healing professions, analogies between the two groups came easily during the 1832 epidemic. Up until modern times, with the development of Western professionalized medicine, most doctors occupied an uncertain middle ground between science and religion. Indeed, priests often stood in for physicians when they were not available, offering advice as well as herbal cures when necessary.[38] With the development of methods like the "moral treatment" in the earliest days of French psychiatry, meanwhile, doctors borrowed a "talking cure" from the Catholic practice of confession.[39]

Thus, doctors who normally voiced contempt for religious superstition nonetheless had some historical precedent for comparing themselves to priests when they wanted to stand upon higher moral ground during the 1832 epidemic. When city officials tried to obtain information from doctors about antigovernment rioters treated in the emergency first-aid stations for cholera victims, for example, physicians claimed that this would violate doctor-client privilege. In an editorial entitled "Outrage against Medical Morality," the respected journal *Gazette des hôpitaux* compared the role of doctors to that of priests. "Imprudent men," the article asked, "would you even dare expect a father confessor to divulge secrets from the tribunal of penitence? Would you dare ask him to sacrifice his conscience and his duty?" Concluding "certainly not," the editorial went on to liken the doctor to a father confessor.[40] France's leading medical journal, the *Gazette médicale de Paris*, used similar impassioned rhetoric, arguing that "in this instance the doctor is like the priest; the [priest] would never unburden the conscience of the guilty person only to hand him over to justice a purer soul, just as the [doctor] would never save [the guilty man] from death just to leave him in better shape to face the executioner."[41] Even if many doctors had rejected religious explanations for cholera, the authority of the priest still carried enough cultural weight to serve as a powerful justification for medical autonomy from administration policy.

Alongside the heated conflict between religious and secular responses to the frightening epidemic, then, lay important areas of intersection, often at an unconscious level. Rhetoric and juxtaposition of advertisements, as well as similarities in recommendations, indicated the extent to which the worlds were not rigidly divided. Both remained powerless in the face of cholera, both struggled to find a place within the changing political and cultural equilibrium, and both borrowed from one another. Catholicism continued to provide key points of reference for interpreting the disaster, even when increasingly secular bourgeois culture had publicly and ideologically rejected it. Parisians, it seemed, had rejected religious authority only superficially, while the Church supported sanitation measures in an attempt to accommodate itself to secularization and the political realities of the early July Monarchy. The relationship between religious and secular authority in the face of cholera could be divided roughly into two parts, one based on the conflict displayed by the rigid rhetorical stance taken by each side, the other based on syntheses of language, style, and sometimes even substance. Nowhere would these conflicts and intersections emerge more clearly than in discussions of charity, the one response to cholera that promised the possibility of immediate positive results.

CHARITY AND THE AFFAIR OF THE TWELVE THOUSAND FRANCS IN 1832

"The administration is jealous," one writer quipped; "it fears that its dead are being enticed away. It is anxious about an agony that might not pass through its hands, or about a convalescent snatched from its care [*d'une convalescence soustraite à sa police*]."[42] To be sure, the collection and distribution of relief occupied a central place in the 1832 epidemic partly because private donations accounted for the major source (more than two-thirds) of funding for fighting the disease.[43] Control over resources thus translated into an unprecedented amount of power in the day-to-day struggle against cholera. The battles over who should manage charity also grew out of a fundamental conflict between the Church, which sought to reestablish its traditional place in French society, and the administration, which was expanding its authority into previously uncharted areas in the turbulent post-revolutionary era.

Until the revolution of 1789, much of the history of charity in France was intricately tied to the history of the Catholic Church. Since the Middle Ages, parishes throughout the country had been the guardians of both the rural and urban poor, providing assistance in the form of food, clothing, lodging, and crude forms of medical attention. Unlike England, where Church-controlled charitable efforts declined as early as the 1500s to be replaced by increasing state intervention in the following century, France depended largely upon Catholic principles of volunteerism even after Enlightenment ideas had condemned the practices and called for government involvement. According to this belief, born of the Catholic Counter Reformation and enhanced by ecclesiastics' prodding, wealthier citizens should take it upon themselves to contribute alms either to the local parish or to a needy individual. Meanwhile, the Church managed and staffed both *hôpitaux généraux* and *bureaux de charité* to house the indigent, aging, sick, and infirm. As much scholarship has demonstrated, however, such institutions, as well as the system in general, remained a long way from meeting the needs of the growing masses of the poor.[44]

Paris presented an especially difficult problem in the years prior to the arrival of cholera. The city experienced an unprecedented flood of immigrants from the countryside seeking work and shelter in the capital, which placed enormous strains on limited housing facilities while taxing the fragmentary remains of the Church charity system. Moreover, the tremendous influx of poor came at a time of heightened tensions between religious and secular authority; the state would not take full charge until the early part of the twentieth century, while the Church had neither the financial means nor the political position to become more fully involved.

In the context of this apparent vacuum, the cholera epidemic of 1832 marks a significant moment in the history of charity. Not only did it represent a crisis of unprecedented magnitude, but it also came at a time when the Church, the state, and the medical profession all struggled to find a place within the changing bourgeois social and cultural equilibrium. The 1832 outbreak marked the first time that many new—and decidedly secular—ideas were being implemented. As we have seen, the sanitary commissions of the medical bureaucracy, the *bureaux de secours* and hospitals, as well as the distribution of the *instructions populaires*, all were attempts at establishing new forms of state control over a major crisis.

The issue of charitable relief, made public by scandals such as what became known as the Affair of the Twelve Thousand Francs, provides an especially good example of the expanding role of secular authority during the 1832 epidemic. When, in the spring of 1832, the conservative writer Chateaubriand offered twelve thousand francs for cholera victims on behalf of the Duchess of Berry (the mother of the rival Bourbon pretender to the French throne, Henry V), the prefect of the Seine abruptly refused the money. "Behind an apparent act of charity one sees a political calculation against which the entire Paris population would protest by its refusal [to take the money]," the prefect explained in his response to Chateaubriand.[45] News items, editorials, pamphlets, and archival documents describe how the Duchess of Berry's twelve thousand francs went on a veritable odyssey through the Paris administrative system, generating controversy wherever they surfaced. After the prefect's rebuff, Chateaubriand approached the mayors of each arrondissement directly. According to the donor, about half the mayors accepted his gift but promptly returned it after being reprimanded by their superiors.[46] Moreover, when mayors shunned the contribution, the prefect of the Seine sent each a letter of praise.[47] Only the mayor of the ninth arrondissement (the district with the highest proportion of cholera victims) opted to ignore his superiors and keep the gift; he was promptly dismissed. Chateaubriand's philanthropic odyssey finally led him to the archbishop of Paris, who gladly accepted the money, distributing it among the city's individual parishes. "Charity, like Faith, is universal [*catholique*]," the archbishop explained to Chateaubriand; "[it is] a stranger to the passions of men, independent of their movements."[48]

The story of the twelve thousand francs became an obsession in the Parisian press, especially once rumors began circulating that the money could be traced (albeit circuitously) to the Catholic Church. According to the story, which first appeared in the antigovernment but moderate *Courrier français,* Madame de Berry's money had been raised in a convent where, as a patron, she had left part of her wardrobe as a contribution. When the right-wing, pro-Catholic Carlists learned of this gift, they urged the mother superior to put the clothes up for auction, thus raising the infamous sum. Taking advantage of the good sister's naïveté, the story explained, the Carlists talked her into testing the political waters by offering the money for cholera patients on behalf of her benefactor, the Duchess of Berry.

Comments in the press followed political lines, roughly divided between supporters and opponents of the July Monarchy. Those in favor of the regime generally defended the administration's refusal, pointing out that if the duchess simply wished to make a contribution, she had only to give the money anonymously.[49] The *Journal de Paris* argued that the donation represented something more than an ordinary rich woman's simply bestowing a gift on the poor because "it is the Duchess of Berry who wants to offer alms to France." The country does not need charity from anyone, the editors explained, "and even less that of princes it has ousted."[50]

No article made anticlerical political motives more obvious, however, than *Le Bonhomme Richard*'s retelling of the incident as a play that took place in a mayor's office. A figure dressed in black (the symbol of a priest) came to offer the mayor a thousand francs, which the mayor refused once he learned that it came from the Duchess of Berry. At that point, a poor widow from the 1830 revolution entered, asking for charity because her eldest son had fallen sick with cholera. The priest hurriedly stuffed his money back into his pocket, saying that "Heaven is finally getting revenge for the barricades," and he announced that he was leaving to present the sum "to the neighborhood parish priest, who will not refuse to distribute the money of legitimate King Henry to his flock." The play ended with the mayor giving the woman the necessary money.[51]

The fanciful retelling of the Affair of the Twelve Thousand Francs can be read as the July Monarchy's idealized effort to counter an embarrassing public faux pas. First, the play had inverted the story so that the villains were reversed; the priest refused to give the needy woman money, an accusation opponents of the July Monarchy had actually leveled against the regime. Second, in the play the administration won, for it had already assumed the traditional function of the Church; not only had the woman elected to come to see the mayor first, but also her inclination was correct, for it was the city official—not the member of the clergy—who saved her from destitution. In this reversal of the story, the administration could emerge victorious.

But, for the most part, the government's refusal met with public outrage from both the left and the right. Louis Blanc called it "a coup d'état against charity," while the Count Rudolphe Apponyi described it as "gauche."[52] Commenting on the scandal, a parish priest reportedly said that even if he found a gold piece from the old regime hidden in his altar, he would rinse it in the baptismal font, make the sign of the cross, and spend it on bread for the poor because "one must accept alms from every hand, even from the clutches of the devil."[53] *Le National,* the country's largest left-wing daily, offered a blanket condemnation of motives of any kind. "If in your administrative actions you are forced to depend on the promptness of private donations," the paper urged, "throw a veil on the motives; take from all hands, and hurry!"[54] The Catholic daily *La Quotidienne* preceded its reprint of the story with the disclaimer that it "did not contain a single true word" and provided an editorial that took a sarcastic approach, commenting that "since the July revolution [of 1830] the French are too happy and too rich to need help."[55]

Chateaubriand himself defended his position on a number of occasions. He sent a letter to *Le Courrier français* in which he disavowed full knowledge of the money's origins.[56] Shortly thereafter, he responded to the event and its accompanying publicity by publishing a pamphlet, "Brief Explanations regarding the 12,000 Francs Donated by Mme la Duchesse de Berry to the Indigent Stricken by Cholera."[57] In it, he attempted to place charity above politics by appealing to tradition: he invoked the Bourbons' history of charitable donations before their overthrow in the revolution of 1789, boasting that the blood of Saint Louis flowed in their veins.[58] He also attacked the administration's callousness, citing letters from the poor who complained that only people who were well-fed, warmly clothed and adequately housed—in short, "people without any needs"—could afford to reject charity.[59] "What would Europe think of the solidity of a government that trembled in the face of alms from a woman?" he asked.[60] By emphasizing Berry's gender, Chateaubriand sought to trivialize the political dimension of charity. What he failed to mention, however, was a fact known to most Parisians: the duchess played an active role in trying to amass support outside France to overthrow the July Monarchy.[61]

When placed in its broadest historical and cultural context, a small event like the Affair of the Twelve Thousand Francs amounts to much more than a petty conflict between warring political rivals. Obviously, by refusing the twelve thousand francs, the government official acknowledged the political power of charity; as the mother of the rival Bourbon pretender to the French throne, the duchess constituted a conspicuous threat to the Orleanist July Monarchy. However, Chateaubriand's gift and the prefect's rejection must also be understood in the context of a larger struggle for cultural authority exacerbated by the arrival of cholera. In fact, responses to the scandal showed that contemporaries were learning to see politics itself as consisting of ideas and actions that had previously been considered outside its influence. The haggling over Chateaubriand's money helped drag the seemingly lofty concept of charity into the muddy waters of scheming and manipulation on the part of both the administration and its opponents. What gave the scandal political significance beyond party or even ideological conflicts was contemporaries' growing awareness of the state's expanding authority, namely into areas previously dominated by the Church. The state, it seemed, was becoming increasingly dominant not only in the practical matter of running relief operations but also in the more ephemeral realm of influencing the world view and spiritual outlook of French citizens as they faced a new epidemic disaster.

The issue of charitable relief made public by scandals such as that of the twelve thousand francs provides an especially good example of the expanding role of secular authority. Sensitive to the state's infringement on what had traditionally been ecclesiastical turf, the Catholic press recorded its disapproval. "Religious work has been entirely isolated from government work," *La Quotidienne* complained early in the epidemic,[62] while *L'Ami de la religion* urged the administration to put aside political motives and take advantage of religious volunteers by using them in the city-run emergency first-aid stations and hospitals.[63] In spite of some attempts on the part of city officials to accommodate members of the clergy within the civil relief efforts, the administration pushed forward with its own program, which was aimed at consciously establishing authority independent of the Church and the right-wing legitimists who supported it.

But a clean break with charity's religious past proved virtually impossible for secular officials at the height of the epidemic crisis. The urgency of the situation forced the July Monarchy to fall back upon familiar religious responses, language, and tactics to solicit charity and to reassure the public. In an intriguing predicament secular authority used the old ideas and values it attacked most vehemently to establish its new bases of authority independent of tradition. To meet this challenge, officials borrowed strategies from their pious predecessors while taking advantage of such new resources as the popular press.

Within the first week of declaring the epidemic in late March, for example, the *Moniteur* began calling for charitable donations from Parisians. Charity took many forms, the most common practice being to contribute to government, newspaper, or—to a lesser extent— Church subscriptions specially set up for the purpose. Administration officials strongly believed that city-run relief would be more efficient and effective than comparable services supervised by the Church.[64] Under this system, organizations called for contributions that they would publicize and eventually distribute to the needy. Gifts could include money or volunteer work as well as materials: foodstuffs, wood, clothing, linens, beds, chlorine (for disinfection), medications, and even buildings could be used by hospitals and emergency first-aid stations.[65]

The press played a particularly important role in setting the tone of confidence that the government sought to relay. In the earliest days of the epidemic papers followed the lead of the *Moniteur*, which had started taking note of charitable contributions. Within a week Parisian papers began publishing the long columns of generous donors that became characteristic of the 1832 epidemic. Printed daily, the lists contained the name, sometimes the address, and always the amount of the contribution, giving the total and previous day's total (until the contributions began falling, at which time the *Moniteur* confined itself to printing only a cumulative amount). Accompanying the lists, a series of descriptive notes discussed specific good deeds. The paper encouraged contributors to "make their names known" and typically each list began with a variation on the statement, "It is hoped that these acts will find numerous imitators in the wealthier classes of the capital." Here, the press used a religious model—soliciting charity—but gave it an undeniably secular flavor.

In addition to the lists of worthy donors and the running tallies of their contributions, papers printed narrative accounts of specific individuals and their donations designed to serve as lessons by example. The appeals reached out to people from different classes. On April 11, for instance, the *Moniteur* told of six workers who presented themselves to officials in the Observatoire district; they had come to furnish a complete bed and to offer their services in aiding administrators and doctors. Side by side with these accounts, newspapers provided a particularly conspicuous display of the royal family's generosity. The duc d'Orléans made a well-publicized visit to the Hôtel Dieu, where "he approached each patient's bed; with interest he informed himself of their condition, and addressed them with words of consolation."[66] Rather than flee to one of their many summer residences, the king and queen remained in the capital, where, amidst much ceremony and fanfare, they provided funds and supplies in addition to daily food rations for the homeless. Through its good example, the royal family was to teach French citizens that they had nothing to fear from facing the epidemic and making direct charitable contributions.

Because contributions from bourgeois Parisians were far more likely than contributions from the poor, papers solicited their help through a growing genre of articles that relied on obvious melodrama to convey social and political values. For example, *Le Bonhomme Richard*, a patronizing upper-class paper whose name invoked the thriftiness espoused in Benjamin Franklin's *Poor Richard's Almanac*, printed the tale of an aristocratic young couple, Louise M*** and Adolphe de B*** who were soon to be married. Louise spent her days dreaming of the wedding gifts she would receive, especially the finery that would bring her even closer to the man she loved. In the days before the wedding, however, she began accompanying her mother into the poor neighborhoods of Paris where people were dying of cholera. Moved by their misery, she decided to give up her wedding presents to charity. Her big fear remained how to break the news to her fiancé, but the story ended with a happy coincidence, for he too had chosen to give away his presents. The young couple fell into one another's arms, were married, and, instead of luxurious gifts, the guests all gave generously to charitable subscriptions for cholera patients.[67] Clearly, just as the wedding guests had learned from the example of the young couple, so too readers of *Le Bonhomme Richard* should reach into their pockets and contribute to the poor victims of cholera.

While secular papers printed such stories more often than their Catholic counterparts, the tales had a clear moral tone. But rather than invoke Christian duty directly, the anticlerical press did so implicitly by invoking a morality detached from the specific mention of a higher power. By implication, the state now assumed this traditional place of authority. In other words, secular culture had appropriated one of the oldest instruments of Catholic motivation— guilt—and translated it into the unreligious language of public assistance. But, most important, stories such as that of the self-sacrificing newlyweds could not have had resonance if Catholicism had not prepared the French cultural imagination for internalizing this particular conception of morality.

At the same time that imitation can be seen as a product of religious values, the concept might also be linked to a set of secular ideas that received special emphasis during the cholera outbreak. The use of lessons by example, conveyed through both numbers and narrative, provided an unconscious behavioral model of contagion not unlike the epidemic itself; one could (and indeed should) "catch" charity rather than a disease. So deeply had these similarities permeated the manner of thinking about charity that the lists of contributors looked very much like the daily mortality bulletins. While the newspapers that printed them never made explicit references to the fact, the two sets of data were in direct competition with one another. In the ultimate blend of religion and science, the administration had in effect set up charitable contributions as a rival "contagion" for combating cholera.

The awkward claims that the religious and the secular had each made upon the concept of charity in 1832 reveal the complex nature of bourgeois cultural authority in the early 1830s. To understand this complexity, it is instructive to examine the different layers of meaning inherent in a scandal such as the Affair of the Twelve Thousand Francs. At the most basic level, the event represented little more than another skirmish in an ongoing battle between competing party interests. The flurry of letters and editorials in the daily press pitted Bourbons against Orleanists, Catholics against anticlericals, as each sought to legitimate their claims. Moreover, while accounts of the scandal usually appeared amidst the more staid columns describing political news, the prevailing tone of the stories suggested that few took the duchess, Chateaubriand, the prefect (or anyone else, for that matter) all that seriously. The tainted money, the naive mother superior, the discredited royalty, and the hypocritically righteous administration all became part of a political soap opera that served as a welcome distraction from the daily horrors of the epidemic.

At the same time, however, the scandal and responses to it indicated that the idea of charity itself was undergoing a fundamental transformation in its public image. While alms had long been associated with maintaining class distinctions and social order, the idea of giving had also developed within a rhetoric that placed it on high moral ground. Chateaubriand's twelve thousand francs helped take this apparent innocence out of charity, integrating it more explicitly within the realities of competing party politics. In the swirling controversy generated by the money, every donation appeared suspect and immediately became subjected to close scrutiny from spite alone, if not always from deeper convictions.[68] This transparency of charity revealed a greater public awareness of politics and motives on the part of both secular and religious authorities. In addition to serving as a battleground for a conflict of party interests, then, the Affair of the Twelve Thousand Francs helped redefine politics by exploiting the political dimension of charity.

This blatant politicization of charity would not have been possible had the scandal not occurred during a period of deep tensions between religious and secular authority, tensions exacerbated by the arrival of the 1832 epidemic. For the state and medical profession in particular, the mysterious disease presented the first major test of secular legitimacy in the aftermath of revolutions that had defeated Church authority in 1789 and 1830. Officials' rejection of the twelve thousand francs could thus be seen in the context of a government trying desperately to remain in control of a crisis while extending its authority into new areas.

At the most fundamental level, the friction generated by the twelve thousand francs raised the larger question of who had the authority to determine whether a secular or religious world view would prevail in the turbulent decade of the 1830s. No clear winner had yet emerged in this critical transitional moment in the history of cultural authority. Cholera remained a mystery, the Church still held considerable power, and the state had not fully established itself. Such an unresolved state of affairs created a situation that enabled an intriguing blend of religious and secular imagery and language to thrive at the height of the 1832 epidemic. In the practices of daily life and in the appeals for conformity, faith, and support that surfaced in everything from popular newspapers to official pronouncements, both religious and secular authorities had to rely upon similar strategies, hence the frequent overlaps in the means used to achieve seemingly contradictory ends. Relying on the power of language as well as the shared political structures at their disposal, the Church and the French state each *needed* the cultural backing of the other in order to continue exercising power. Both the Church and the state drew upon the same sources for cultural authority while using these sources to establish their distinctive character and purpose.

SHOWERING THE ARCHBISHOP
WITH FLOWERS IN 1849

Two striking images demonstrate the magnitude of the change that occurred in attitudes toward the Catholic Church over the course of the July Monarchy: in 1831 angry mobs sacked the St. Germain l'Auxerrois church and the archbishopric in Paris, while, after the 1848 revolution, similar crowds asked bishops to bless the "liberty trees" commemorating the new republic. Although such *gestes historiques* run the risk of broad generalization and oversimplification,[69] they reveal a fundamental transformation in the complex dynamics among the Church, state, and French citizens by the time of the second cholera epidemic. Not only had the open animosity toward Catholicism that had resurfaced in the 1830 revolution declined markedly, but also—as the blessing of the liberty trees revealed—religion had become more fully integrated into popular culture as a progressive force. At the same time, bourgeois Parisians seem to have abandoned their open hostility to Church authority, and they even called upon religious leaders to help maintain order after 1848. Despite some first-rate scholarship on the Church in nineteenth-century France, however, the reasons for the change remain somewhat of an enigma, especially where the issue of urban religiosity is concerned.[70] For purposes of argument, I shall briefly summarize some possible explanations here.

Most important, a complex religious revival had taken place during the July Monarchy, a revival linked to changes coming "from below" much more than from the Church hierarchy. In the years since the 1830 revolution, romanticism, socialism, and a general disenchantment with the legacy of 1789 had created a climate conducive to borrowing ideas of Christian spirituality and reappropriating them for use by the left.[71] Disillusioned with violence and looking for spiritual fulfillment in an era when many of the formal practices of the Catholic Church remained discredited, many workers and their leaders turned to Jesus as the embodiment of what they sought.

At the same time, after 1848 the middle classes began to look increasingly to the Church as a defender of order and stability. In light of the two thousand deaths and eleven thousand arrests resulting from the recent and eerily familiar revolution, the Parisian bourgeoisie sought whatever allies they could find against socialism, even if members of the group did not immediately turn pious. "As for what is today called the *bourgeois class,* so hostile [to the Church] before February [1848], I do not think it has returned to a better state of mind . . . ," the vicar of St. Eustache wrote in November 1848. "It will support us as a counterweight to the doctrines it finds disturbing, and as a kind of spiritual police force whose role is to inculcate respect for laws which are in its interest. But that is the limit of its respect for and trust in us."[72] Put another way, even if bourgeois Parisians could not bring themselves to support the Church intellectually or culturally, they saw its value as a potential political and social ally.

Whether seen as a deep-rooted revival or merely a decline in hostility to clerics,[73] the more active role of religion in 1849 was a result of a new relationship between the Church and politics. Since the defeat of the Bourbons in the revolution of 1830, the Church had become a political "outsider." For bourgeois Parisians, this new status for the Church meant that members of the clergy received fewer political and financial favors, and thus inspired less resentment.[74] Moreover, events in 1830 marked a definitive break between many forms of Catholicism and royalism. Given the discrediting of their former Bourbon benefactors and given the animosity expressed by the July Monarchy as it struggled to establish authority independent of the Church, French Catholics found themselves in need of new political allies.[75]

Within the context of this new relationship between religion and politics, the "social question" played an important part in redefining the position of the Church and bourgeois attitudes toward it. Suggested by the hygienists' forays into the urban environment and given terrifying relevance by the arrival of the first cholera epidemic, the issue of what to do with the urban poor had become a problem of pressing concern that exploded in the 1840s. This problem had a twofold impact on attitudes toward the Church. First, the existence of increasing poverty and urban decay called into question the economic and social policies of the July Monarchy, a regime whose stagnation had already begun to alienate its most arduous bourgeois supporters.[76] Clearly, something was not working, and, as a result, any potential solution could not be overlooked. As an outsider, the Church found itself in a position of offering what were perceived to be new options. Second, the discovery of the displaced, suffering lower classes reopened a world of concern where, as the traditional guardian of the poor, the Church had once enjoyed sole influence. In other words, the articulation of the social question both created a need for greater Church participation and also discredited the regime that most violently objected to it, thus paving the way for ecclesiastics to play a more visible—and popular—role in French society.

The full impact of the social question on the religious revival during the July Monarchy must be understood in relation to the rise of socialism and a "Christianization of the left."[77] As the left-wing response to the problems of urbanization and industrialization in the 1820s and 1830s, French socialism would initially appear to have little in common with Catholic attitudes. For one thing, both came to the problem from vastly different philosophical and political traditions. Ideologically, the Church accepted social and economic inequality as a basic given, while socialists placed all forms of equality at the center of their program.[78] According to Church doctrine, the social balance depended on a clearly defined system of reciprocity between the haves and the have-nots, in which each group fulfilled a basic, necessary function. As the vicar of the Paris charitable institution St. Vincent de Paul put it, "The poor person is necessary to the rich because without the pauper the rich person derives no merit from his wealth; and the rich man is necessary to the poor one because without kindness and generosity the pauper would find no resources to quell his misery.''[79] In such a context, any calls for equality threatened the social equilibrium defined by Catholicism. Moreover, as the historical keeper of the poor and downtrodden, the Church sought to revive its *ancient* position vis-à-vis government authority while the socialists were consciously building a *new* ideology and power base.

Despite these fundamental differences, however, Christianity and socialism had important similarities that would soon influence responses to the 1849 cholera epidemic. Even if they came from distant ends of the political spectrum, both voiced their opposition to the regime of Louis Philippe and both took an active interest in the sufferings of the lower classes. When the social question made the weaknesses of the July Monarchy increasingly clear, both groups courted the lower classes as potential political allies.[80] Moreover, because of their similarities, they could borrow easily from one another. In light of Catholics' traditional role toward the poor, for example, it was not surprising that socialists found much religious imagery and rhetoric useful for making their appeal. They quickly seized upon the image of Jesus as the first republican-revolutionary and as providing a striking and compelling model for the experiences of the modern world; in 1848 revolutionaries sang a popular song called ''Jésus républicain,'' while a daily newspaper was named *Le Christ républicain*.[81] Many left-wing groups such as the *démocrates-socialistes* had learned to harness traditional religious culture for progressive political purposes, especially in the years immediately after the 1848 revolution.[82]

Catholics also drew inspiration from their apparent rivals. Socialist ideas—in practice, if not in theory—helped push some segments of the clergy further to the left and enabled Catholics to translate their message into rhetoric targeted at the lower classes. Meanwhile, left-wing ideals of egalitarianism influenced the structure of the Church, at least within the rank and file of the clergy, where many relationships became less hierarchical.[83] A vocal minority of priests did push openly for social reforms in spite of opposition from the Church elite of bishops, who deplored the links between socialism and Catholicism.[84]

Finally, even the revolution of 1848 helped enhance the strength of the Catholic Church before the second cholera epidemic. By discrediting the socialists, events such as the failure of the National

Workshops and the bloody June Days created an environment where only Catholicism remained to court the disenchanted lower classes. Given its broad appeals to the people of Paris and its distance from both the socialists and the July Monarchy, the Church seemed an attractive ally to the increasingly conservative bourgeois politicians of the young Second Republic. Thus, the new relationship between religion and politics, the posing of the social question, and the threat of socialism combined to create a new place for the Catholic Church in French society by the time cholera returned to Paris in the summer of 1849. Together, these factors inspired bourgeois Parisians to see and court the less-fortunate classes as an unprecedented political force.

—m—

On the surface, reactions to the new outbreak suggested that the religious climate had changed little since 1832. "The moment will have come, however, to humble oneself under the vengeful hand of the Creator," one Catholic paper proclaimed as cholera deaths climbed into the hundreds per day in June 1849. "This unceasing spectacle of Death that runs through the city . . . randomly harvesting the most humble victims; will not death shatter your pride, does it not speak to your hearts?" The author lamented the lack of young people entering into the service of the Church, estimating that for every hundred cholera patients at least eighty were unable to receive the attention of a priest. "Religion is lost in Paris and in the surrounding dioceses," he argued. "In the current situation it is [not] a matter of keeping things the same [*conserver*] but above all of bringing about a revival [*faire revivre*], and we're not even managing to keep things the same."[85]

Moreover, as in 1832, some anticlerical attitudes did surface, mostly in the left-wing press. Yet even here the tone had changed. In *La Démocratie pacifique,* for example, a story appeared about the wife of a worker "who died suddenly" (a euphemism for cholera) and was refused a funeral service and a proper burial. Indignant residents of the neighborhood took the body to the local church, the paper explained, where "the recalcitrant clergy [that was] hardly charitable was actually obliged to receive [the woman's body] in order to appease public exasperation." Commenting on the story, the editors wondered, "In light of such behavior, how can the clergy complain of unbelief and the population's estrangement?"[86] More significant than the attacks on the clergy, however, was the indignation Parisians voiced at the woman's failure to receive a proper religious burial. Clearly, even readers of the left-wing press expected the Church to execute this basic rite of passage.

Convictions of impiety on the one hand and anticlericalism on the other did not enjoy the unanimity they had during the first epidemic.[87] For the most part, Parisians seemed aware that the religious climate of their city had improved. "This return to religion is an auspicious omen and suggests a hopeful future," *L'Union* (formerly *La Quotidienne*) wrote at the beginning of the second epidemic.[88] No longer did one speak of cholera as a "scourge of God" or a punishment for impiety but rather as a valuable lesson, one that helped explain this heightened fidelity. "In effect, this terrible scourge had allowed the clergy to demonstrate the power of charity, therefore drawing souls to God," wrote L. F. Guérin, who published a two-volume study in 1852 about religious attitudes during the 1849 epidemic. "Within the ranks of lay people it has brought about much greater Christian devotion; at last it has excited a consoling and salutary burst of faith and piety."[89] No longer a symbol of religious decay, cholera was now seen as capable of encouraging religious fervor.

The image of the Church in Paris had also improved, as reflected in the more positive popular response to the city's new archbishop, Msgr. Sibour. Whereas Quélen had encountered considerable hostility during the first epidemic, Sibour's activities received glowing praise in both the religious and secular press. One notable account that appeared in several papers described Sibour walking through the place Maubert, greeted by a crowd of women who worked the market stalls, showering him with flowers as he returned from saying a mass in honor of cholera patients.[90] At the height of the epidemic rumors circulated that he himself suffered from cholera, having caught it after saying a mass at the Eglise St. Etienne-du-Mont, thus making him a kind of popular martyr.[91] One group of workers even petitioned the archbishop to say more prayers for bringing an end to the epidemic. "Horrified by the terrible scourge that so cruelly ravages the population of Paris," the worker who wrote the petition said in a letter to the editor of the popular paper *L'Opinion publique,* "I had the idea of appealing to God, asking Him to bring an end to the ravages of the disease." He noted that the petition was one "proletarians had signed with an eagerness which proves that not all faith has been extinguished in them."[92] In 1832, when Catholicism had been more on the defensive, it would have been virtually unthinkable for the religious or secular press to devote attention to a worker's petition to Church officials.

Along with this popularity, the Catholic Church had gained significant political influence among bourgeois Parisians as a defender of order in the aftermath of 1848. Church authorities held enough sway in the Second Republic, for example, to convince the president, Louis Napoleon Bonaparte, to send troops to defend the Pope in Rome, thereby violating a directive of the national constitution.[93] Meanwhile, Frédéric Falloux, the minister of public instruction and religious affairs (who would soon introduce a series of laws that would give the Catholic Church an unprecedented role in post-revolutionary French education), issued a letter to bishops throughout the country asking them to give the necessary orders so that a *Te Deum* could be sung in commemoration of the first meeting of the Estates General in 1789.[94] Since Sibour's response opened with the phrase, "In accordance with the government's wish asking us to see Religion," we can assume that the minister had been quite explicit in his request.[95] More remarkable than the cooperation itself was the *extent* of that cooperation; clearly the government *needed* the approval of the Church in order to legitimize even the most secular activities—ironically, in this case, the confirmation of the revolution that had swept away the traditional bases of Church authority.[96]

Not surprisingly, then, religion seemed to assert itself more openly and boldly during the second epidemic. While Catholic newspapers observed that charitable donations would be distributed "in conforming with a general ordinance of the twelve mayor's offices [*mairies*] of Paris,"[97] the archbishop proclaimed publicly that civil resources would not suffice. "Public charity could never either understand [*connaître*] or calm all suffering," he explained in a widely distributed pamphlet. "State revenues will be exhausted, and [the administration] will still remain far from the noble goal that it hopes to attain! [State relief] needs to be supported and supplemented by private Charity. . . . Let us be aware of our gratitude to the government for everything that it does; but let us remain convinced that this cannot prevent us from coming to the aid of our brothers."[98]

Such a critique came out of a certain self-confidence rather than from the political antagonism that had characterized the Church response during the first epidemic. Religion also enjoyed greater self-confidence partly because doctors failed to offer any new compelling explanations about the nature of cholera, a fact that made medical professionals more modest. "It must be repeated, it must be very humbly and painfully acknowledged," the *Gazette médicale de Paris* admitted after the epidemic had reached its peak, "cholera-morbus from India remains unknown to us, in terms of its logic [*principe*] and in terms of its mode of propagation, [and] even less in terms of its ability to be cured."[99]

Perhaps it was this new position of relative security vis-à-vis medical professionals and administrators that gave Catholic officials the courage to publish a religious alternative to the secular *instructions populaires*.[100] Entitled "Everyman's Instructions," the pamphlet had a format and vocabulary similar to the administrative *instructions*, with easy-to-read sections on diet, drink, and moderation, as well as reiterations of the hygienists' recommendations to air out rooms, avoid overcrowding, and wear flannel. But despite its close resemblance to the official *instructions*, the Catholic brochure conveyed an explicit religious message, complete with inspirational passages from the Bible. In a section entitled "Tranquility of the Soul," for example, the pamphlet made it clear that religion and medicine now worked hand in hand. "Doctors recommend the [tranquility of the soul], everyone preaches this," it proclaimed, "but this is in vain unless one looks for it from God." Such a presentation conveyed the message that medicine had given its blessing (literally in this case, as the vocabulary suggested) to the Catholic enterprise; not only had doctors advocated the tranquility of the soul as a legitimate scientific measure for combating the epidemic, but medicine provided the conceptual model for the religious *instructions*.

Elsewhere in the pamphlet the intersections between religion and medical authority became even more apparent. "Don't wait for this terrible moment to reconcile yourself with God," it warned at one point and then drew an intriguing analogy between sinners and individuals sick with cholera. "Know, however, that just as the patient cannot hope to be cured unless he presents himself to a doctor and follows the prescribed remedies, the sinner cannot hope to be pardoned, to live in peace, and to find salvation unless he presents himself to the Savior."[101] Whereas Church writings in the first epidemic would have been more likely to equate the victim with the sinner, the analogy drawn in the religious *instructions* revealed a less critical attitude toward both the patient and the disease. No longer meant to be taken literally, the image was now invoked metaphorically, an indication that Catholic views had been influenced by secular ones.

The very appearance of an explicitly religious pamphlet so closely resembling the official *instructions populaires* implied a new association between religious and secular authority, which was also apparent in medical documentation. When *L'Union médicale,* the most highly respected medical journal of the second epidemic, condemned the administration for its failure to set up *bureaux de secours* quickly enough, for example, it praised the ongoing but overextended charitable efforts run by the Church.[102] In a later issue it even suggested having local priests explain health measures, an idea it described as "an ingenious means for reassuring the population."[103] The *Gazette des hôpitaux civils et militaires,* another respected medical journal, printed a letter signed merely "X" that praised the measures being taken by the archbishop. In reference to Sibour's first statement about the epidemic, the writer explained:

> This circular is not only a wise Christian exhortation based on the thoughts of an elevated philosophy [but] also an excellent hygienic instruction in which the venerable shepherd limits himself to recommending a moderate [*sage*] and regulated life, without having encroached upon the domain of science, as is too often the case of those in his church. Voilà, my dear colleagues, a manner of practicing religion that cannot fail to find an echo in all hearts.[104]

Such a letter would never have appeared in the country's leading medical journal in 1832.

Moreover, the official government report for the epidemic implied that religion may have influenced the calmer popular responses to the second outbreak. "If [the epidemics of 1832 and 1849] bring to mind an era of pain and sacrifice," the report explained, "they have also shown us how both charity and religion have blossomed; both [epidemics] have also shown us the eagerness of charity and religion . . . to hold the hand of the most unfortunate sufferer." Ignored by the 1832 report, religion now occupied a valuable role in helping to avoid the catastrophes and chaos so characteristic of the first epidemic.[105] Most significantly, it did so in a forum previously dedicated to celebrating the triumph of a new scientific paradigm.

In addition to influencing secular discourse, religion entered charity discussions more publicly, reflecting a return to the old Catholic notion of a reciprocal relationship between rich and poor. Two articles that appeared in the popular Catholic paper *Le Journal du peuple* demonstrated this relationship clearly. The first, titled "Call to the Rich" (which in fact meant the bourgeois who had come to dominate Parisian economics and society during the July Monarchy), encouraged charitable donations in a conciliatory rather than a patronizing manner.[106] "Have the poor forgive you your wealth and your luxury by making the poor profit from your luxury and wealth," the paper urged the better-off. Pointing out that the poor had remained calm during both the epidemic and the threat of civil disorder, the editorial maintained that it was now time for the rich to fulfill their part in the unstated bargain. "Rich people—we say to you—in abstaining [from revolt] the People fought for you. They fulfilled their obligation. Fulfill yours." The appeal was blunt and purely pragmatic, if also couched in religious rhetoric. "Don't forget that every worker to whom you give bread by giving him work is a soldier that you pull out of the army of insurrection! Dream at last, reflect above all upon this sublime verse of a grand poet: 'He who gives to the poor loans to God!'" Unlike the case in 1832, when charity meant specific contributions of alms—food, blankets, clothing, lodging—the new charity consisted of providing *work* so that individuals could provide these necessities on their own. Here, even in a right-wing Catholic paper, we see a revival of older Catholic ideas to some degree influenced by socialism and the experiment of the 1848 revolution: the poor deserved more than material gifts, for now they needed work and education. Moreover, their newfound pride now required respect. "Emergency!" the paper pleaded, "Urgency for all positive measures that bring about popular improvements! . . . Give daily bread to the families of the people by providing them with work, educating their children, supporting their elderly; this is what is truly urgent!"

The following week, *Le Journal du peuple* printed its "Appeal to the Poor," a plea that called on the lower classes never to lose the

Catholic faith.[107] In the context of post-1848 Paris this appeal meant one thing in particular, and the paper masked this request only thinly: avoid being influenced by the socialists. "Unlike your flatterers, we don't seek to mislead you [by promising] the monstrous utopia of *social equality*," the article explained, "but we dream of a true equality for you, an equality within reach, that of work, education, morality, and well-being." Not only did such rhetoric condemn the socialists, but it also attempted to circumvent their authority with promises of achieving these dreams through education. Thus, the paper's appeal looked both backward to the traditional relationship between the donor and the recipient and also forward to promoting a social balance in which everyone's basic needs for work and happiness were fulfilled.

Even though the post-Enlightenment and post-revolutionary rhetoric employed by bourgeois medical professionals, administrators, and journalists frequently attacked the Catholic Church, the institution played an important role in shaping perceptions of cholera, its messengers, and the Paris environment during both outbreaks. In 1832 it provided something concrete against which bourgeois Parisians could react. By attacking unsuccessful medical and administrative measures, as well as by presenting cholera as the wrath of a punishing God, Church responses helped emphasize an underlying level of animosity between the secular and the sacred as each struggled to articulate a new place within the changing political, social, and cultural equilibrium during the early July Monarchy. Particularly in the area of charity, both sides came into open conflict as they fought at the most superficial level of party politics as well as over the deeper question of whether a bourgeois world view could or should prevail. At the same time, the constant overlapping of rhetoric and style indicated that both sides were drawing upon similar experience and expertise in the face of a mysterious crisis that no one could understand or contain.

By the time of the second epidemic, the political, social, and cultural landscape of the relationship between religious and secular authority had changed significantly, even though no medical breakthroughs had established the cause or cure for cholera. Over the course of the July Monarchy, the legitimists, the pro-Catholic conservatives who had posed such a strong threat to the newly liberated Parisian bourgeoisie in 1832, declined significantly in power and influence. As a result, by 1849 supporting the Church was no longer a political liability for a class that now felt a stronger challenge from the left. Moreover, the Church itself had undergone a revival that made it see the less-fortunate and their relationship to disease in a new light. The Church's new conceptualization of the poor provided a vocabulary and image that would enable the bourgeois to counter the socialists' appeal with at least a rhetoric of compassion.

At the same time that the Church became less of a threat, the Parisian bourgeoisie was becoming more secure in its own sense of identity. Because of the greater collaboration among medical professionals, government officials, and journalists, which revealed a stronger sense of cohesion during the second epidemic, secular authorities could turn openly to the Church in 1849 in a way that would not have been possible seventeen years earlier. Even if the stalemate and stagnation of the July Monarchy, along with the terror inspired by yet another bloody working-class revolution in 1848, had profoundly shaken bourgeois authority and confidence, solid foundations for this authority had been laid during the reign of Louis Philippe and his ministers. When secular and religious authorities responded to cholera in 1849, then, they did so as allies who openly acknowledged their mutual support. To contrast the impact of unstable bourgeois authority in 1832 with the greater confidence it enjoyed by 1849, let us now turn to a close discussion of particular moments when disease and social unrest intersected during both outbreaks.

5

Disease and Social Unrest

"God has struck us with the same scourge in the wake of two revolutions," a newspaper editorial in *Le Crédit* announced at the height of the French capital's second great cholera epidemic in 1849. The paper pointed to distinct parallels between the first outbreak in 1832 and the current crisis, explaining, "Just at the time when political and social disturbances threaten everyone's existence, [God] has willed that we be threatened yet again by the mysterious influences of nature, [influences that are] stronger than all human prudence and resistance."[1] Referring to the aftermath of revolutions in 1830 and 1848, the Parisian daily saw profound links between what it considered to be failed revolutions and the arrival of cholera epidemics less than two years later. What the authors of the June 11 article did not anticipate, however, was an even more immediate connection between the current outbreak and urban unrest; two days later, on June 13, just after mortality figures from cholera had peaked, Paris experienced its most significant uprising since the bloody June Days.

Having explored the complex interactions among cholera's messengers, their bourgeois messages, and how they articulated them, we can at last return to the strands of disease and revolution that opened this book. This final chapter examines the concrete moments when intersections between cholera and social unrest became most apparent. In April 1832 large numbers of ragpickers took to the streets to protest the government's introduction of a new street-cleaning policy, while days later rumors that the epidemic was actually a government assassination plot caused a series of brutal murders. Several weeks later crowds again clashed with National Guard troops during the funeral of General Lamarque, a popular leader who died of the disease. In 1849 opponents of the government's intervention in Italian foreign policy prompted the worst unrest since the previous year's bloody June Days, an insurrection that coincided directly with the period of highest mortality from the second outbreak. Combined with the threat of death from cholera, these moments of revolutionary violence caused Parisians to take stock of life in the capital and to articulate their feelings in dramatically different ways in 1832 and 1849.

By contrasting bourgeois discussions surrounding specific moments of social unrest that accompanied each epidemic, this chapter sets out to understand the silence of 1849 in the context of urban social relations in mid-nineteenth-century France. In the first outbreak, the hygienists' investigations, Church proclamations, Paris malade, and cholera's apparent preference for less-fortunate neighborhoods all combined with the capital's revolutionary tradition to influence bourgeois perceptions of the urban poor as inherently "revolting" in every respect. Even though seventeen years later cholera still remained a medical mystery and Paris had been through yet another major revolution, issues such as the "social question," a religious revival, and socialism, as well as a more firmly entrenched Parisian bourgeoisie combined to soften the rhetoric describing the capital and its poor inhabitants. While most lower-class Parisians probably never came to trust their social superiors, over the course of the 1830s and 1840s they had at least developed enough faith in medical professionals and government officials not to accuse them of an assassination plot. With the less-fortunate demonstrating such restraint, bourgeois Parisians altered their understanding of the relationship between disease and revolt, and consequently their presentation of a new epidemic reality. To give a full sense of the contrast between the two epidemics, then, let us begin in 1832 with an analysis of what bourgeois Parisians found to be the most disturbing cholera stories of all.

THE BRUTALITY OF DETAIL

Within less than a week after the declaration of the 1832 epidemic, two forms of popular violence erupted throughout the capital, both of them indicative of cholera's profound challenge to the precarious balance of social order: uprisings by ragpickers and riots against suspected poisoners. Although the disturbances began for different reasons and followed distinct trajectories, both became fused in the mind of the bourgeois. Together, they provided concrete examples of a hidden world of poverty and depravity brought to the surface for the first time by cholera. By exploring each of these events and responses to them in some depth, it is possible to arrive at a greater understanding of the deeper forces that may have inspired bourgeois Parisians to describe them as they did.

In keeping with the hygienists' idea that putrid miasmas constituted a major threat to the health of Parisians, the city government introduced a new means of removing garbage from the streets in late March of 1832. The large, cumbersome carts were replaced by smaller *tombereaux* drawn by a single horse. According to the plan, the vehicles would be able to enter the smallest streets and would collect refuse more frequently, with a second round at dusk added to the normal collection earlier in the day. While the officials who designed the plan may not have been fully aware of it, in a sense the new system very much resembled the hygienists' investigation of urban space; for the first time ever, the smaller carts could now penetrate the narrowest streets of the capital's poorer neighborhoods in a systematic and thorough manner. Like the medical investigations (and like the disease itself), city authority was extending into areas previously untouched. Though the plans to implement the new cleaning policy were not in direct response to cholera, they had unfortunately been slated to take effect the same week that thousands of Parisians in the poorer neighborhoods began collapsing in the streets with painful cramps, vomiting, and diarrhea.

In the first few days of April, police reports and the popular press described a series of riots protesting the implementation of the new system. Beginning on April 1, angry groups of men and women seized several of the *tombereaux,* ceremoniously throwing them into the Seine while setting others on fire.[2] The disturbances lasted approximately four days, destroyed more than sixty carts, and resulted in the arrest of 225 people, nearly all of them from the lower classes. The riots took place in traditional areas of popular violence, areas also devastated by high rates of cholera mortality: the faubourg St. Antoine, the place de Grève, and the Conservatoire des Arts et Métiers. Most sources blamed the *chiffonniers,* the ragpickers.[3] As the poorest segment of the Parisian lumpenproletariat, a group that made its livelihood by scouring piles of garbage in search of valuable items for resale, the *chiffonniers* had the most to lose from the new system. Because people usually became ragpickers out of economic desperation, the additional collection rounds meant a fundamental attack on their means of subsistence because they would reduce the amount of refuse available for possible re-sale.[4] The *tombereaux,* and their more frequent passage, proved to be a blatant betrayal of a long-standing agreement that had allowed ragpickers a specific "grace period" [*heure de tolérance*] to make their rounds before an army of sweepers removed the daily accumulation of garbage. In the words of one petition that boasted "ten thousand signatures and as many crosses of approval," the ragpickers urged Gisquet, the prefect of police, to remember "the permission that had been granted us to exercise a recognized profession."[5]

Not surprisingly then, the more sympathetic public discourse describing the riots focused on the immediate financial interests that had been the traditional right of the ragpickers. According to the German writer and reporter Heinrich Heine, the *chiffonniers* de-fended their turf in much the same way as had nobles, guild mas-ters, professors, and others since the Middle Ages.[6] Another writer mentioned the existence of "*chiffonniers-négociants* who are said of-ten to make fortunes of this traffic."[7] And the urban investigator H. A. Frégier would later describe the *chiffonniers* as having their own financial empire, replete with *marchandise, maître-chiffonniers,* and *chiffonniers-entreposeurs,* an empire that had begun to crumble with the new system of smaller carts.[8] Even the prefect of police felt compelled to issue a circular which said that, contrary to popular opinion, "the [new] service should not change anything that would affect their interests."[9] And indeed the ragpickers' own petition had appealed to Gisquet as members of a "recognized profession," an acknowledgment of the credibility that professions were coming to enjoy in the capital.[10] The destruction of the carts, then, could be seen as a concrete response to the challenges that the new street-cleaning policy posed to the ragpickers' ancient profession and eco-nomic livelihood.

But even though the riots could be interpreted in financial terms comprehensible to some of the most respectable members of the Parisian bourgeoisie, less sympathetic observers found deeply trou-bling implications in the events. A part of the urban environment since the old regime, the *chiffonniers* had usually been viewed as liminal men, women, and children, quaint figures[11] characterized by the fact that they dressed in tatters and used a pole with a kind of

hook on the end to deposit desired bits of garbage into their *hottes,*
or baskets.[12] Once home, they carefully and industriously (as the
middle-class lore had it) sorted through the rubbish in order to sell
different parts to appropriate middlemen. The destruction of the
garbage carts during the first days of the cholera epidemic helped
reshape the portrait of the *chiffonnier* from a harmless figure of urban folklore to one more intricately tied to that of Paris malade.
When treating cholera patients in the faubourg St. Denis, for example, one doctor clearly felt that he had in fact discovered a terrifying
unknown race. "[The chiffonniers] sort through the product of their
daily rounds," he wrote with the clear, disapproving stamp of a
hygienist; "then they pile it up in every corner, even under their
beds [*couchettes*]. . . . [They collect] bones with bits of putrefying
flesh still clinging to them [which they] wrap in old mud-soiled
rags; moreover, fetid miasmas continually emanate from these bits
of garbage, making ragpickers' dwellings permanent homes of infection."[13]

These stark images of urban depravity had been safely hidden
away until the outbreak of cholera and the accompanying social
unrest had, as one police official put it, transformed ragpickers from
a group "that nobody ever saw in normal times" to one "that
seemed to emerge suddenly from beneath the pavement."[14]
Brought into public view by both the hygienists' investigations and
the ragpickers' unprecedented violence, the *chiffonniers* were dangerous precisely because they epitomized the hideous underworld
of revolutionary disorder and Paris malade revealed by the cholera
epidemic. Their existence, their new visibility, served as an unfor-
gettable image of a sick, "revolting" city that extended well beyond
the few riots in which the ragpickers participated. Their private
depravity had become undeniably and emblematically public.

The ragpickers' new visibility helped articulate the precise
boundaries within which respectable Parisians should act.[15] Just as
hygienists defined health in terms of what it was *not,* so too the
portrait of a ragpicker emerged in terms of how he or she failed to
measure up to an unwritten bourgeois ideal; because the portraits
appeared in private memoirs and published investigations, it is
likely that the portraits were not intended to better the *chiffonniers*
themselves. "They know no laws, country nor justice," wrote one
observer; "a kind of hermaphroditic race, they do not belong to

nature because they do not resemble savages, nor to society because they are not policed.''[16] Another writer, an Englishman, also commented on the ambiguous gender of the ragpicker, noting that ''if we were to judge by habiliment, feature, complexion, voice, or even beard, we might occasionally find it very difficult to determine the age or sex of any given specimen.''[17] This anxiety regarding the ragpickers' ambiguous gender anticipated concerns with documenting and maintaining sexual difference that would become much more prominent among the middle classes later in the century.[18] In the early 1830s, however, they spoke more to concerns that men, women, and even children were essentially performing the same tasks at a time when work was becoming increasingly differentiated by gender.

Not only did the ragpickers raise issues of gender confusion, but they also offended the bourgeois sense of order in their relationship to both space and time. Spatially, the *chiffonniers* blurred the cherished distinctions between work and domestic life. Those fortunate enough to have dwellings inspired criticism because they performed too many different tasks within a single tiny room.[19] Those who lived on the streets or slept in the fields distressed bourgeois observers because they carried the sum of their belongings in their *hottes.* ''The ragpicker's basket not only serves as the receptacle for the objects he collects for his livelihood,'' Frégier noted with a mixture of astonishment and disgust, ''but . . . is also where he keeps his household belongings. Among the rubbish that he exploits he finds his own personal effects.''[20] Thus, the very symbol of the ragpicker, the *hotte,* could be linked with broader cultural developments reflected in more clearly delineated roles for men and women as well as a growing architectural trend to designate specific functions for individual rooms in the middle-class dwelling.[21]

Temporally, the ragpicker lived in a liminal world between light and dark, following a clock that refused to conform to bourgeois convention. ''The hours they keep are such as are unknown in the civilized world,'' a contemporary explained; ''theirs is neither a working nor an astronomical day. It is an anomalous period, which, so to speak, has neither beginning nor end, and we can only describe it as a *cercle vicieux* in which they are constantly moving.''[22] Or, in the simple, passing remark of another writer who did not need to explain the transgression to respectable Parisian readers:

"The ragpicker has his breakfast at nine in the evening [and] his large meal at three in the morning."[23] In a world where a growing number of etiquette manuals made bourgeois Parisians critically aware of the need for following proper daily rituals, the transgression of the ragpickers inspired particular anxiety.[24] When these criticisms were combined with the fact that the ragpickers' genderless households prevented them from fulfilling the proper roles of men and women, the negative portrait was virtually complete.

By seeming to thwart bourgeois social conventions with their gender ambiguity and cultural nonconformity, the *chiffonniers* increasingly prompted police officials and urban investigators to try to find other means of fixing them concretely within the prevailing social order. Thus, in 1832 there were calls to revive enforcement of an 1828 police ordinance that, in an attempt to reduce crime, had taken the unprecedented step of requiring ragpickers to purchase a copper medallion to be worn on the back of their baskets in plain view.[25] The oval plate had to give a description [*le signalement*] of the individual, as well as "the initials of his Christian names, his name and his nickname, if he has one."[26] The preamble of the document made a special point of asking officers to pin down nicknames, considering that "the majority of ragpickers do not have a permanent residence, that instead of using their real names, most have more or less bizarre nicknames by which they are known, and that in this ambiguous and uncertain position they easily escape every sort of investigation and surveillance."[27] Describing children who had apparently abandoned their families for the world of ragpicking, Frégier found their lost patrimonial identity almost more disturbing than their flight itself. "Within a matter of years they have become so estranged from their families," he wrote, "that they have forgotten the name and address of their fathers, remembering only their own first names."[28] Thus, along with a permanent dwelling, a full family name provided a means of fixing the cultural coordinates of an individual within the rapidly changing social order of Paris. Both forms of *address* helped to establish an outward, traceable individual identity at a time when contemporaries perceived that immigration had dramatically increased the capital's rootless population.[29] By thwarting these identifying characteristics, the *chiffonniers* once again highlighted their differences from the middle classes. At the same time, their outrageous violence hammered home the urgency of establishing social boundaries through fixed cultural identities.

Objectively speaking, such classifications could seem quite arbitrary, as can be seen from the similarities and differences between the *chiffonniers* and their apparent rivals, the hygienists.[30] On the one hand, both groups gathered material, classifying it within specific categories of value and usefulness. On the other hand, this mysterious, unclassifiable race collected and brought into its hovels the very garbage that the hygienists sought to remove from the streets as the prime causes of infection. Moreover, the *chiffonniers* defended themselves by using arguments based on their traditional proprietary and economic rights, while the hygienists based their own claims to legitimacy on their role as scientists bringing new, progressive ideas antithetical to that tradition.

At a time when the perceived fluidity and instability of Parisian life made the middle classes especially eager to establish social and cultural boundaries between themselves and those beneath them, the "transgressions" of the ragpickers served as a vivid reminder of how tenuous most boundaries really were. No longer romanticized by folklore, the *chiffonniers* occupied a position at the bottom rung of the city's socioeconomic ladder, which placed them outside the familiar structures of classification and power and, by definition, outside of local authorities' control. Without gender, without status, and without a place in either a savage or civilized state, the ragpickers underscored middle-class values by giving bourgeois Parisians something to define themselves against. At the same time, however, the ragpickers had tremendous power and significance as outsiders. Like the mysterious disease that had brought them out from beneath the pavement, they presented a formidable challenge to a society newly committed to quantification and classification as a means of curing Paris malade. In the spring of 1832, as the steam of fiery *tombereaux* rose from the waters of the Seine, however, the victory of science and bourgeois values was by no means assured.

An even greater and more violent threat to the Parisian sense of order and rationality came just days later, on April 4, as attention shifted from the *tombereaux* to a series of grisly disturbances provoked by rumors that the epidemic was part of an assassination plot. "Killing rages through the streets," the entertainment paper *Le Bonhomme Richard* announced. "People believe in an infamous plot; they want to take justice into their own hands, and [they] attack several peaceful citizens upon the simplest suspicion of crime."[31] Partly because cholera's violent symptoms bore some resemblance to the effects of poisoning, and more likely because the massive, sudden deaths needed a scapegoat, rumors spread rapidly among the poorer classes that someone—usually a wine merchant or a doctor—was trying to rid the city of unwanted elements. Although probably no more than five or six individuals died at the hands of angry mobs in the disturbances that rocked the capital, the scenes and their subsequent publicity in the press generated considerable discussion and anxiety. Moreover, by coming so closely on the heels of the ragpicker riots, the disturbances compounded bourgeois anxiety by implying that, like disease, urban violence could be contagious.

Associations between poisoned wells and pestilence had long been in the lexicon of responses to epidemic diseases, with outcast groups such as Jews, gypsies, or witches receiving most of the blame.[32] Like their early-modern counterparts, those who rioted during the 1832 epidemics raged against authorities such as doctors and government officials. After all, Western medical wisdom had constantly created analogies between poisons and the hypothetical agents of disease.[33] But unlike the situation during the old regime, now the press played an unprecedented role in compounding, perpetuating, and even giving a certain legitimacy to rumors. The newspapers were influential not just among the members of the upper classes, who were more likely to read, but also among the less-literate lower classes who listened in cafés and public squares, and who (before the explosion of the popular press in the mid-1830s) were more likely to equate printed documents with the voice of outside authority. Moreover, after the killing of the king, the Terror, and images of angry crowds from 1789–95, the idea of violence took on enhanced *political* significance with national as opposed to local or regional implications.

Potent episodes of social unrest inspired by poison rumors accompanied cholera outbreaks from the very beginning.[34] In the early 1830s the fear of "body snatching," the quest by anatomists to find corpses for dissection, caused a series of bloody upheavals in

Great Britain. Like France, meanwhile, Russia, Germany, and parts of Italy experienced violent riots in the wake of stories that cholera resulted from a government plot to poison the undesirable lower classes. These uprisings persisted into the 1890s and have been viewed as the growing pains of modernization or resistance to state authority, though contemporaries looked upon them as uncivilized acts of barbarism.[35]

The French response to cholera both drew upon past experiences and broke with precedent. In Paris, the poison rumors and accompanying unrest occurred only during the 1832 epidemic despite subsequent cholera outbreaks in 1849, 1854, 1866, and 1884. As elsewhere in Europe, factors such as heightened population density, the need to find a tangible explanation for a mysterious disease that would make sense to the lower classes, a growing animosity to outside intervention, and resentment toward the wealthier classes no doubt all played a part. But France was also different. Major changes in regime in 1789 and 1830 prompted bourgeois Parisians to interpret and describe the unrest linked to the epidemic as a part of a revolutionary tradition. Though the current of change had been instrumental in bringing them to power, many middle-class Parisians felt profound ambivalence about being part of such a tradition, particularly when the violence turned ugly, as it did during the 1832 cholera epidemic. Thus, in France more than elsewhere in Europe, the poison riots forced the middle classes to confront the lives of the poor within the context of an increasingly threatening revolutionary tradition, a fact that threw their sense of control into question.

In order to understand how Parisians tried to make sense of the poison riots, it is first necessary to look at how the story unfolded. Never a linear narrative with a beginning, middle, or ending, the violence achieved coherence through the repetition of different stories that were told, retold, and embellished or excerpted along the way. Unless one was reprinted verbatim from another newspaper, no two accounts were ever exactly alike. Certain details such as a location, name, profession, poisoned substance, weapon, or the fate of a victim recurred with some frequency, but not in identical combinations and not in every story. Moreover, because of the chaos and confusion, descriptions by doctors, police, and journalists operated freely within the same narrative field as gossip and innuendo. With no clearly perceived legitimate bearer of Truth, all accounts could easily feed one another. Even if no one living in Paris during the first cholera epidemic got the same accurate story, all the details converged to create a prevailing mood of instability and fear inspired by the return of a particular kind of "barbarian" violence now associated with revolutionary excess. Rather than attempt to reconstruct what "really" happened, then, I shall focus on the most conspicuous themes that surfaced as Parisians came to terms with the events.

Rumors about merchants, doctors, and other unspecified suspects circulated loosely among terrified lower-class Parisians, and these rumors were often canonized in the ink of the popular press. Interestingly, no account at the time specifically used the word *bourgeois* in conjunction with lower-class accusations, though in accounts written after the fact the charge surfaced.[36] Nearly all the people charged were men, and in several cases Jews were singled out, though open anti-Semitism went no further.[37] Many accounts shied away from making specific accusations, relying upon the passive voice to explain an act. Stories also circulated about vaguely defined "innocent bystanders," such as the good Samaritan who stopped to help a sick man on the street by offering to fetch him a glass of wine; when he returned, a "menacing" crowd had gathered to warn the sick man that the wine was in fact poison. The only thing that saved the good fellow from being torn to pieces by the crowd, the article explained, was his presence of mind to drink the wine himself.[38]

Physicians faced particularly vicious attacks, in part because of their new visibility as a profession and in part because many lower-class Parisians saw them as the dreaded representatives of an increasingly imposing outside authority.[39] "I'll never forget the impression I had when, while making every effort to comfort and save . . . the unfortunate [victims of cholera], I read in their disturbed faces, their taciturn moods, and their empty words [*propos sourds*] that they suspected me of poisoning them," the exalted Dr. Magendie told students in one of his lectures about cholera.[40] Dr. Poumiès felt physically intimidated. "More than once I was threatened, insulted, treated as a poisoner; I worked under extreme danger, [and] some of my colleagues were grossly mistreated." He wondered how many times he had heard the cry: "Down with doctors!" And describing a riot in front of the Hôtel Dieu, he remained convinced that "if at that moment someone had revealed my profession, I would have been torn to pieces."[41]

Most often, riots focused attention on hospitals because of the alleged maltreatment patients suffered inside.[42] Because only the wealthy could afford the services of a private physician, the large and unsanitary institutions had become the repository of the forgotten poor, places equated with disease and death at the hands of strangers. Contemporary descriptions, fed by constant stories in the press, told of typhoid outbreaks as well as countless casualties from disease and neglect.[43] "The appearance of hospitals was a horrible sight," one observer recalled, noting that in a single day as many as thirteen people had died in the same bed at the Hôtel Dieu:

> What torments filled these long halls of suffering that housed the disease! In a tone of voice that no ear has ever heard before, some give off piercing and raucous cries in the midst of horrible convulsions that signal the hour of their deaths. Others fall prey to fainting spells, syncopes, [and] bouts of dizziness without even uttering a last gasp, for they haven't run the gamut of their suffering. Others shiver and clench their teeth; others raise themselves up from their beds as if lifting themselves from their crypts.[44]

Indeed, it had been deemed a major public health coup when the revolutionary government passed laws declaring that there should be one patient per bed and that each bed should be separated by at least three feet. But many idealistic reforms carried out during the Revolution were abandoned, and the stories of mistreatment persisted through much of the century.[45]

Such rumors about the dangers lurking in hospitals emerged with particular force during the 1832 epidemic, when many of the poor refused to enter treatment facilities of any kind. More than usual, their fears had transformed these unsavory institutions into "a vast arsenal of poison."[46] At the height of the epidemic a doctor in the twelfth arrondissement described the typical story of an elderly couple who had been evicted while sick with cholera. Because they had nowhere else to sleep, he suggested the Hôtel Dieu, but they resisted violently, saying that they "preferred to die rather than enter a hospital."[47] To further complicate the picture and make the hospitals even more threatening, the city government had passed a law prohibiting visitors in the cholera wards and also establishing a military post in front of the Hôtel Dieu to guard against violence.[48] As a result, the poor might easily see the institutions as representing the imposing power of an outside authority, one that delineated a conscious and forceful boundary between them and those above them in the capital.

With such fears circulating freely, it is not surprising that so many riots took place outside of hospitals. In one notable clash, which received much attention in the press, a crowd of angry workers came to the Hôtel Dieu and tried to force their way into the building. Convinced that cholera was a hoax and accusing doctors of "a plot to get rid of the less fortunate," the crowd blocked the entrance and demanded admission from a doctor who had just arrived with a patient. Indignant, the doctor called the mob "as barbarous as the Russians,"[49] and grabbing one of the most violent protesters while uncovering the patient, shouted: "You don't want to believe in cholera? Well! just look at a real cholera victim!" According to the newspaper accounts, "Upon seeing the appearance of this livid and decomposed face, the crowd recoiled in horror." Such a dramatic story of revelation and medical triumph in the face of the literal personification of cholera was intended to go a long way in shaping concrete impressions of the epidemic, as evidenced by the appearance of this story in several different accounts.[50]

However, some fared even worse; the real terror of the poison riots came from stories where suspected assassins were literally torn to pieces at the hands of angry mobs. The highly respected *Gazette médicale de Paris* reported that on the Quai de la Féraille "one unfortunate victim was knocked to the ground and then ripped to shreds by dogs that were told to attack. Finally he was tied to a fir plank and thrown into the river so that everyone on the bridges and quays could see what punishment was inflicted on poisoners."[51] The reality of these five or six highly public, violent deaths in 1832 raised the revolutionary hysteria to a level not seen since the Terror. "Nothing is so horrible as the anger of a mob when it rages for blood and strangles its defenseless prey," Heine wrote to readers of the *Gazette d'Augsbourg* in mid-April. He described "a dark sea of human beings in which, here and there, workmen in their shirt sleeves seemed like the white caps of a raging sea." On the rue de Vaugirard he witnessed a group of old women who removed their clogs (the shoes of the lower classes) to smash in the head of a suspected poisoner. "I saw one of the wretches while he was still in the death rattle," Heine reported. "He was naked and beaten and bruised, so that his blood flowed; they tore from him not only his clothes, but also his hair and cut off his lips." A man came up to the body and tied a cord around its feet and dragged it through the streets crying, "Voilà le choléra-morbus!" The story concluded with the final blow delivered by "a very beautiful woman, pale with rage, with bare breasts and bloody hands. She laughed to me and begged for a few francs reward for her dainty work which with to buy a mourning dress because her mother had died a few hours before of poison."[52]

As a writer and foreign reporter, Heine used early-modern images of barbarism to considerable dramatic advantage, particularly regarding women,[53] but he was not alone. Much like the traumatized Edmund Burke writing about events in 1789, the Austrian cultural attaché seemed to echo the thoughts of many when he wrote of the riots, "The populace of Paris is in the process of proving that the people will always be the people and that in all countries of the world and under the same circumstances they will partake of the same excesses."[54] Meanwhile, Jules Janin, the voice of the conservative, comfortable bourgeois, described the riots with sensational effect in the opening pages of his *Paris depuis la révolution de 1830* (1832) as "the voice of the people that has spoken" and asked rhetorically, "How did this formidable voice speak? It spoke like the voice of the people speaks, through iron, through blows, through abuse, through murder, through blood, through all forms of anger and violation."[55] Though he had a different political agenda, the left-wing socialist Louis Blanc used similar rhetoric. "And thus for an instant from the eyes of the rich the veil was lifted that hides the hideous base of the social world that they want to possess," he began, remembering the events in his memoirs. "Suddenly, out from the shadows of these neighborhoods where misery allows itself to be forgotten, there emerged masses of men with bare arms, somber faces, [and] a look full of hate [ready] to inundate the capital. What were they looking for? What did they ask for? Nothing *said* it, except that they explored the city with a defiant eye and become agitated with ferocious murmurs."[56] Even as he mocked the naïveté of the Parisian upper classes, Blanc drew on images that had been circulating throughout the capital: the muscular arms of angry workers, their sudden emergence from some dark nether place, and the power of raging waters, all occurred with varying frequency in other accounts.

For nearly everyone who commented on them, then, the poison riots called into question the essence of Parisian life, the nature of class conflict, and the legacy of revolution. Perhaps *L'Ami de la religion* captured the fears of many when it sarcastically observed that "these foolish rumors contain the stuff to humiliate us a bit." The editors could not understand how stories "can create such dupes in Paris in the nineteenth century, in the midst of all the torrents of enlightenment that inundate us, [especially] after two revolutions that have made such rapid steps toward social perfection."[57] Perhaps more than the arrival of the disease itself, the barbaric behavior of the lower classes thwarted the belief that Paris represented the essence of beauty, enlightenment, and rationality. Put another way, the events suggested that the revolution had not yet ended and that the social unrest associated with the outbreak of cholera might mean that revolution was somehow endemically and viscerally a part of Parisian life.

To counterbalance explanations that emphasized the inherent barbarism of humanity, many commentators who supported the *juste milieu* of the July Monarchy blamed the events on manipulation by troublemakers from both extremes of the political spectrum. The *Journal des débats* reported crowds gathered along the quays and the bridges leading to the Hôtel Dieu and asserted that they represented an "alliance between the credulity of the poor and the false insinuations of the agitators."[58] In a front-page editorial *Le Courrier français* wondered, "Is it an infernal plot that, to serve political grudges, wants to provoke violence at any price from a people who made the July Revolution and from the government that died as a result?"[59] The mayor of the fourth arrondissement posted a circular that accused some poisoners of encouraging violence "to avenge the defeat of Charles X."[60] Noting that "in the invasion of a cruel epidemic, the enemies of public peace find a new opportunity to excite the indigent against the wealthy classes," an official of Louis Philippe gave the mayor of the tenth arrondissement one hundred francs to help provide services for cholera patients.[61] The daily police reports also suggested that authorities were keeping a close watch on political opponents, notably right-wing Carlists and left-wing republicans.[62]

In one dramatic instance, Gisquet's fear of opposition right-wing groups actually heightened the violence associated with the poison scare by giving official credibility to the rumor. On April 2 a circular signed by the prefect of police appeared in all the major newspapers and on posters throughout the capital; it proclaimed that the epidemic had provided "the eternal enemies of order a new opportunity to spread infamous slander against the government among the population" and explained:

> To substantiate atrocious suppositions, wretches have come up with the idea of roaming the cabarets and butchers' stalls with flasks and packets of poison, in order either to throw them into fountains and spits, and onto meat, or even to give the impression of this happening. [They then] get themselves arrested in the very act by accomplices who, after having pretended to be from the police, help them escape. [This sets] things in motion for demonstrating the reality of the odious accusations against authorities.[63]

In his zeal to battle the political opposition, the prefect of police instead helped heighten social tensions by suggesting that individuals actually did spread poison. By arresting suspected poisoners, police officials further confirmed the rumors' validity.[64]

Opposition political groups, however, could not be blamed for everything, and at bottom lay a fundamental fear that authorities had lost control of the city. Accordingly, after the prefect's fiasco the government went to considerable lengths to link denials of the poison rumors with hard medical evidence. Publishing numerous statements and results of tests by doctors, the papers sought to assure the public that the poison stories were unwarranted. "Even though it is surely unnecessary to belabor the point among thinking people regarding the unlikelihood and impossibility of the poisonings that have preoccupied Paris," the *Moniteur* announced, "the Administration has not stopped carrying out research and calling for analysis of all substances that might be the object of suspicion." A lengthy and detailed description of one investigator's analysis of 246 different suspicious products followed—substances that included wine, milk, bonbons, sausage, tobacco, and butter with mysterious green spots. In the end, all of them proved benign. "Almost all of the beverages submitted for testing were natural and generally of very high quality," the article noted, concluding with a direct reference to the class-specific nature of the rumors, "especially those [substances] found in the neighborhoods within the interior of the *barrières*."[65]

The *Moniteur* and other major dailies made frequent use of such reports to dispel the rumors with hard scientific evidence in much the same way that they used statistics and detailed descriptions of the emergency first-aid stations.[66] On April 8, for example, a statement appeared on the front page of the paper in which the doctors of the large Hôpital St. Louis denied that cholera was contagious or caused by poisoning. The printed investigations offered incredible details of each product, the suspicious substance, and the results of tests. Such reports were presented to the public as the height of scientific knowledge and expertise and, according to the government's claims, represented "the most active research." Many prominent doctors and chemists signed the various statements. Battling the irrationality of raw violence with the zealous rationality of "public health," administrators and health officials tried to link knowledge and power to recapture the city.

THE COFFIN AND THE FLAG

Just two months after the ragpicker and poison riots another major disturbance rocked the capital, an urban insurrection that came closer than any other to toppling the still-unstable July Monarchy. "It was one of the most tragic events of history," wrote one observer of the events in June, "to see the funeral torches of the contagion illuminating the blood spilled in the civil disorders of Paris."[67] The *Moniteur* seemed less moved and described the situation as "the development of a conspiracy that hides behind [the] coffin."[68] In early June General Lamarque, a former military leader under Napoleon, died of cholera. Extremely popular among both the middle and lower classes, the general appealed to the growing nostalgia for the firm leadership of the emperor while also championing the ideals of Belgian and Polish national self-determination. Although wary of his particular popularity as a deputy and leading orator of the left, government officials agreed to allow the funeral procession to march through Paris. But, as predicted, opposition political groups used the event to stir up agitation against the July Monarchy. Thus began two days of political upheaval marked by the familiar emblems of the revolutionary tradition: flags, bloodshed, barricades, combat between the National Guard (composed principally of members of the bourgeoisie[69]) and civilians, as well as songs and slogans harking back to the glory of 1789.

Lamarque's funeral and the subsequent unrest it inspired provide an instructive contrast with the April riots for understanding the relationship between disease and revolution in 1832. Now, unlike the case during the ragpicker and poison riots, "high" politics—that of factions and parties—entered more prominently into the rhetoric of newspaper analyses, police correspondence, government reports, and even the content of the insurrection itself. Coming so soon after the morbid April events and accompanied by an increase in cholera deaths, the unrest in June once again forced Parisians to reflect upon the role that disease and revolt played in their lives. This time, however, revolution became the dominant fear. In an ironic sense, life almost seemed to have returned to "normal," and yet cholera had made an irreversible impact on how bourgeois contemporaries interpreted the events.

Fearing trouble from "members of all popular associations and generally all the artisans of disorder," officials initially believed they could keep the funeral under control. Gisquet arranged for two battalions of troops from the Garde Municipale to accompany the coffin and had others stationed at various strategic and sensitive points throughout the capital.[70] In addition, the prefect believed in an important distinction between political expression and the popular protest revealed during the poison riots that he hoped would help maintain public order. "It is more reasonable to think," he reported the day before the funeral, "that the major men of the opposition will themselves use all their influence so that this ceremony takes on the character of a lofty political demonstration without dishonoring it with popular excesses."[71] As a term frequently used to describe lower-class behavior during the April riots, "popular excesses" still carried a specific meaning for officials; clearly Gisquet feared any fusion between these excesses and "high politics." Believing the unpredictable and mysterious biological dangers associated with the epidemic to have passed, he hoped the seemingly more rational political forces familiar to him would keep the situation under control.

Several hours into the procession, however, trouble erupted when a group of agitators called for carrying the body of the general, as a revolutionary hero, to the Panthéon. In the ensuing confusion someone—none of the sources could agree on whom—fired a shot into the crowd.[72] Open clashes between some of the twenty-four thousand spectators and ten thousand troops quickly spread along the funeral route, and at one point it was not clear that the general's body would arrive safely at its final resting place in the provinces. By nightfall most of the city's shops had closed, and fighting persisted particularly in the poorer sections, the rues St. Antoine, St. Denis, and St. Martin. The following day, June 6, unrest continued but soon focused on a single neighborhood around the Cloître St. Méry, a working-class section of central Paris ravaged by cholera and characterized by narrow alleys and winding passages, territory according to one eyewitness "chosen by preference for uprisings."[73] Here insurgents began prying loose cobblestones and building barricades as government troops cordoned off the area to prepare for battle.[74] Police sources reported over one thousand arrests in conjunction with the events of June 5 and 6, and in the end estimates placed the number of dead and wounded at approximately nine hundred.[75] The day after the disturbance, authorities declared the capital under a state of siege.

More than the April riots, the revolutionary imagery and rhetoric of June 5 and 6 at the funeral of General Lamarque once again placed Paris at the center of the European political stage. "It was beautiful and touching yesterday to contemplate the Italian and Spanish tricolor banners [mixed in] with the two colors of Poland," *Le Corsaire* reported, "and the funeral flag of the refugees escorting our tricolor banners from France."[76] All accounts of the procession mentioned the frequent republican cries of "Liberty or Death!" "To arms!" "Long Live Liberty!" as well as expressions of solidarity with "our unfortunate brothers of Poland." The crowd even defied the government by drowning out the watered-down "La Parisienne" with the true song of revolution, "La Marseillaise."[77] In contrast to the barbaric and bloody images of the poison riots, the prominence of traditional revolutionary symbols and slogans gave the events of June 5 and 6 a consciously political tone but, more important, a tone invoked by a familiar script from events in 1789 and 1830.

It is difficult to discern who the participants actually were, though the press and police reports pointed to deliberate agitation from opposition political groups rather than a spontaneous uprising by the unruly lower classes. As the vocabulary used to describe the instigators suggested, the accusations ran the social and political gamut. One paper blamed the disturbances on "the entrepreneurs of social disorder," while the *Moniteur* described the conflict as one "between the anarchists and the troops of the line."[78] Reflecting the most commonly held view, police reports suggested that the events emerged from a conspiracy between two groups on opposite ends of the political spectrum, the Carlists, legitimists who sought a return of the Bourbon royal family guillotined during the Revolution, and the Republicans, a collection of left-wing groups who wanted broad popular participation in government. This "Carlist-Republican faction," police reports argued, took advantage of the funeral to incite popular agitation aimed at overthrowing the July Monarchy.[79] Meanwhile, the list of those accused of the disturbances around the Cloître St. Méry consisted mostly of workers, all but one of them men well below the age of forty.[80]

Even though it would be difficult to establish a direct causal relationship between the events of early June and the presence of cholera, certain objective correlations did exist and ultimately fed contemporary perceptions of the relationship. Chronologically, the unrest in the wake of Lamarque's funeral came less than two weeks before a major recrudescence of the epidemic, thus supporting claims that the disease reappeared because of the "heated passions" inspired by the funeral.[81] After the initial peak in early April, when cholera deaths reached more than seven hundred a day, the figure declined and remained below one hundred per day for the month of May and early June. But on June 18 mortality jumped to over three hundred per day and remained significant for over a month.[82] Moreover, the areas of greatest agitation correlated with neighborhoods hit hard by the disease, particularly that of the Cloître St. Méry. Here, population density was especially high, and mortality figures ran well above those of most other districts of the capital.[83] The official report for the epidemic discounted any connections between the events and cholera, but as we shall see in looking at a comparable situation in 1849, mentioning the possibility of a correlation at all was significant.

Nowhere was the chronological and geographical proximity between disease and revolutionary activity more apparent than in the emergency first-aid stations around the Cloître St. Méry. Because of the area's large number of potential cholera victims, the city administration maintained the *bureaux de secours* in a constant state of readiness, thus making them a likely place to treat any number of health emergencies. Accordingly, on June 6 the prefect of the Seine sent a letter to the mayor of each arrondissement urging him to make the *bureaux* and stretchers used for cholera patients available for wounded soldiers of the insurrection.[84] Ultimately, however, these institutions treated political insurgents as well as government troops and cholera patients, creating an environment with what Antoine Métral described as "the wounded of the civil war mixed in . . . with the victims of the contagion."[85]

In this context, doctors had to care for casualties of both crises, a dual responsibility that police officials quickly sought to exploit. Just after the June uprising, the prefect invoked an edict from the year 1666, as well as an ordinance from November 4, 1788, requiring that all health officials provide each patient's name, address, age, and occupation, and the circumstances of the injury. Information about wounded insurgents would be collected by the same officials responsible for the *bulletins du choléra*. Retroactive to June 4, the requests were obviously aimed at locating participants in the political unrest so that they might eventually be brought to trial based on the testimony of a medical professional. Clearly, the hygienists' practice of collecting information and detail had broadened administration officials' understanding of how to use power. Medical personnel, as well as their *techniques* of gathering facts, could be used as a source of knowledge about political agitators. The dual crises of cholera and revolution had created the environment that made such a conceptual link between medicine, power, and politics possible.

But whereas doctors seemed willing to provide data in the name of health and hygiene, they vigorously protested requests in matters of politics. As we saw in the previous chapter, doctors compared themselves to priests, and many decried the violation of doctor-patient privilege accusing the administration of exploiting doctors' services for political rather than medical ends. In the influential *Gazette des hôpitaux* a lead editorial entitled "Outrage against Medical Morality" condemned the new policy. Arguing that there was nothing wrong with information about the wounds themselves, the paper objected to the requirement that the *circumstances* of an injury be stated as part of the medical record.[86] The *Gazette médicale de Paris,* meanwhile, lashed out against "the ordinance that prescribes that doctors violate secrets" and asserted that no doctor would be willing to give up "the sole advantages that remain his: independence and dignity."[87] This sparring represented part of the ongoing struggle between medical professionals and the administration that we encountered in the earlier discussion of the *bureaux de secours.* In the eyes of many doctors, the prefect had pushed the fusion between politics and medicine too far.

Beyond the objective chronological and geographical links between the June uprising and the epidemic, then, contemporaries had assimilated each event into their understanding of the other. Frequently and not always consciously, for example, the vocabulary describing the events of early June invoked images of cholera symptoms. Writing of the tense buildup to Lamarque's funeral, for example, one observer explained that once the cry "To arms!" had been raised, "in an instant Paris *vomits* the entire torrent of its population onto the boulevards."[88] Meanwhile, *Le Bonhomme Richard*'s conservative editorial about the uprising discussed agitators in much the same way that the previous months' newspaper accounts had described the epidemic and the behavior of the lower classes. "They have thus shown the pistols and fists that they kept hidden; [they] spread themselves throughout several points in the capital and partook of the most grave excesses."[89] The *Gazette médicale de Paris* made the most explicit link of all; the depiction of the wounded being treated in Paris hospitals was a conscious imitation of the somber, ongoing cholera reports published in the *Moniteur* and other daily papers. "All of these wounded are gravely stricken," one article proclaimed. After describing a number of gruesome wounds it concluded that "the state of these patients is generally quite grave. Already a great number of deaths has been counted."[90] And, as we saw earlier, cholera overlapped with the events of June 5 and 6 in numerous spoofs of the daily mortality bulletins in the popular press.[91]

While ultimately arguing that no correlation could be established, the official government report for the epidemic nonetheless found it important to analyze the relationship. "The commission has carefully followed the march of cholera in the very areas that were the scene of the events of June 5 and 6," the reporter explained in the conclusion to the chapter that examined the role of living and working conditions in cholera mortality, "and at this time it did not observe any increase in cases or deaths from cholera in the buildings along the rue et du cloître St. Méry."[92] More specifically, the report sought to dispel the common wisdom that the fear, agitation, and fatigue caused by the political events had somehow encouraged cholera's recrudescence in late June by lowering the body's resistance:

> [The fighting of June 5 and 6] had absolutely no effect on the disease, whose activity had already been much reduced. [This can be explained] either because political commotions, generally of a passing nature, produce a terror less profound in people's minds than the presence of a terrible scourge . . . or else because in effect the horror that [the events] first inspired was subsequently diminished to the extent that people accustom themselves to danger.[93]

Even though political insurrection bred fear and panic (generally listed among the predisposing causes of the disease), the report implied that, as a fleeting and familiar phenomenon, urban unrest did not inspire the same fear as a mysterious plague. Revolution, they seemed to argue, could not cause cholera.

But could cholera cause revolution? Like most bourgeois observers, the report did not attempt to interpret the June uprising as a consequence of the epidemic that had been raging in the capital since late March. In fact, the report concluded that political unrest and the epidemic posed unrelated threats to the social order. Even when pointing to the "close alliance between the physical and the moral," the authors only probed the relationship between the impact of the insurrection on the later recrudescence, not mentioning that the misery and high mortality in the early part of the epidemic could have accounted for subsequent social discontent. Put another way, the official report, whose title promised a discussion "On the Progress and *Effects* of Cholera," took up the issue of urban unrest in a chapter about living and working conditions without addressing the possibility that the disease could have social and political ramifications. Officials' appraisal of the events ignored the needs and views of the lower classes; perhaps because the experts had come to define the disease so broadly in terms of Paris malade, the victims themselves had become symptoms of a far greater urban malady.

FROM ''BARBARIANS'' TO ''CITIZENS''

At first glance, it appears that by 1849 the links Parisians noted between disease and social unrest strongly resembled those of 1832. "The influence of great gatherings of men and political commotions on the progress of cholera is so well established," one doctor wrote, "that one wonders if it isn't possible to ask if its appearance in Europe, and its subsequent progress, might not have been slowed, and perhaps even prevented, without the state of anxiety and agitation in which the people of Europe find themselves for many years now." Pointing to the example of cholera's recrudescence after General Lamarque's funeral in 1832, the doctor argued that any public gathering could be a possible source of infection because of the overexcitement caused by heated political debate.[94] *L'Union* (formerly the Catholic *La Quotidienne*) attributed the increased mortality in mid-June 1849 to a sudden rise in temperature as well as to "the aftermath of revolutions that have frightened persons incapable of guarding themselves against the strong emotions that result from the scourge."[95] *Le Crédit*, meanwhile, wrote of "this triple infection in France," arguing that "misery" and "civil war" represented greater threats than the disease that had ravaged the capital.[96] Some commentators also saw the second epidemic as a consequence of the 1848 revolution. One pamphleteer, for example, found the parallels between 1830–32 and 1848–49 so obvious that the writer thought it possible "[to] predict a new epidemic for the next revolution."[97]

More often, however, bourgeois Parisians now tended to define the relationship between disease and revolt less literally than they had in 1832. "[The feeling in] Paris is one of disappointing tranquility, as if a formidable revolution had not just broken out in its midst," a lead article in *Le Courrier français* told readers in late March 1849.[98] The epidemic, which had begun two weeks earlier, had claimed approximately sixty victims per day until the middle of

May when deaths nearly quadrupled. Even so, Parisians of all classes greeted cholera's arrival with little of the drama that had accompanied it in 1832. Neither poison rumors nor descriptions of ragpickers reappeared with the mysterious disease, and the most salient images of class hatred seemed to have vanished along with the idea of Paris malade. Meanwhile, the revolutionary tradition appeared to have lost much credibility and force. The one brief moment when disease and revolt did overlap, in the insurrection of June 13, scarcely reenacted the "folklore of violence" from previous revolutionary events, while references linking cholera and 1848 were few and far between. And though occasional metaphors still juxtaposed cholera and urban unrest, they employed a new political rhetoric that sought to incorporate the lower classes in a way that would have been unimaginable just seventeen years before.[99]

A close look at one of the few iconographic images that remains from the 1849 epidemic provides a revealing overview of how attitudes had changed since the first outbreak (see figure 9). Entitled "Two Scourges of the Nineteenth Century: Socialism and Cholera," the lithograph shows cholera, represented by a skeleton, reading *Le Peuple*, a left-wing daily newspaper. With its arm around a sinister-looking figure that plays a bone for a flute, cholera holds a red flag bearing the words "Socialist Republic." Both figures sit upon a dead body, probably from the lower classes because the feet are bare. At the bottom of the picture various other corpses (some of them in National Guard uniforms and others dressed like aristocrats) lie scattered along with the fallen flag of the French Republic, broken Greek columns, and a small cross with two cloaked figures (presumably priests) suspended from it. An enormous guillotine overshadows the entire picture.

The *victims* set this image apart from anything that would have been produced during the first epidemic.[100] The lithograph's immediate symbolism indicates that cholera and socialism had conquered all of France—rich and poor, the Church and the republic—with the aid of revolution. In 1832 bourgeois perceptions had linked the less-fortunate so completely and persuasively with the inherently disease-ridden nature of Paris malade that the poor would never have been granted the privilege of languishing next to an aristocrat or member of the clergy. Put simply, the visceral understanding of disease in the first epidemic made it impossible for the image of a

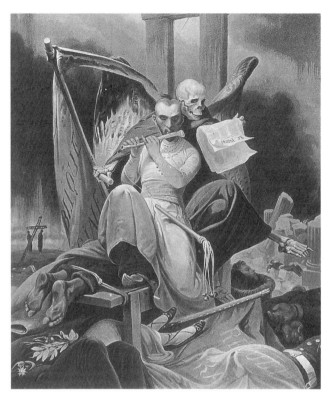

Figure 9. Horace Vernet, "Deux fléaux du XIXᵉ siècle: Le Socialisme et le choléra." Source: Cabinet des Estampes, no. A8126, Bibliothèque Nationale, Paris.

sympathetic lower-class victim to emerge with widespread credibility. Meanwhile, the revolutionary tradition had returned in an ambiguous form. The large guillotine dominating the picture was hardly a subtle depiction of the dangers of revolutionary excess. At the same time, however, the broken Greek columns, which invoke the dramatic art of the republic in 1789 and 1848, the victims from different classes, along with the damaged republican flag, suggest that revolutionary ideals had been thwarted as well. Finally, the central place of a popular newspaper, Pierre Joseph Proudhon's *Le Peuple*, underscores a double threat of a different nature from that of disease and revolt: socialism and the political left-wing press. Both represented *political* rather than visceral biological challenges to the prevailing order, threats that coincided with cholera but did not automatically merge inextricably with it to create an even more terrifying conception of disease and Paris malade.

In order to understand just how differently the cartoon depicted the connection between disease and revolution, it is worth examining the insurrection of June 13, the one moment in 1849 that inspired Parisians to explore the relationship.[101] Here, a political crisis prompted by President Louis Napoleon's unconstitutional decision to fight against Italian nationalists in Rome coincided almost exactly with the period of highest mortality from cholera. Nearly two months after the disease's arrival, just when left-wing deputies in the National Assembly called for a massive public demonstration to save the constitution and impeach the president because of "The Affair of Rome," the number of deaths jumped to levels seen in 1832, with nearly seven hundred on June 10 alone.[102] Three days later a large crowd of between six thousand and thirty thousand[103] marched toward the National Assembly, but shots of unknown origin sent groups scattering throughout the city, where they erected barricades and violently clashed with government troops. Like the riots associated with General Lamarque's funeral in 1832, the disturbances during the second epidemic focused on neighborhoods in the poorer, cholera-stricken sections of the city, with barricades and battles along the rue St. Denis, the rue St. Martin, and particularly the area around the Conservatoire des Arts et Métiers.[104] National Guardsmen rapidly put down the insurgents in most parts of the city, and officials declared the capital under a state of siege, suspending all left-wing newspapers. In the end, authorities arrested 450 citizens, all but 3 of them men and most not native Parisians. Analyzing the arrests as part of "our political history," *Le Journal du peuple* noted that this group (mostly between the ages of twenty-five and thirty-five) was older than participants in the 1830 revolution, the riot at Lamarque's funeral, or the revolution in February and June 1848. The paper, like much of the contemporary literature, pointed out that the insurgents included more professionals and fewer members of the lower classes than in previous events.[105]

Despite the fact that the June 13 insurrection coincided with a major increase in cholera deaths, few bourgeois Parisians commented on the geographical and chronological correlations between the disease and social unrest, which had been such a staple of discussions in 1832. The official report, which compared responses in both outbreaks, made no mention of the phenomenon at all, even though, as we saw earlier, the first study had at least explored the problem, even if ultimately to dismiss it.[106] No account of events that compared the two outbreaks mentioned anything about the ragpicker or poison riots. And despite the growing sympathies with the plight of the urban poor over the course of the 1840s, still no one thought to raise the possibility that cholera might inspire revolt.

When bourgeois Parisians did discuss the relationship between the epidemic and the events of June 13, they most often presented the situation as a simple product of political provocation to which cholera formed only the backdrop. The virtual disappearance of *Paris malade* marked a shift from seeing urban social relations as the product of uncontrollable biological forces to a view that placed greater emphasis on politics and the bourgeois belief in humans' power to shape outcomes. Even when discussing "the social sickness," the pro-government press attacked a political ideology rather than a threatening malady somehow intrinsic to the urban environment. "In vain, state pundits [*philosophes d'Etat*], doctors in politics, want to provide a cure for this miserable condition," the editors of the conservative *Journal du peuple* proclaimed at the height of the second epidemic on June 9. "The wisdom of their consultations has triumphed over our fears more and more each day. All the same, we still succumb to the influence of the revolutionary scourge."[107] A political conception of the relationship between disease and revolt also emerged in metaphors that used images of urban pathology to critique society. "Finally, are we not certain to perish sooner or later from this evil that reddens us [with socialism] and that we have endured until now [as ones who are] perpetually stricken?" *Le Courrier français* asked. The editors even went so far as to proclaim that "June 13 proved that society has nothing to fear from the savage passions and mad doctrines that declare war on it."[108]

The rhetoric inspired by the June 13 insurrection indicated that, like *Paris malade*, the idea of a revolutionary tradition had lost its charge. To be sure, the uprising stimulated the use of the characteristic revolutionary images and slogans from 1789, 1830, and 1848, such as when left-wing opponents of the government referred to themselves as "the Mountain" or when agitators tried to excite the crowds with the cry "To Arms!" But, for the most part, the event never captured revolutionary passions. From one end of the political spectrum to the other, the events of June 13 emerged as an embarrassing mediocrity, a fact that influenced prevailing views of cholera and the Parisian revolutionary tradition as a whole. Karl Marx termed the insurrection "a caricature, as laughable as it was futile, of June 1848."[109] Meanwhile, echoing Marx with a touch of Tocquevillian snobbery, a pro-government paper lamented the prevalence of "very mediocre intelligences" and compared 1849 unfavorably with past experience. "When Mirabeau, Danton, [and] Robespierre made revolutions, it was a science, talent, the work of intelligence that they brought with them," the paper complained, whereas "this time the revolution was made by democratic talent against incapacity [and] aristocratic Cretinism."[110] Editors of a somewhat less conservative paper, *Le Courrier français,* responded to the insurrection by declaring, "Enough already! This game of revolutions is beginning to dishonor our country as much as it ruins us."[111] Unlike critics in 1832, who condemned the revolution of 1830 for its outcome, those in 1849 denounced the revolutionary experience itself, an experience that most bourgeois were more eager than ever to put behind them.

In many cases, bourgeois Parisians saw socialism, a political ideology that directly challenged their raison d'être, as presenting a far greater danger than the dread disease. Not only had the fiasco of the National Workshops in 1848 discredited the idealism of the left, but the bloody June Days had linked it inextricably with violence and chaos. Now, the socialists had replaced the reactionary Carlists as the enemies of public order, a fact mirrored by the connections drawn between cholera and politics in the popular press. Linking the decline in mortality and controls placed on the socialist press after the June 13 insurrection, for example, two papers concluded that "the sanitary and moral state of Paris has improved in a noticeable manner. Thus there are grounds for hoping that the two scourges that afflict us at the same time will soon disappear completely, the one taking the other with it."[112] Papers such as *Le Corsaire* glibly defined the disease as "socialism put into action," while *Le Journal du peuple* referred to the left-wing opposition as "social cholera," an illness described throughout the bourgeois press as having symptoms, mortality, and cures.[113] "We dream of remedies that could still fight, with efficiency, the social cholera that devours us and that in our eyes is a thousand times more dangerous than the

Asiatic plague," the editors of the conservative paper characteristically told readers in a diatribe against socialism.[114] Following elections in May 1849 that had polarized French politics, a popular joke circulated in the salons of Paris in which a moderate republican tries to curry favor with a wealthy woman by saying that, truth be told, he could compare the invasion of socialism only with that of cholera. "Oh, Monsieur, what are you saying!" the woman exclaims, catching the republican off balance and prompting him to ask why she fails to share his opinion. "I find that you insult cholera!" she replies.[115] Obviously, the metaphors and jokes had resonance because left-wing agitation had become a more conspicuous threat since the 1848 revolution. At the same time, however, this coupling of socialism and cholera suggested that Parisians now saw politics itself as a more potent force than it had been in 1832.

As further proof that politics posed a greater threat than disease, several observers in 1849 actually believed the epidemic to be an antidote to revolution. "I never would have thought that cholera could be good for something and that it could save us from a day of disorder," the Austrian cultural attaché wrote in his diary as tensions mounted toward the June 13 insurrection. "The faubourgs Saint-Antoine, Saint-Denis, Saint-Marceau are so decimated that all the preoccupations of the populace are turned in this direction."[116] Describing reactions in the twelfth arrondissement, a rapidly growing lower-class neighborhood with considerable cholera mortality in 1849, one observer wrote of workers' resistance to political prodding. "Today the reds wanted to stir things up; the workers, dreading cholera, don't want to budge."[117] One paper went so far as to suggest divine intervention. "Battered spirits no longer find the motivation to respond to revolutionary excitations," *L'Opinion publique* noted in a lead editorial, "and the plague, this scourge of God, has become a preservative against this other scourge called civil war."[118] Seen through the eyes of conservatives, the disease represented a possible cure for socialism and urban unrest, a marked contrast with 1832, when bourgeois Parisians had feared the disease as the epitome of the depravity intrinsic to their city. Revolution, a product of human activity, now posed the greatest threat.

Analyses that no longer interpreted cholera through the lens of Paris malade also revealed that the enmity of bourgeois Parisians had softened. Despite the fact that mortality figures showed that the less-fortunate still died in far greater numbers, accounts of how they had used sound and reasoned judgment to resist political agitators had replaced discussions of predisposition, responsibility, and suspect behavior.[119] For example, even the most conservative accounts presented the workers as somehow knowing that revolution was not in their better interest. As one Catholic paper catering to the lower classes put it, "A terrifying memory of the bloody June days [in 1848]" had combined with "the somber and mournful preoccupation with cholera," prompting one worker to climb to the top of a barricade and proclaim, "Civil war has never been good for the worker."[120] Meanwhile, the bourgeois paper, *Le Journal des débats*, one of the fiercest critics of lower-class behavior during the first epidemic, reported that "the large population . . . remained peaceful and calm," and speculated that "this attitude no doubt foiled the plans of the agitators, who, as in June [1848], counted on pushing [the population] to the most deplorable extremes."[121] When writing of "this cool, reflective attitude of the people," *La Bonne Foi* had come a long way from descriptions of "the voice of the people that had spoken . . . through iron, through blows, through abuse, through murder, through blood, through all forms of anger and violation."[122]

Not only did bourgeois rhetoric applaud lower-class restraint, but it also suggested that these unfortunates might one day learn good values themselves. "The people," Louis François Lélut wrote in a report to the Academy of Moral and Political Sciences in 1849, "is the part of the nation that calls out most urgently for the concern of the State; it is [that part] that owns the least, knows the least, must be gradually encouraged [*menée*] to possess, to know [*savoir*], and, through this, to want more." Moreover, according to Lélut, the state should assume a greater role in the process.[123] While few bourgeois had embraced the less-fortunate residents of the capital as true social, economic, or political equals, they now employed a more inclusive, if often condescending rhetoric that claimed to speak in their interest. Trying to dissuade the workers from answering the call to revolt in what would become the June 13 insurrection, for example, *Le Corsaire* pointed to what it considered to be the more serious matters of foreign affairs and the presence of cholera in the capital, and finally appealed to them on financial grounds: "Parisians! Think about it seriously; it concerns the treasures of your marvelous city. Every barricade mounted in your streets costs you a million. Every attempt at insurrection strikes at the heart of your commerce, once the most flourishing in Europe."[124] Such an appeal to economic interests and investment invited the less-fortunate to follow in the footsteps of —by implication—their powerful and successful bourgeois betters. It would have been virtually unthinkable for the self-respecting bourgeois in 1832 to have either the confidence or the inclination to make such an appeal to the barbarians they had perceived before them. So while articles printed about the poor in 1832 revealed a certain voyeuristic fascination that focused on brutal differences, those in 1849 spoke more to similarities inherent in a universalizing bourgeois message. Put simply, the rhetoric that described the lower classes in 1849 revealed a surprising optimism about the possibilities of change.

The new relationship between the haves and the have-nots emerged with particular clarity in the pages of the expanding popular press. The existence of papers such as *La Bonne Foi* revealed that the lower classes now enjoyed an acknowledged, if not strictly egalitarian, place in the changing field of political participation. No longer banished to the margins or viewed as a mysterious menace to the Parisian environment, the lower classes were now courted by a popular press that had expanded remarkably in numbers and diversity as well as in circulation and influence.[125] Since the revolution of 1848, and especially after June 13, when new censorship laws took most of the opposition press out of circulation, a considerable number of small publications flourished under government protection in the capital. Papers with titles such as *Good Faith: Journal of Popular Interests, The Journal of the People: Moral and Material Improvement in the Condition of the Popular Classes*, and *Political Opinion* all carried features and editorials designed to capture working-class attention with a powerful blend of conservative politics and grass-roots Catholicism. In addition to circumventing the popularity of socialism, the small papers also represented an open admission that the lower classes constituted a visible and viable political force that could be tamed or even used.

The small papers and their content reflected new attitudes toward poverty and the poor that had been emerging over the course of the July Monarchy. Realizing that the problems associated with industrialization and immigration were not likely to disappear and that the socialists sought to profit from the alienation of the growing numbers of poor, concerned officials were coming to understand that not everyone had the financial or physical resources to answer Guizot's famous invitation, to "get rich." One doctor, a contributor to the Abbé Migne's massive theological encyclopedia, articulated the problem with particular clarity. Writing of the *instructions populaires* issued during the 1849 epidemic, he described the poor as victims of circumstance. "One cannot help but be moved with compassion," he explained, "for the popular classes without fortune and for the worker without work who, despite the best intentions that they can muster to make these beneficial instructions profitable, are more or less blocked by *a multitude of circumstances not within their control.*" In the years since the first epidemic, perceptions of the lower classes had changed in such a way as to give the doctor the insight to understand a certain hypocrisy inherent in measures such as the *instructions populaires* for fighting cholera, prompting him to ask, "Can the pauper destroy walls and partitions to air out his apartment, he who has but a small, narrow room? Can he defend himself against dampness when rain leaks through the roof? Can he dress warmly when he has but rags to cover his nudity?" The doctor answered his own questions with a definitive "No, and it is because he is not able." Such an observation would not have been possible in 1832, when most everyone accused the lower classes of refusing to follow health measures out of ignorance and even spite.[126]

This new understanding of the poor in turn had implications for how medical professionals, administrators, and journalists understood and presented the epidemic reality in 1849. In an article entitled "The Influence of Narrow Streets on the Development of the Epidemic," editors of the *Gazette des hôpitaux* argued that streets should be widened not so much as a precaution against cholera but to make working-class districts more faithfully resemble airy bourgeois neighborhoods.[127] Writing after the 1849 outbreak, a group of doctors saw the problem quite pragmatically. "It is up to society to defend itself," they noted. It "must demonstrate to the suffering classes that men of order and reason can effectively combat misery . . . only gradually and with perseverance, without which nothing great, useful, or viable has a base." They called for organizing and attaching morality to public assistance, explaining that "by diminishing misery, one reduces unrest."[128] Or, put another way, the environmentalist explanation for cholera had received a human face.

Implicit in this new environmentalism was a more nuanced understanding of cholera's relationship to different social classes. As we have seen, the *instructions populaires* issued for the second epidemic urged that "all individuals, regardless of their social position," should take precautionary measures.[129] When discussing different mortality rates for different days of the week (a veiled reference to working-class intemperance, which was notorious on Sundays and Mondays), the *Rapport sur les épidémies cholériques de 1832 et de 1849* almost blatantly disagreed with the class bias of its counterpart for 1832. "We do not share the same opinion in this regard," the authors stated, blaming the discrepancy on the hospitals' policy of recording weekend admissions during the early part of the week.[130] Unlike the case in 1832, accounts by doctors, the mainstream press, and government officials suggested that lower classes did not *cause* cholera but were merely likely victims.[131]

—◊◊◊—

The most striking part of the 1832 cholera epidemic for Louis Canler, a former police official, was the social unrest. In one story he described a *chiffonnier* who accused a man of trying to poison him by paying him with throat lozenges instead of cash.[132] Canler's blending of the two sets of April riots (and without mentioning Lamarque's funeral) into his cholera tableau reveals how the uprisings had become intertwined with one another, and how both merged with memories of cholera itself. While the discussions of the *tombereaux,* the *chiffonniers*, and the poison riots epitomized the most disturbing issues raised by the unprecedented arrival of the epidemic, they also made the event even more terrifying. In reality, both cholera and angry mobs randomly took the lives of innocent victims. More than the thousands of ugly deaths from the disease itself, however, the few grisly murders of suspected poisoners captured the public imagination, as the butchering of a few came to represent a complete collapse of human rationality and social order. For a brief moment, description, exposure, vulgarity, and outrage merged as a single act of collective defiance; the tormented body of the suspected poisoner itself became the physical symbol, the *personification* of cholera, as well as a threat to the wavering boundaries between the worlds of the haves and the have-nots, health and unhealth, civilization and barbarism, disease and revolt. For the bourgeois reading the accounts in the papers, popular justice became synonymous with danger as it emerged in the double-edged sword of brutality and disease. At the most basic level the brutality of detail could be lost on no one who witnessed garbage carts and human bodies quite literally torn apart.

Even though the uprising that accompanied General Lamarque's funeral seemed to be played out under vastly different circumstances from the earlier unrest of the 1832 epidemic, responses to the April and June riots revealed that Parisians located all of these uprisings within the context of a particularly close association between disease and revolt. Whether viewing events through the lens of Paris malade or whether creating an interpretive framework by piecing together chronological and geographical correlations, medical professionals, administrators, and journalists in 1832 sought connections because they *believed* them to exist. Such preconceptions would shape not only how they perceived the disease but also how they told the epidemic story. Widely circulated and publicized through medical reports, circulars, and articles in the professional and popular press, the symbiosis between cholera and social unrest seemed virtually complete in the understanding of the epidemic reality in 1832. In just seventeen years, however, the two concepts had begun to follow separate cultural and political trajectories that would greatly influence responses when cholera returned.

Interpretations of the relationship between social unrest and epidemics in 1832, then, revealed the interplay between two seemingly contradictory sets of concerns for bourgeois Parisians. On the one hand, there existed a fear of lower-class unrest, a fear grounded in the recent experience of the great revolution of 1789 and its bloody aftermath in the Terror of 1793–94. Here, the urban poor threatened the bourgeois social order through their role as participants, as actors who could be manipulated by other human actors. On the other hand, the outbreak of cholera introduced an element of greater unpredictability into the Paris environment, for it represented a mysterious crisis over which no human could have control. The ragpickers' terrifying transgression of so many boundaries and the shredded bodies of suspected poisoners gave this unpredictability a human form. Combined, the political threat of lower-class violence and the biological menace of a mysterious disease reinforced one another, ultimately contributing to a conception of urban social relations in which the nature of the violence was both familiar and new. In the spring of 1832, just as cholera had absorbed the revolutionary tradition, so too the tradition had absorbed the disease.

By 1849, however, the strands of disease and revolution had been disentangled so completely that just months after the terrifying spectacle of class warfare in the bloody June days bourgeois Parisians applauded the reason of workers and introduced a rhetoric of compassion. When rioters took to the streets using familiar revolutionary images and slogans, few observers thought to draw comparisons with cholera. Rather, contemporaries likened the disease to socialism. While events in 1848 suggested to bourgeois Parisians that this growing doctrine of the left posed a fundamental threat to them and their values, their fears were grounded primarily in political and social anxieties rather than in the visceral biological ones that had shaped their reactions just seventeen years before. Articulating new views of the urban poor, bourgeois Parisians had also reformulated their impressions of cholera.

Conclusion

As we have seen, the explanation for the "silence of 1849"—the more restrained, less hysterical approach to the second epidemic— is not a simple one. The differing responses to each cholera epidemic must be understood in relation to a distinct dynamic between revolution and bourgeois identity in 1832 and 1849. During the first outbreak, revolution and urban social unrest caused greater anxiety among bourgeois Parisians. The regime that claimed to speak in their interest had come to power only two years earlier amidst much doubt and uncertainty. The early years of its rule had been riddled with conflict both between classes and among various segments of the middle classes themselves. And even though 1789 had ushered in an era of bourgeois rule, the return of revolution in 1830 provided a mixed message, for it reminded bourgeois Parisians just how precarious their newly secured power might be. Thus, when cholera arrived in the spring of 1832 bourgeois Parisians saw it not just as an inexplicable natural disaster but also as a crisis inherently bound up with the general malaise that many felt toward the Paris environment and its growing legions of poor.

Such anxieties reinforced one another in all genres of literature dealing with cholera, from assertions in medical treatises to accounts in the popular press. By presenting the outbreak as a product of environmental conditions in 1832, for example, the anticontagionists made it more possible for the bourgeois Parisian to draw links between disease and revolt. Now, virtually anything undesirable could be considered a part of Paris malade. Combined with the realization of the dangers inherent in rapid urbanization, the capital's formidable revolutionary tradition set the stage for heightened fears that further expanded the nonmedical definition of disease. While much of cholera's potency came from its novelty in 1832, the fact that it arrived in a city already agitated by revolutionary turmoil made it even more threatening. The violent precedents in 1789, 1793, and 1830, for example, enabled middle-class Parisians to interpret the poison riots so closely tied with the first outbreak as a similar challenge to the social order. Catholic depictions of the capital prior to 1832 as the city of revolution, vice, and impiety also contributed to an expanded view of cholera in which disease and politics became intertwined to create a single great urban malady.

By 1849 bourgeois Parisians no longer drew such close rhetorical links between disease and revolt. Though they may have continued to feel some uneasiness in the aftermath of the 1848 revolution, several factors contributed to the demystification of cholera for them. Forces that would help change attitudes toward the lower classes had been gathering through much of the July Monarchy. A Catholic religious revival and the rise of socialism had created a climate in which it became politically advantageous to appeal to the lower classes with a more conciliatory rhetoric. In 1832, descriptions of barbarians and Paris malade were widely equated with the dangers of cholera, but in 1849 these same lower classes became objects of pity, as urban investigators, religious leaders, and social commentators began addressing the "social question." Having experienced socialism's powerful appeal to the workers in 1848, prudent bourgeois understood that it made more sense to include the very people they had dismissed just seventeen years earlier. Whether or not they truly believed the portrait, they painted the lower-class population as cowering in the face of disease and far too reasonable to resist government initiatives. The depiction of the potentially dangerous classes as solid, hardworking people served as a rhetorical strategy for defusing the tensions that had reached a peak with the overthrow of the July Monarchy in the spring and summer of 1848. Meanwhile, a revived Catholicism provided an alternative rhetoric for appealing to the poor; after 1848 not only did the Church pose a smaller institutional threat to the Parisian bourgeoisie than it had in 1832, but it also provided a less menacing alternative than the open and hostile provocations of socialism. Cholera could then become an ally against socialism as bourgeois Parisians sought a different method for preventing revolt.

This new strategy for approaching the less-fortunate Parisians in turn influenced perceptions of cholera. Once the rhetoric describing the poor as barbarians had been replaced by one of conciliation, the strands of disease and revolution could no longer be so tightly interwoven. Disentangled from Paris malade and urban poverty, cholera in 1849 took on a narrower meaning devoid of its earlier social charge. While the disease still presented an immediate crisis, it had been demystified as something no longer intricately tied in with a broader set of more terrifying images from the Paris environment.

The silence of 1849 can also be explained by a more developed sense of shared identity among bourgeois Parisians. The growing influence of bourgeois values played an important part in shaping how contemporaries saw the disease, largely because of the prominent role played by members of the middle classes in the professions most actively engaged in fighting it. The medical professionals, administrators, and journalists who each played a key role in shaping perceptions of both epidemics only fully came of age during the 1830s and 1840s. In 1832 these groups, like the bourgeoisie as a whole, had been very much on the defensive as they fought for professional recognition and respect. Doctors and—to a lesser extent—journalists waged their major battles for professional status during the 1840s. The greater sense of identity that resulted from these consolidations made cholera's messengers less likely to engage in the kinds of conflicts that hampered their collaboration during the first epidemic. By 1849 they could afford to present a more unified front in the face of cholera, even though they knew little more about the disease than they had seventeen years earlier.

The greater sense of confidence and cohesion that emerged after the economic, political, and social consolidation of the Parisian bourgeoisie helps explain how perceptions of cholera had changed so dramatically over such a relatively short period of time. As a class on the defensive in 1832, bourgeois Parisians saw the disease and the accompanying social unrest as direct threats to their position, thus making it advantageous for them to use cholera to define themselves in contrast to its victims. By 1849 bourgeois identity had solidified, giving the Parisians who responded to the epidemic a greater sense of who they were and what role they should play during the crisis. While in 1832 they protected themselves by using cholera to show differences with the working classes, in 1849 cholera did not need to serve as a means of creating distance between the haves and the have-nots because bourgeois Parisians seemed less preoccupied with fears that they would be pulled into the ranks of the less fortunate. Put another way, by the time of the second outbreak the Parisian middle classes could afford to define themselves in terms of who they *were* rather than in terms of who they were not.

Such confidence had an important impact upon how bourgeois Parisians saw and treated the poor during the second epidemic, a fact that no doubt contributed to the "silence" of the lower classes themselves. By appeasing their enemies with promises of universal male suffrage and a rhetoric of greater compassion, the men who ruled the capital after 1848 hoped to head off future revolt. More than spontaneous uprisings, they feared that the socialists might soon regain their influence over the hearts and minds of the Parisian workers. A greater sense of bourgeois confidence also made Catholicism appear less threatening than it had been in 1832. The decline of the right-wing Carlists as a political threat made the Church more palatable to some bourgeois. In fact, the Church had become a formidable ally. To combat socialism and cholera, for example, bourgeois Parisians appealed to the lower classes with a rhetoric inspired by Catholicism within the pages of a growing genre of newspapers that spoke more directly to them.

Just as medical professionals, administrators, and journalists influenced perceptions of cholera and the lower classes, so too the epidemics strengthened a sense of bourgeois identity. First, the crises called for far greater involvement of health and administration officials—members of the middle classes—in the exercise of state power. While examples of cooperation between doctors and the administration had been evident previously in Paris, events in 1832 provided a unique catalyst for an even more extensive form of collaboration at a time when both medical knowledge and administrative efficiency had made unprecedented advances. By creating crises that affected the health of the city's population, cholera made the services of doctors, police officers, and bureaucrats indispensable in a way they never had been before. The press, meanwhile, served as an increasingly important vehicle for presenting the information that these groups sought to convey.

Second, cholera also contributed to the creation of an urban bourgeois identity by helping reformulate ideas of public and private. In the eighteenth century the wealthy led public lives in the ritualized existence of the royal court, while in the nineteenth century, thanks in part to the investigations of the hygienists, the lower classes became the objects of public scrutiny. With the new visibility of the poor, the bourgeois sought to become invisible both as charitable donors (giving anonymously) and as cholera victims (protesting their names being listed in mortality statistics). As bourgeois sources such as the hygienists and newspapers made the lives of the poor increasingly part of public discourse, privacy became desirable. Moreover, the penetration of urban space through inquiry and policies such as collecting garbage with smaller carts, turned urban space inside out; while the belief in contagion had closed the world in on itself, the bourgeois approach opened it up, with light becoming synonymous with knowledge, and darkness with disease. In order for urban space to become safe from cholera, public and private had to be redefined so that the lives of the lower classes, representing a prime cause of infection, could become more visible. Unlike the aristocrats of the previous centuries, nineteenth-century bourgeois Parisians believed that seeing took precedence over being seen. From another perspective, the bourgeois were obsessed with what was hidden, a fact that would influence how they defined "health" and its relationship to their sense of well-being throughout the rest of the century. When investigators explored the darkest corners of Paris, they understood that disease needed to be unmasked, brought into the open.

Within France, the 1832 and 1849 epidemics had a distinctive French, even Parisian, flavor. The country's revolutionary tradition, along with the unique relationship between socialism and Catholicism set Parisian responses to cholera apart from those elsewhere in Europe and North America. Rumors of body snatchers in London and the disturbing riots against suspected poisoners in places as diverse as Germany, Italy, and Russia never equated cholera with revolution, even at the height of panic in 1832. And even in the aftermath of 1848, when other European cities had followed Paris into revolution, only officials in the French capital responded to cholera as heirs of an increasingly well-defined and evolving revolutionary tradition; fears that the less-fortunate might be co-opted by a distinct brand of French socialism, for example, inspired bourgeois Parisians to employ the kind of conciliatory rhetoric that might build key bridges between the haves and the have-nots. Ironically, however, the revolutionary tradition that inspired so much fear had also brought bourgeois Parisians to power and helped them to maintain it. Because of 1789 and its aftermath, bourgeois Parisians were the only European elites to greet cholera as a class that was simultaneously on the defensive and on the offensive.

Although France did not suffer disproportionately when the first great cholera pandemics swept through Europe and North America during the 1830s and 1840s, the French experience would have international repercussions. Because of the Paris medical school's prominence in the first half of the nineteenth century, France played an unusually large role in determining how cholera was seen and defined elsewhere. Ideas about contagion, predisposition, class-specificity, and milieu had all been articulated by French medical professionals and provided a blueprint for how others responded to the disease. In 1849, for example, the city of New York paid a significant sum to translate and publish the definitive *Rapport sur la marche et les effets du choléra-morbus* (1832). "It is only by a perusal of the Report itself," the translation's preface explained, "that we can learn to do justice to the patient industry, close research, varied science, and clear judgement manifested in the execution of an arduous, disagreeable, but necessary duty, the ultimate effect of which cannot but prove highly beneficial to suffering humanity."[1] Such an ambitious translation revealed the perceived importance of the Parisian medical profession for understanding cholera. At the same time, it demonstrated the process by which the techniques of the hygienists were transported beyond French borders to influence approaches to the disease.

Exploring the Parisian experience of the 1832 and 1849 cholera epidemics has some intriguing broader implications that I hope will be taken up by future scholars. First, in order to understand it in all its complexity, bourgeois identity must be examined as something fluid, as a constant process of changes and responses to them. Politics, social position, and economic status tell only part of the story. Analyzing values and ideas during a crisis such as a cholera epidemic provides not just another perspective or privileged moment for understanding raw emotions but also a different methodology for approaching an older historical problem of class-identity formation. A simple definition of terms such as *bourgeois* or *middle class* has been evasive in large part because we have shied away from making complexity, contradiction, and ambiguity *the* central characteristics of how we understand the bourgeois's simultaneous quest toward the universal and the individual.

Second, the cultural dimension of the history of medicine can teach us much about how a given society perceives itself, not just in relation to attitudes toward health and disease but also in relation to issues that may appear to have little to do with medicine at all. The interweaving of cholera and revolution suggests that medical ideas played a crucial and complex role in shaping political ideas and the dynamics of urban social relations. In other words, medicine need not always be a separate field of study and analysis. It might even provide an entirely new perspective on older issues such as the rise of absolutism, the development of a national identity, and, of course, the formation of class consciousness.

Third, and finally, this study raises the obvious questions of what—if anything—cholera in nineteenth-century Paris can teach us about our relationship to epidemics today. It seems inadequate, almost hollow, to recount mechanically the ways twentieth-century encounters with AIDS or Ebola do or do not repeat the experience of people who lived before, particularly since this is a matter open to considerable individual interpretation based on particular social and cultural contexts. But universal issues such as scapegoating, denial, fear, and the fervent desire to take stock of the most fundamental social values remind us that the lessons of the past raise valid and disturbing questions, questions that will haunt every future study of epidemic disease.

Notes

AA   Archives de l'Archevêché de Paris
AAP   Archives de l'Assistance Publique
ADS   Archives du Département de la Seine et de la Ville de Paris
AN   Archives Nationales
APP   Archives de la Préfecture de Police

INTRODUCTION: THE "SILENCE OF 1849"

1. F. L. Poumiès de la Siboutie, *Souvenirs d'un médecin de Paris* (Paris, 1910), 237–38.

2. The actual death is brought on by heart and kidney failure resulting from a depletion of vital chemicals and electrolytes that accompanies dehydration. Richard J. Evans, *Death in Hamburg: Society and Politics in the Cholera Years, 1830–1910* (London, 1990), 227.

3. Administration Générale de l'Assistance Publique, *Rapport sur les épidémies cholériques de 1832 et 1849* (Paris, 1850), 152 (hereafter referred to by its title). The report cites this figure, as do most other official sources. Chevalier suggests, however, that the number of deaths may have been higher because of inaccuracies in government statistics. See "Paris," in Louis Chevalier, ed., *Le Choléra: La Première Epidémie du XIXe siècle* (La Roche-sur-Yon, 1958), 4, 10.

4. There has been almost no secondary scholarship on the 1849 epidemic in Paris, with the exception of B. Bezine, "Le Choléra à Paris de 1849" (thesis, Faculté de Médecine, Paris, 1921). Written by a medical student, this work focused on modes of transmission and epidemiology.

5. Figures compiled from the indexes of the *Moniteur universel,* 1829–66.

6. My research indicates that *L'Ami de la religion* published 115 articles on cholera in 1832 and 26 in 1849. Impressionistic evidence from other Parisian newspapers of the time suggests comparable discrepancies.

7. The story of the street's original name had an aura of mystery, thus giving rise to several variations, all of which attempted to correct the popular association between the street and death by invoking the name's more "credible" origins. "Contrary to what many believe," one of the city's earliest dictionaries claimed, "its name comes not from the number of murders committed there, but from a family of bourgeois named Mortelier who once

lived there." *Dictionnaire historique de la ville de Paris* (1830), Bibliothèque Historique de la Ville de Paris, ms. 42.

8. *Bulletin municipal officiel de la ville de Paris*, 7 June 1958, 1100.

9. The epidemic killed fifty-three people per thousand on the rue de la Mortellerie compared with seven per thousand on the rue des Champs-Elysées. See Lucien Lambeau, "La Rue de l'Hôtel de Ville: Ancienne rue de la Mortellerie," *La Cité* (June 1924): 28–37.

10. ADS Collection Lazare, D1 Z, 1085–87; Jean Deville, *Histoire médicale du choléra-morbus dans le quartier de l'Hôtel de Ville* (Paris, 1833), 18; Jean Deville, *Compte-rendu des travaux de la Commission centrale de salubrité du quartier de l'Hôtel de Ville depuis son installation jusqu'à l'invasion du choléra-morbus et depuis cette époque jusqu'au 30 août 1832* (Paris, 1832), 20, 32; Georges Hartmann, "Les ravages du choléra dans le quartier de l'Hôtel de Ville en 1832," *La Cité* (January 1933): 293–96. For a discussion of the significance of Parisian street names as a literary trope in the nineteenth century, see Priscilla Parkhurst Ferguson, *Paris as Revolution: Writing the Nineteenth-Century City* (Berkeley and Los Angeles, 1994), 11–35.

11. Chevalier, *Le Choléra*, 13.

12. *Le Courrier français*, 5 April 1832, 1.

13. Figures cited in Gordon Wright, *France in Modern Times*, 4th ed. (New York, 1987), 134. It has proved remarkably difficult to find agreement on these figures. I thank Mark Traugott for a valuable detailed discussion that ultimately led me back to Wright.

14. Unfortunately, it has been virtually impossible to find sources that represent anything but the point of view of the upper classes. Problems of literacy, along with the fact that often members of the working classes had neither the time nor the space to leave written records, make it hard to know exactly how the majority of the Paris population thought about the epidemics. In a few cases it has been possible to use smoke and mirrors to read popular attitudes through bourgeois texts, but this approach invariably raises questions about authenticity and interpretation.

15. Ange-Pierre Leca, *Et le choléra s'abattit sur Paris, 1832* (Paris, 1982).

16. George David Sussman, "From Yellow Fever to Cholera: A Study of French Government Policy, Medical Professionalism, and Popular Movements in the Epidemic Crises of the Restoration and the July Monarchy" (Ph.D. diss., Yale University, 1971); William Coleman, *Death Is a Social Disease: Public Health and Political Economy in Early-Industrial France* (Madison, 1982); Jacques Piquemal, "Le Choléra en France et la pensée médicale" (thesis, Institut de l'Histoire des Sciences et Technologies, Université de Paris, 1959); Robert Pollitzer, *Cholera* (Geneva, 1959); Jacques Sellier, "Le Choléra à Paris au XIXe siècle: Essai de topographie biologique" (thesis, Académie de Médecine de Paris, 1979).

17. Louis Chevalier, *Laboring Classes and Dangerous Classes in Paris during the First Half of the Nineteenth Century*, trans. Frank Jellinek (Princeton, 1973), 344–49; Chevalier, *Le Choléra*, 3–10; S. H. Preston, "Urban French Mortality

in the Nineteenth Century," *Population Studies* (Great Britain) 32, no. 2 (1978): 275–98.

18. This list is by no means exhaustive. By far the best source is Chantal Beauchamp, *Délivrez-nous du mal!: Epidémies, endémies, médecine et hygiène au XIXe siècle dans l'Indre, l'Indre-et-Loire et le Loir-et-Cher* (Maulevrier, 1990), which investigates cholera and other nineteenth-century diseases through a cultural and intellectual study of elite and popular attitudes in the provinces; on cholera, see esp. 83–143. (I thank Jean-Pierre Peter for this reference.) See also Catherine Rollet and Agnès Sauriac, "Epidémies et mentalités: Le Choléra de 1832 en Seine-et-Oise," *Annales: Economies, sociétés, civilisations* 29, no. 4 (July/August 1974), 935–66. Also, Chevalier, *Le Choléra,* contains an uneven collection of articles dealing with the epidemic in other major French cities.

19. Patrice Bourdelais and Jean-Yves Raulot, *Une Peur bleue: Histoire du choléra en France, 1832–1854* (Paris, 1987). I found Bourdelais's thesis, which served as the basis of the book, to be more focused and engaging: "Le Choléra en France, 1832 et 1854: Essai d'épistémologie historique" (thesis, Ecole des Hautes Etudes en Sciences Sociales, Paris, 1979).

20. Sussman, "From Yellow Fever to Cholera."

21. Chevalier, *Le Choléra,* 12.

22. François Delaporte, *Disease and Civilization: The Cholera in Paris, 1832,* trans. Arthur Goldhammer (Cambridge, 1986).

23. Ibid., 61.

24. In addition to reading his books and interviews, I had the opportunity to discuss my research with M. Foucault the year I was beginning serious work on my dissertation. Just before his death, he taught a small seminar at the University of California, Berkeley. I am grateful to him for his early support of my work and for the many casual insights that have no doubt found their way into the more significant pages of this book.

25. Michel Foucault, "The Politics of Health in the Eighteenth Century," in *Power/Knowledge: Selected Interviews and Other Writings, 1972–1977,* ed. and trans. Colin Gordon et al. (New York, 1980), 166–82; Michel Foucault, *The History of Sexuality,* vol. 1: *An Introduction,* trans. Robert Hurley (New York, 1980); Michel Foucault, *The Birth of the Clinic: An Archaeology of Medical Perception,* trans. A. M. Sheridan Smith (New York, 1973).

26. Michel Foucault, *Discipline and Punish: The Birth of the Prison,* trans. Alan Sheridan (New York, 1977); Foucault, *History of Sexuality.*

27. Foucault, *History of Sexuality,* 92–102.

28. My discussion is inspired by Lynn Hunt's introduction to the volume she edited, *The New Cultural History* (Berkeley and Los Angeles, 1988), as well as by exchanges with my fellow graduate students at the University of California, Berkeley, and more recently with colleagues at the University of California, Davis.

29. The breakthrough works were the following: Foucault, *History of Sexuality;* Joan Wallach Scott, "Gender: A Useful Category of Historical

Analysis," in her *Gender and the Politics of History* (New York, 1988), 28–50;
Edward W. Said, *Orientalism* (New York, 1978).

30. Beauchamp, *Délivrez-nous du mal*, 13.

31. *Rapport sur les épidémies cholériques*, 162.

32. C. P. Tacheron, *Statistique médicale de la mortalité du choléra-morbus dans le 11ᵉ arrondissement de Paris* (Paris, 1832), 51.

33. *Gazette médicale de Paris*, no. 15 (14 April 1849): 275.

34. Vivian Nutton, *Theories of Fever from Antiquity to the Enlightenment* (London, 1981); James C. Riley, *The Eighteenth-Century Campaign to Avoid Disease* (Houndmills, England, 1987), x–xv; Margaret Pelling, *Cholera Fever and English Medicine, 1825–1865* (Oxford, 1978), 3–10; John V. Pickstone, "Dearth, Dirt and Fever Epidemics: Rewriting the History of British 'Public Health,' 1780–1830," in *Epidemics and Ideas: Essays on the Historical Perception of Pestilence*, ed. Terence Ranger and Paul Slack (Cambridge, 1992), 125–48.

35. Riley's *The Eighteenth-Century Campaign to Avoid Disease* provides an in-depth intellectual history of the environmental approach to disease. For a detailed discussion of the competing medical theories, see Delaporte, *Disease and Civilization*, 115–37.

36. *Rapport sur la marche et les effets du choléra-morbus dans Paris et les communes rurales de la Seine, année 1832* (Paris, 1834), 139–40.

37. The Englishman Dr. John Snow linked the disease's origin to a contaminated water supply. To prove his point, he removed the handle from the famous Broad Street Pump, and cases of cholera in the neighborhood around it plummeted. He blamed the rapid spread of the epidemic on poor hygienic conditions and sanitary carelessness, as the disease traveled easily from those who changed bed linens of cholera patients and went on to other tasks without washing their hands. Three decades later, the German scientist Robert Koch isolated the responsible bacillus with the aid of advances such as the microscope and techniques for staining cells. Ultimately, the discoveries of Snow, Koch, and others resulted in the "germ theory of contagion," in which the spread of infectious diseases was attributed to bacteria or other microorganisms. However, it would take nearly a decade more, and the experience of the Hamburg epidemic of 1892, for these ideas to gain universal acceptance in the scientific community. The most extensive broad history of cholera remains Pollitzer's *Cholera*.

38. Evans, *Death in Hamburg*, 227.

39. On the transformation of Paris during the July Monarchy, see Philippe Vigier, *Nouvelle histoire de Paris: Paris pendant la monarchie de juillet* (Paris, 1991), 177–227; David H. Pinkney, *Napoleon III and the Rebuilding of Paris* (Princeton, 1972), 3–24. On the sewers, see Donald Reid, *Paris Sewers and Sewermen: Realities and Representations* (Cambridge, 1991), 25–27. For a good summary of the artistic representation of Paris in paintings, lithographs, and maps, see Dennis Paul Costanzo, "Cityscape and the Transformation of Paris during the Second Empire" (Ph.D. diss., University of Michigan, 1981), 1–49.

40. Chevalier has inspired a lively scholarly debate about the impact of immigration on the Paris population during the first half of the nineteenth century. By juxtaposing figures from Paris with those of the Department of the Seine as a whole, a more recent contributor to the debate, Le Mée, argues that the capital may not have in fact experienced the dramatic increase of immigrants documented by Chevalier. R. Le Mée, "Les Villes de France et leurs populations de 1806 à 1851," *Annales de démographie historique* (Paris) (1989): 382. The key point for our story is that many contemporaries believed that population and misery were both increasing at an alarming rate. I thank Ted Margadant for this reference.

41. *Le Crédit,* 13 June 1849, 3.

42. Louis Chevalier, *La Formation de la population parisienne au XIXe siècle* (Paris, 1950), 45–50.

43. Chevalier, *Laboring Classes and Dangerous Classes,* 194–95.

44. *Rapport sur les épidémies cholériques,* 149–68.

45. Administration Générale de l'Assistance Publique, *Rapport sur l'épidémie cholérique de 1853–54, dans les établissements dépendant de l'administration générale de l'assistance publique de la ville de Paris* (Paris, 1850), table 40 (hereafter referred to by its title).

46. *Journal des débats,* 11 April 1849, 2.

47. The *Rapport sur les épidémies cholériques* seemed especially impressed by the marked difference in expenditures: "whereas the first epidemic carried along expenditures of several millions, that of 1849 only cost several hundred thousand francs," 158.

48. Review of Eugène Roch's *Paris malade,* in the *Journal des débats,* 29 September 1832, 3–4.

49. Perhaps the best way to understand the persisting fears of Parisians in the 1840s is to consider fears of earthquakes in twentieth-century California. Californians who experienced the Loma Prieta earthquake in 1989 live in denial about the next "Big One," but each new earthquake above 6.0 on the Richter scale invariably produces a flurry of anxious articles in local newspapers.

50. Karl Marx was one of the earliest commentators to point this out in *The Eighteenth Brumaire of Louis Bonaparte,* trans. (New York, 1963), esp. 15–60.

51. Hatin, one of the earliest chroniclers of the history of the press in France, ends his eight-volume study with a glowing account of the liberty achieved under the July Monarchy. Eugène Hatin, *Histoire politique et littéraire de la presse en France,* vol. 8 (Paris, 1861), 547–616. More will be said of the July Monarchy and the press in Chapter 2.

52. Rémond makes a convincing case that the July Monarchy was essentially conservative. René Rémond, *The Right-Wing in France from 1815 to de Gaulle,* 1954; trans. James M. Laux (Philadelphia, 1966), 123–24.

53. Claude Bellanger et al., *Histoire générale de la presse française,* vol. 2 (Paris, 1969), 102; Charles Ledré, *La Presse à l'assaut de la monarchie, 1815–1848* (Paris, 1960), 129.

54. *L'Union médicale* and the *Gazette médicale de Paris* criticized the administration in numerous articles from the beginning of the epidemic in mid-March until early June. See Chapter 13, 133–35.

55. Odile Krankovich, an archivist at the Archives Nationales who has written extensively about censorship during the mid-nineteenth century, knows of no evidence suggesting government interest in witholding information about the 1849 epidemic.

56. Irene Collins, *The Government and the Newspaper Press in France, 1814–1881* (London, 1959), 109; Bellanger et al., *Histoire générale de la presse,* vol. 2, 229–30. Official censorship tended to be linked more explicitly to attacks on the July Monarchy in the printed media and caricature, as well as theater, especially after the assassination attempt against King Louis Philippe in 1835. James Smith Allen, *In the Public Eye: A History of Reading in Modern France, 1800–1940* (Princeton, 1991), 87. For a discussion of censorship in the first half of the nineteenth century, also see Robert Justin Goldstein, *Censorship of Political Caricature in Nineteenth-Century France* (Kent, Ohio, 1989), esp. 119–79; L. Gabriel-Robinet, *La Censure* (Paris, 1965).

57. On the obstacles to literacy in France, see Allen, *In the Public Eye,* 61–70.

58. Several works have engaged with the idea of a revolutionary tradition in France. See, for example, François Furet, *Revolutionary France, 1770–1880,* trans. Antonia Nevill (Oxford, 1992); Ferguson, *Paris as Revolution;* François Furet and Mona Ozouf, eds., *The Transformation of Political Culture, 1789–1848,* vol. 3 of *The French Revolution and the Creation of Modern Political Culture,* ed. Keith Michael Baker (Oxford, 1989); Maurice Agulhon, *Marianne into Battle: Republican Imagery and Symbolism in France, 1789–1880,* trans. Janet Lloyd (Cambridge, 1981); William H. Sewell, Jr., *Work and Revolution in France: The Language of Labor from the Old Regime to 1848* (Cambridge, 1980). While these works have branched out beyond institutional histories, no one has fully explored the role of an unlikely element such as disease.

59. Here I am in essential agreement with Furet, who argues that "in France class consciousness was a legacy of the French Revolution before it became the product of industrial development." Furet, *Revolutionary France,* 343. The French Revolution is perhaps *the* most studied event of all modern history. For contemporary surveys of the literature, see Jack Censer, "Commencing the Third Century of Debate," *American Historical Review* 94, no. 5 (December 1989): 1309–25; Lynn Hunt, *Politics, Culture, and Class in the French Revolution* (Berkeley and Los Angeles, 1984), 1–10. The classic text for a Marxist interpretation is Albert Soboul, *The French Revolution, 1787–1799,* trans. Alan Forrest and Colin Jones (New York, 1974), while the revisionist position was staked out by François Furet in *Interpreting the French Revolution,* trans. Elborg Forster (Cambridge, 1984).

60. On Parisian social unrest during the revolution and early nineteenth century, see the following: Sewell, *Work and Revolution in France;* George Rudé, *The Crowd in the French Revolution* (London, 1959); Albert Soboul, *The Parisian Sans-Culottes and the French Revolution* (London, 1964); David H.

Pinkney, "The Crowd in the French Revolution of 1830," *American Historical Review* 70 (October 1964): 1–17; Edward Shorter and Charles Tilly, *Strikes in France, 1830–1968* (Cambridge, 1974).

61. On this rhetoric, see Sewell, *Work and Revolution in France.*

62. The literature about middle-class identity formation is vast and often contradictory. Most useful have been the following: Adeline Daumard, *Les Bourgeois de Paris au XIXᵉ siècle* (Paris, 1970); Stuart Blumin, "The Hypothesis of Middle-Class Formation in Nineteenth-Century America: A Critique and Some Proposals," *American Historical Review* 90 (1985): 299–338; Karl Marx, *The Class Struggles in France, 1848–1850,* trans. (New York, 1964); Marx, *The Eighteenth Brumaire of Louis Bonaparte;* Anthony Giddens, *The Class Structure of the Advanced Societies* (London, 1973); Peter N. Stearns, "The Middle Class: Toward a Precise Definition," *Comparative Studies in Society and History* 21 (1979): 377–96. Rémond, *The Right-Wing in France,* 108–17.

63. Marx himself never provided a basic or consistent definition of the bourgeoisie in his vast writings on the proletariat and capitalism.

64. Daumard, *Les Bourgeois de Paris,* 20–22, 39–76.

65. This was somewhat the situation of Tudesq's *grands notables,* a term he expanded from contemporaries' usage to describe the fuzzy border between the nobility and the bourgeoisie. André Tudesq, *Les Grands Notables en France: Etude historique d'une psychologie sociale,* 2 vols. (Paris, 1964). On the ascent of the Parisian bourgeoisie and its struggle with the aristocracy, see Jean L'Homme, *La Grande Bourgeoisie au pouvoir, 1830–1880* (Paris, 1960), esp. 18–42.

66. Henri Gisquet, *Mémoires de M. Gisquet, ancien préfet de police, écrites par lui-même,* vol. 1 (Paris, 1840), 247.

67. Stuart Blumin, *The Emergence of the Middle Class: Social Experience in the American City, 1760–1900* (Cambridge, 1989), 2.

68. In the following pages it is not my goal to provide a definitive sociological model or definition for the middle classes. Rather, I wish to provide enough information for a working, albeit impressionistic, image to emerge. For purposes of argument, then, I am taking the liberty of consolidating a number of more complex arguments to create this artificial composite schema. See Daumard, *Les Bourgeois de Paris,* 125–46; Peter N. Stearns, *Paths to Authority: The Middle Class and the Industrial Labor Force in France, 1820–1848* (Urbana, 1970), 108–9; Arno J. Mayer, "The Lower-Middle Class as Historical Problem," *Journal of Modern History* 47 (September 1975): 409–36.

69. Marx refers to a similarly constituted group as the country's "ideological representatives and spokesmen, . . . [its] so-called talents." Marx, *Class Struggles in France,* 34.

70. Daumard, *Les Bourgeois de Paris,* 124–36; Vigier, *Nouvelle histoire de Paris,* 385–93.

71. Daumard, like Marx (*Class Struggles in France,* 37), argues that the differences within the middle classes accounted for some of the turmoil in the 1848 revolution as people from the disillusioned and disenfranchised

lower strata of the middle classes bonded with the lower classes against the stagnant bourgeoisie of the July Monarchy. Daumard, *Les Bourgeois de Paris,* 344.

72. Gender differences no doubt had an impact on the definition and experience of bourgeois culture. Since this book concerns the creation of a *public* epidemic reality more than a private one, I focus almost exclusively on qualities and values characteristic of bourgeois men. Women obviously suffered from the ravages of the disease, but even those who worked as nurses or collected charitable contributions did not have the opportunity to serve in the same capacity as the medical professionals, administrators, or journalists who would tell the official epidemic story.

73. On the July Monarchy and its bourgeois label, see Pamela M. Pilbeam, *The 1830 Revolution in France* (London, 1991), 132–33; Vigier, *Nouvelle histoire de Paris,* 338–46.

74. Pilbeam, *The 1830 Revolution in France,* 128–29. Daumard's study *Les Bourgeois de Paris,* which essentially covers the period 1815–48, treats the topic thematically rather than chronologically, an indication of the minimal tangible difference she perceives between the two regimes.

75. The pioneer for such an approach is Daumard, who toward the end of her exhaustive quantitative study of *Les Bourgeois de Paris,* 321–27, pauses to consider "l'âme de la bourgeoisie parisienne." More recent works, such as Alain Corbin's *The Foul and the Fragrant: Odor and the French Social Imagination,* trans. (Cambridge, 1986), and Jean-Pierre Goubert's *The Conquest of Water: The Advent of Health in the Industrial Age,* trans. Andrew Wilson (Princeton, 1989), like Chevalier's *Laboring Classes and Dangerous Classes,* discuss bourgeois values by implication. A notable exception is Katherine A. Lynch, *Family, Class, and Ideology in Early Industrial France: Social Policy and the Working-Class Family, 1825–1848* (Madison, 1988), which contrasts the discussions of moral economists and social catholics related to industrialization in northern France.

76. On the history of private hygiene, see Georges Vigarello, *Le Propre et le sale: L'Hygiène du corps depuis le Moyen Age* (Paris, 1985), 207–16; Goubert, *The Conquest of Water,* 82–102; Corbin, *The Foul and the Fragrant,* 161–64.

77. Norbert Elias, *The Civilizing Process,* vol. 1: *The History of Manners,* trans. (New York, 1978); Dominique Laporte, *Histoire de la merde: Prologue* (Paris, 1978); Peter Stallybrass and Allon White, *The Politics and Poetics of Transgression* (Ithaca, 1986). I am grateful to Richard Evans for pointing out the cholera connection in his discussion of responses to the 1892 cholera epidemic in Hamburg. Evans, *Death in Hamburg,* 229.

78. Jürgen Habermas, *The Structural Transformation of the Public Sphere: An Inquiry into a Category of Bourgeois Society,* trans. Thomas Burger (Cambridge, 1989), traces how the bourgeoisie eventually gained power at the end of the eighteenth century by appropriating the public sphere of the state, thereby creating a context in which a market economy and government power became synonymous. I have taken Habermas as a point of departure for defining *public* in such a way that it refers to the liberal public sphere in order

to describe the dissemination of bourgeois values; at the same time, the *plebeian* sphere was part of the bourgeois's intended audience.

79. On this legacy, see Alan B. Spitzer, *The French Generation of 1820* (Princeton, 1987).

80. For the basic class-based analysis of the bourgeoisie's rise to power during the French Revolution, see Georges Lefebvre, *The Coming of the French Revolution*, trans. R. R. Palmer (Princeton, 1947); Albert Soboul, *The French Revolution, 1787–1799*, trans. (New York, 1975).

81. I am building on Giddens's model, which divides the concept of "class consciousness" into three layers, from least to most developed: (1) a concept of class identity based on class differentiation; (2) a conception of class conflict, where perceptions of class unity are linked to a recognition that an outside class or classes have opposing interests; and (3) a "revolutionary" class consciousness, which involves the belief that deliberate class action can bring about change for the benefit of that class. Giddens, *The Class Structure*, 112.

82. This was the number of people who died in the hospital, a telling barometer of poverty at a time when only the least fortunate died there. Vigier, *Nouvelle histoire de Paris*, 262–63. Daumard corroborates these dramatic figures by citing reports published in the late 1820s: of 224,000 Parisian households, 136,000 were in a state of indigence, with 36,000 bordering on it. Daumard, *Les Bourgeois de Paris*, 18–19.

83. Vigier, *Nouvelle histoire de Paris*, 286.

84. Figures from Daumard, *Les Bourgeois de Paris*, 42.

85. Karen Halttunen, *Confidence Men and Painted Ladies: A Study of Middle-Class Culture in America, 1830–1870* (New Haven, 1982); Blumin, *The Emergence of the Middle Class*.

86. Stallybrass and White, *The Politics and Poetics of Transgression*; Leonore Davidoff and Catherine Hall, *Family Fortunes: Men and Women of the English Middle Class, 1780–1850* (Chicago, 1987).

87. In the nineteenth century, like today, the words *nous* (we) or *on* (one) translated into the "royal we" in English, thereby denoting individual as opposed to collective agency. This was particularly true of medical reports concerning the epidemics.

88. These power dynamics resemble those outlined in Said's *Orientalism*. As we shall see, the medical investigations, academic writings, fiction, and other forms of cultural expression used to describe and define the lower classes find modern counterparts in descriptions of how "the West" approached "the Orient."

89. On the bourgeoisie and the National Guard, see Daumard, *Les Bourgeois de Paris*, 306–7; Vigier, *Nouvelle histoire de Paris*, 395–400. The most thorough study of the National Guard remains Louis Girard, *La Garde nationale, 1814–1871* (Paris, 1964). On the role of the National Guard as a supplementary police force, see Patricia Ann O'Brien, "Urban Growth and Public Order: The Development of a Modern Police in Paris, 1829–1854" (Ph.D. diss., Columbia University, 1973), 69–71.

90. Scholars have made the same assertion about European identity vis-à-vis the rest of the world. See Denys Hay, *Europe: The Emergence of an Idea* (Edinburgh, 1968).

91. Blumin's work drew my attention to this paradox. See *The Emergence of the Middle Class,* 9–10. Daumard argues that the Parisian bourgeoisie "is individualistic, yet lucid enough to be aware that the power of individuals is a function of that of the group." Daumard, *Les Bourgeois de Paris,* 357.

92. David H. Pinkney's *Decisive Years in France, 1840–1847* (Princeton, 1986) makes a convincing case for the 1840s marking the end of the old regime. Moreover, it provides a good overview of such major developments as the proliferation of railroads, the consolidation of the professions, and the beginnings of industrial capitalism in France.

93. In *Work and Revolution in France,* Sewell indirectly supports this point by arguing that the working classes had to create their republic "independently, outside the structures of the bourgeois state," 273.

CHAPTER 1. THE EPIDEMIC AND REVOLUTIONARY TRADITIONS OF PARIS

1. For a broad discussion of the role of diseases in the old regime, see Fernand Braudel, *The Structures of Everyday Life: Civilization and Capitalism 15th-18th Century,* vol. 1 (New York, 1979), 78–92.

2. The terms and information are taken from Matthew Ramsey, *Professional and Popular Medicine in France, 1770–1830: The Social World of Medical Practice* (Cambridge, 1988), pt. 2; on attitudes toward physicians, see 65–69.

3. Marc Bloch, *The Royal Touch: Sacred Monarchy and Scrofula in England and France,* trans. J. E. Anderson (London, 1973); Ernst H. Kantorowicz, *The King's Two Bodies: A Study in Medieval Political Theology* (Princeton, 1957).

4. George Rosen, *A History of Public Health* (1958; reprint, Baltimore, 1993), 148–52; Theodore M. Porter, *The Rise of Statistical Thinking, 1820–1900* (Princeton, 1986).

5. It is telling that unless they are specifically about medicine, the vast number of books on the development of the French absolutist state devote almost no attention to matters of public health. On health policies under absolutism, see Rosen, *A History of Public Health,* 57–106, and "The Fate of the Concept of Medical Police, 1780–1890," in George Rosen, *From Medical Police to Social Medicine: Essays on the History of Health Care* (New York, 1974), 142–75. For a more specific study of France, see Edward M. Solomon, *Public Welfare, Science, and Propaganda in Seventeenth-Century France* (Princeton, 1971).

6. The secondary literature about the Marseille plague is surprisingly sparse. For a start, see Françoise Hildesheimer, *La Terreur et la pitié. L'Ancien Régime à l'épreuve de la peste* (Paris, 1990); Charles Carrière, M. Courdurié, and F. Rebuffat, *Marseille ville morte. La peste de 1720* (Marseille, 1968); Jean-Noel Biraben, *Les Hommes et la peste dans les pays européens et méditerranéens,* 2 vols. (Paris, 1975–76).

7. Quoted in Daniel Roche, *The People of Paris: An Essay in Popular Culture in the Eighteenth Century*, trans. Marie Evans and Gwynne Lewis (Berkeley and Los Angeles, 1987), 64.

8. The picture is obviously far more complex than this one, which I have painted in rather schematic form for purposes of contrast. See, for example, Olwen Hufton, "Towards an Understanding of the Poor in Eighteenth-Century France," in *French Government and Society, 1500–1850: Essays in Memory of Alfred Cobban*, ed. J. F. Bosher (London, 1973), 145–65; Colin Jones, *Charity and Bienfaisance: The Treatment of the Poor in the Montpellier Region, 1740–1815* (Cambridge, 1982); Kathryn Norberg, *Rich and Poor in Grenoble, 1600–1814* (Berkeley and Los Angeles, 1985); Roche, *The People of Paris*, 64–77.

9. Denis Diderot, *L'Encyclopédie ou dictionnaire des sciences, des arts et des métiers* (Paris, 1762; 1969 facsimile reprint), vol. 13, 88–103 (hereafter referred to as *Encyclopédie*).

10. Hufton, "Towards an Understanding of the Poor," 147–48. The essay critiques the philosophes' condemnation of Catholic charity. For a discussion of medical theories and practices during the Enlightenment, see Riley, *The Eighteenth-Century Campaign to Avoid Disease*.

11. Charles Coulston Gillispie, *Science and Polity in France at the End of the Old Regime* (Princeton, 1980), 194–256; Caroline Hannaway, "Medicine, Public Welfare, and the State in Eighteenth-Century France: The Société Royale de Médecine of Paris, 1776–1793" (Ph.D. diss., Johns Hopkins, 1974).

12. Rosen, "Mercantilism and Health Policy in Eighteenth-Century French Thought," in Rosen, *From Medical Police to Social Medicine*, 206.

13. *Encyclopédie*, vol. 3, 364.

14. *Encyclopédie*, vol. 5, 788.

15. Eugène Roch, *Paris malade: Esquisses du jour*, 2 vols. (Paris, 1832).

16. Ibid., vol. 2, 361. Apart from this occasional refrain, however, the massive work seemed to be wholly without either plot or obvious point, describing the 1832 cholera epidemic from the perspective of *la vie quotidienne*. In the preface to the second volume the author claimed that the success of the first had invested him with "the duty not to allow this work to remain incomplete." No records exist to indicate that the work was either performed or printed as a newspaper serial.

17. Quoted in Roche, *The People of Paris*, 10. For an excellent discussion of this background, see Chevalier, *Laboring Classes and Dangerous Classes*, 147–51.

18. Sauval, quoted in Chevalier, *Laboring Classes and Dangerous Classes*, 148.

19. Restif de la Bretonne, *Les Nuits de Paris*, 7 vols. (Paris, 1788); see also L. S. Mercier, *Le Tableau de Paris*, 12 vols. (Amsterdam, 1781–88).

20. See, for example, Robert A. Nye, *Crime, Madness, and Politics in Modern France: The Medical Concept of National Decline* (Princeton, 1984), 72, 76, 81, 85, as a start.

21. Chevalier, *Laboring Classes and Dangerous Classes*, 182.

22. *Nouveau tableau de Paris au XIXe siècle,* vol. 3 (Paris, 1835), 2.

23. Corbin, *The Foul and the Fragrant,* esp. 111–27; Reid, *Paris Sewers and Sewermen,* esp. 18–83. The nature of the urban investigations will be taken up in more detail in the next chapter.

24. *L'Ami de la religion,* 3 April 1832, 421.

25. *La Gazette d'Auvergne,* quoted in Chevalier, *Le Choléra,* 19.

26. Writing a letter to *Le Courrier français,* a pharmacist complained that a prefect's ordinance in the Basses Alpes forced him to be quarantined for two weeks only because he had arrived from the capital. "While I was waiting, I was banished to the countryside," he fumed; "no one dared to come near me, and they looked upon me as a victim of the plague." For the benefit of the Parisian audience, the paper reprinted the prefect's decree, along with the pharmacist's assertion that the quarantine policy would do little good. *Le Courrier français,* 3 May 1832, 4.

27. Charles Duveyrier, "La Ville nouvelle ou le Paris des St. Simoniens," in *Le Livre des cent-et-un,* vol. 8 (Paris, 1834), 304.

28. Antoine Métral, *Description naturelle, morale et politique du choléra-morbus à Paris* (Paris, 1833), preface.

29. *Rapport sur la marche et les effets du choléra-morbus* (Paris, 1834), 190.

30. Roch, *Paris malade,* vol. 1, 210.

31. Napoléon Henry, *Le Choléra-morbus, sa nature, son siège et son traitement* (Paris, 1832), 30.

32. Fascinating stories remain to be told about the relationship between disease and revolution in other areas of the world, particularly in Latin America, where both cholera and revolt have been important parts of political life. I thank Julyan Peard, a specialist in "the new medical history" of nineteenth-century Brazil, for pointing out that even the literature concerned with medicine, society, and culture remains focused largely on issues of development. The epidemic of scholera has been most widespread in Britain and France, with excellent individual studies for Germany and North America as well. Among the most influential works are the following: Bourdelais and Raulot, *Une Peur bleue;* Asa Briggs, "Cholera and Society in the Nineteenth Century," *Past and Present* 19 (1961): 76–96; Chevalier, *Le Choléra;* Delaporte, *Disease and Civilization;* Michael Durey, *The Return of the Plague: British Society and Cholera, 1831–2,* (London, 1979, 1983); Evans, *Death in Hamburg;* Charles M. Godfrey, *The Cholera Epidemics in Upper Canada, 1832–1866* (Toronto, 1980); Leca, *Et le choléra;* Rodrick McGrew, "The First Cholera Epidemic and Social History," *Bulletin of the History of Medicine* 36 (1966): 61–73; R. J. Morris, *Cholera, 1832* (London, 1976); Pelling, *Cholera Fever and English Medicine;* Charles E. Rosenberg, "Cholera in Nineteenth-Century Europe," *Comparative Studies in Society and History* 8, no. 4 (July 1966): 452–63; Charles E. Rosenberg, *The Cholera Years: The United States in 1832, 1849 and 1866* (Chicago, 1962); Sussman, "From Yellow Fever to Cholera."

33. Here I am borrowing from the term coined by Agulhon: "the folklore of the Republic," broadly defined as "the rituals, customs and ceremonies to which it gives rise." Agulhon, *Marianne into Battle,* 4–5. I have also

been influenced by T. J. Clark, *The Absolute Bourgeois: Artists and Politicians in France, 1848–1851* (Princeton, 1982), particularly the chapter "The Picture of the Barricade," 9–30.

34. Heinrich Heine, *Saemtliche Werke in zehn Baenden*, unter Mitwirkung von Jonas Fraenkel, Ludwig Kraehe, Albert Leitzmann und Julius Petersen herausgegeben von Oskar Walzel, vol. 6 (Leipzig, 1912), 166.

35. *Le Corsaire*, 15 July 1832, 1.

36. Alfred Nettement, *Etudes critiques sur le feuilleton-roman*, vol. 2 (Paris, 1845–46), 112–13.

37. François René Chateaubriand, *Mémoires d'outre tombe*, vol. 4 (1849–50; reprint, Paris, 1968), 63.

38. APP D/A 122, Choléra, pièces diverses. This is unfortunately not a firsthand account but rather a police *commissaire*'s notes taken from another source—probably Paul Thureau-Dangin's *Histoire de la monarchie de juillet*, 7 vols. (Paris, 1884–92)—in anticipation of a later outbreak. Even if the story is difficult to substantiate, however, it is noteworthy that the police *commissaire* or Dangin incorporated this symbol of revolutionary violence into the description, an indication of persisting links between disease and revolution at least until the end of the nineteenth century.

39. The debate over the character and significance of the 1830 revolution continues, though it has received far less attention than 1848 and none of the revisionist study applied to 1789. Since J. L. Bory's study, *La Révolution de juillet* (Paris, 1972), which sees 1830 as a cynical bourgeois play for power, virtually no work has appeared in French. David H. Pinkney, *The French Revolution of 1830* (Princeton, 1972), remains the classic starting point for Anglo scholars (and subsequently French scholars because a translation appeared in 1988). Pinkney argued that it was not truly a revolution at all, except for administrative employees and the change in political regime; agreeing with many contemporaries who wrote about the events immediately afterward, he challenged the subsequent Marxist interpretation that 1830 marked one more step along the road of the bourgeois ascendancy to power. In her study, *The 1830 Revolution in France*, Pilbeam offers a thorough discussion of the historiographical debates (1–12), while suggesting that scholars should place the events within a much larger chronological and geographical perspective.

40. For a detailed discussion of these conflicts, see H.A.C. Collingham, *The July Monarchy: A Political History of France, 1830–1848* (London, 1988), 23–142; A. Jardin and A.-J. Tudesq, *La France des notables: L'Evolution générale, 1815–1848*, vol. 1 (Paris, 1973), 125–46.

41. For a discussion of the complex relationship between the July Monarchy and the right, see Rémond, *The Right-Wing in France*, 79–98.

42. Evans makes a convincing case to support the idea that the 1830 revolution "caused" cholera. He argues that contacts between the military and civilian populations facilitated cholera's entry into western Europe. The movements of large groups of people—both troops and refugees—combined with poor hygienic conditions to spread the bacteria quickly. Richard

Evans, "Epidemics and Revolutions: Cholera in Nineteenth-Century Europe," *Past and Present* 120 (August 1988): 133–35.

43. *La Quotidienne*, 31 March 1832.

44. Métral, *Description*, 5; Louis Blanc, *Histoire de dix ans, 1830–1840*, vol. 3 (Paris, 1867), 197. See also Evans, "Epidemics and Revolutions," 131–33.

45. *La Quotidienne*, 13 April 1832, 1–2.

46. M. Bellemare, *Le Fléau de Dieu en 1832* (Paris, 1832), 5.

47. Ibid., 50.

48. Jules Janin, *Paris depuis la révolution de 1830* (Brussels, 1832).

49. Also see *La Quotidienne*, 13 April 1832, 1–2. Unfortunately, I have not been able to locate any specific background information, though it appears to be part of a genre that emerged during the July Monarchy. See James Cuno, "Charles Philipon and La Maison Aubert: The Business, Politics, and Public of Caricature in Paris, 1820–1840" (Ph.D. diss., Harvard University, 1985), for a detailed discussion of the production and distribution of other images. I thank T. J. Clark for this reference. On caricature under the July Monarchy, see Petra ten-Doesschate Chu and Gabriel Weisberg, eds., *The Popularization of Images: Visual Culture under the July Monarchy* (Princeton, 1994).

50. The cartoons discussed here and elsewhere in the book reflect most of the iconographical material that remains from the early cholera outbreaks. Because I have been unable to track down the context for these cartoons, the readings are by necessity my own. This problem of interpretation does not, however, diminish their value as representations of the epidemic threat since many of the same images also appear in literary depictions. For a broad discussion of cholera's iconography in the nineteenth and twentieth centuries, see Patrice Bourdelais and André Dodin, eds., *Visages du choléra* (Paris, 1987).

51. For a discussion of this literature, see Albert Boime, "Jacques-Louis David, Scatological Discourse in the French Revolution, and the Art of Caricature," in *French Caricature and the French Revolution, 1789–1799* (Berkeley and Los Angeles, 1988), 67–82.

52. On the significance of Napoleon for bourgeois Parisians, see Daumard, *Les Bourgeois de Paris*, 337.

53. This event was immortalized in Baron Antoine-Jean Gross's famous painting of *Bonaparte Visiting the Pest-Ridden of Jaffa* (1804).

54. Roch, *Paris malade*, vol. 1, 64. Interestingly, the Saint-Simonians were among the most explicit on this point. Charles Béranger, "Le Choléra, Napoléon, l'ordre légale," Saint-Simonian pamphlet (Paris, 1832), Bibliothèque Nationale; Maschereau, "Ce que faisait Napoléon pour exciter l'enthousiasme du peuple," Saint-Simonian pamphlet (Paris, 1832), Bibliothèque Nationale.

55. See Chapter 3, p. 110. ADS VD⁴ 3381 Département de la Seine, Commission Centrale de Salubrité, "Instruction populaire sur les princi-

paux moyens à employer pour se garantir du choléra-morbus et sur la conduite à tenir lorsque cette maladie se déclare," 15 November 1831.

56. Métral, *Description*, 5.

57. Unfortunately, no contextual information accompanied the cartoon.

58. The reference to opposition political groups as *fléaux* was a common one. One official went so far as to warn Parisians publicly that "[les] deux fléaux [Carlists and Republicans] se sont unis aujourd'hui entre nous." Marthe-Camille Bachasson Montalivet, "Troubles de Paris—Proclamation" (Paris, 1832).

59. Pilbeam, *The 1830 Revolution in France*, 132–33.

60. Contrast, for example, Pilbeam's discussion of the bourgeois revolution in ibid., 121–49, with Collingham, *The July Monarchy*, 6–21.

61. Roch, *Paris malade*, vol. 1, 391–92.

62. On the economic crisis of 1827–32, see J. P. Gonnet, "Esquisse de la crise économique en France de 1827–32," *Revue d'histoire économique et sociale* 33 (1955); Pilbeam, *The 1830 Revolution in France*, 37–59. On the ominous climate, see Chevalier, *Laboring Classes and Dangerous Classes*.

63. Adeline Daumard, quoted in Georges Duby, ed., *Histoire de la France urbaine*, 5 vols. (Paris: Seuil, 1980–85), vol. 4: Maurice Agulhon, ed., *La Ville de l'âge industriel*, 588.

64. Christine Piette, quoted in Barrie Ratcliffe, "Perception and Realities of the Urban Margin: The Rag Pickers of Paris in the First Half of the Nineteenth Century," *Canadian Journal of History/Annales canadiennes d'histoire* 27 (August 1992): 212. Other figures taken from Vigier, *Nouvelle histoire de Paris*, 262–65.

65. Chevalier, *Laboring Classes and Dangerous Classes*, 206; Duby, *Histoire de la France urbaine*, vol. 4, 587–88.

66. ADS VD^6 669, Epidémies du choléra, Commissions d'Hygiène (1831–32). For a discussion of what such investigations would lead to later in the century, see Ann Louise Shapiro, *Housing the Poor of Paris, 1850–1902* (Madison, 1985).

67. François Marc Moreau, *Histoire statistique du choléra-morbus dans le quartier du faubourg St.-Denis* (Paris, 1833), 45–46.

68. This fact accounted in part for the controversy surrounding the initial publication of the names and addresses of the dead. See Chapter 3.

69. *Rapport sur l'épidémie cholérique de 1853–54*, table 39.

70. *Le Corsaire*, 31 March 1832, 4.

71. *Journal des débats politiques et littéraires*, 28 March 1832.

72. *Le Corsaire*, 4 April 1832, 4.

73. *Le National*, 30 March 1832, 2–3.

74. A.F.M. Rey-Dusseuil, *Le Cloître St. Méry* (Paris, 1832), 60.

75. *François le fataliste* (30 March 1832), quoted in Sussman, "From Yellow Fever to Cholera," 259.

76. *Rapport sur la marche et les effets du choléra-morbus*, 124–25.

77. *La Quotidienne*, 7 April 1832, 2.

78. Métral, *Description*, 15.

79. Roch, *Paris malade*, vol. 1, 418–19.

80. Balzac made the relationship particularly clear by explaining, "Just as there could be a man capable of infamy, there are certain dishonorable streets within Paris; then there are noble streets, then streets that are simply honest; then there are streets where the public has yet to form an opinion on their morality; then the murderous streets, the streets that are older than the most bitter old people, streets that are always dirty, labor streets, working streets, merchant streets." Quoted in Duby, *Histoire de la France urbaine*, vol. 4, 588.

81. *La Quotidienne*, 3 April 1832, 3.

82. Louis François Trolliet, August Pierre Isidore Polinière, and Alexandre Bottex, *Rapport sur le choléra-morbus de Paris* (Lyon, 1832), 15.

83. Ibid., 23.

84. ADS VD⁴ 3381, Département de la Seine, Commission Centrale de Salubrité, "Instruction populaire sur les principaux moyens à employer pour se garantir du choléra-morbus et sur la conduite à tenir lorsque cette maladie se déclare," 15 November 1831, 1. These pamphlets are discussed in detail in Chapter 3.

85. M. F. Magendie, *Leçons sur le choléra-morbus* (Paris, 1832), 240; emphasis added.

86. Tacheron, *Statistique médicale de la mortalité du choléra-morbus*, 53. Most of the statistical descriptions of the epidemic included a breakdown by days of the week, which strongly suggested the links between morality and mortality. See the *Rapport sur la marche et les effets du choléra-morbus*, 142–43.

87. *La Quotidienne*, 4 April 1832, 2.

88. *Gazette médicale de Paris*, 5 April 1832, 156.

89. Moreau, *Histoire statistique du choléra-morbus*, 54–55.

90. Chateaubriand, *Mémoires*, vol. 4, 64.

91. Jacques Boucher de Crevecour de Perthes, *Sous dix rois: Souvenirs*, vol. 5 (Paris, 1863), 9.

92. Rudolphe Apponyi, *Vingt-cinq ans à Paris: Journal du comte*, vol. 2 (Paris, 1913), 162–63.

93. *L'Entracte*, 3 April 1832, 2.

94. Métral, *Description*, 54.

95. *Moniteur universel*, 10 April 1832, 1019; *La Quotidienne*, 10 April 1832, 2. Meanwhile, *Le Globe*, the St. Simonian newspaper, made use of a Prussian medical report which claimed that more people had died in villages than in cities because of inadequate health facilities and less competent doctors. *Le Globe*, 31 March 1832. To substantiate the idea that the rich also died from the disease, *Le Bonhomme Richard* began printing obituaries of wealthy and prominent Parisians, 18 April 1832, 4.

96. More will be said of these protests in Chapter 3.

97. Janin, *Paris depuis la révolution*, 9.

98. Apponyi, *Vingt-cinq ans à Paris*, vol. 2, 177–78.

99. See pp. 73–75 below.

100. Heine, *Saemtliche Werke*, vol. 6, 187.

101. *Le Globe*, 1 April 1832.

102. Blanc, *Histoire de dix ans*, vol. 3, 209. Using almost identical words, Heine made a similar observation. Heine, *Saemtliche Werke*, vol. 6, 186–87.

103. Sussman contests the assertion that the rich fled the city, citing records indicating that the poor left in equally striking numbers. If the wealthy were fleeing the capital, he argued, they would probably go to their summer homes, but mayors from communes where vacation homes were located complained of sluggish charitable contributions because the wealthy Parisians had remained in the capital. Moreover, wealthier residents realized that they could probably receive better health care in a large city, while the poor had greater reason to return to their homes of origin in search of jobs and support. Sussman, "From Yellow Fever to Cholera," 248–51.

104. Described in Apponyi, *Vingt-cinq ans à Paris*, vol. 2, 175.

105. *Moniteur universel*, 10 April 1832.

106. Roch, *Paris malade*, vol. 1, 418–19.

CHAPTER 2. CHOLERA'S MESSENGERS

1. Hunt, *Politics, Culture and Class in the French Revolution*.

2. I use this term in its broad twentieth-century sense, which had no true equivalent during the early part of the nineteenth century. For a discussion of the term, see Jan Goldstein, *Console and Classify: The French Psychiatric Profession in the Nineteenth Century* (Cambridge, 1987), 10–15.

3. According to the *Almanach royal et national pour l'année 1833* (Paris, 1833), there were 1,137 *médecins*, 247 surgeons, and 260 pharmacists. The *Almanach national annuaire de la République française pour 1848, 1849 et 1850* (Paris, 1850) lists 1,432 *médecins* and surgeons combined, and 346 pharmacists.

4. The first woman did not receive a French doctorate in medicine until 1875; women were thus kept outside the formal structures of the medical profession, let alone the official discourse on cholera. Many, however, participated as nurses or lay healers. The records for the medals awarded to zealous citizens during the 1849 epidemic, for example, list dozens of women, notably nuns, for their service. *Moniteur universel*, 2 November 1849. For women and the French medical profession in the early part of the nineteenth century, see Matthew Ramsey, *Professional and Popular Medicine in France*, 219–22.

5. On medical training after the Revolution, see Ramsey, *Professional and Popular Medicine*, 74–77, 108–10; George David Sussman, "The Glut of Doctors in Mid-Nineteenth-Century France," *Comparative Studies in Society and History* 19, no. 3 (July 1977): 287–88; Erwin H. Ackerknecht, *Medicine at the Paris Hospital, 1794–1848* (Baltimore, 1967), 31–44.

6. F. Trelloz, "Les Médecins de Paris," in *Le Livre des cent-et-un*, vol. 11 (Paris, 1831–34), 155–89. Theodore Zeldin describes how this process inten-

sified over the course of the nineteenth century in his chapter on doctors in *France, 1848–1945: Ambition and Love* (Oxford, 1979), 21–42, esp. 30–32.

7. The conflicts between the doctors and health officers resulted because the revolutionary government had set up a two-tiered system of medical care in the hope of making the profession accessible to more people. These conflicts came to a head in the medical congress of 1845, when the officers were finally abolished. George Weisz, "The Politics of Medical Professionalization in France, 1845–1848," *Journal of Social History* 12, no. 1 (fall 1978), 3–30; Jacques Léonard, *La Médecine entre les pouvoirs et les savoirs: Histoire intellectuelle et politique de la médecine française du XIXe siècle* (Paris, 1981), 217–18; Jacques Léonard, *Les Médecins de l'Ouest au XIXe siècle*, vol. 2 (Paris, 1978), 788–822.

8. Léonard, *La Médecine entre les pouvoirs*, 68–79; Ackerknecht, *Medicine at the Paris Hospital*, xiii; Evelyn Ackerman, *Health Care in the Parisian Countryside, 1800–1914* (New Brunswick, 1990), 33–35; Ramsey, *Professional and Popular Medicine*, 122–23.

9. Léonard, *La Médecine entre les pouvoirs*, 109.

10. Archives de l'Académie Nationale de Médecine, liasse 64. According to Léonard, advertisements for formally trained doctors and their cures had been used for only a little over a decade before cholera arrived, and the widespread controversy they generated was a clear sign of the French medical profession's growing pains. Léonard, *La Médecine entre les pouvoirs*, 170–71. Colin Jones has done intriguing work on the early-modern period, "The Great Chain of Buying: Medical Advertisement and the Origins of the French Revolution" (forthcoming in the *American Historical Review*), in which he shows how medical *affiches* intersected with the social concerns of the revolutionary assemblies.

11. For the development of the French medical profession I have relied on the following sources: Léonard, *La Médecine entre les pouvoirs*; Ramsey, *Professional and Popular Medicine in France*; Toby Gelfand, *Professionalizing Modern Medicine: Paris Surgeons, Medical Science, and Institutions in the 18th Century* (Westport, Conn., 1980); Ackerknecht, *Medicine at the Paris Hospital*; Sussman, "From Yellow Fever to Cholera," 184–213. While it focuses on the experience of doctors in western France, Léonard's definitive thesis, *Les Médecins*, also offers particularly rich insights into the French medical profession as a whole.

12. On medicine and the Revolution, see Léonard, *La Médecine entre les pouvoirs*, 11–66; Léonard, *Les Médecins*, vol. 1, 197–231; Ramsey, *Professional and Popular Medicine*, 71–84; Rosen, *A History of Public Health*, 143–47; Ackerknecht, *Medicine at the Paris Hospital*, 33–36.

13. Quoted in Léonard, *Les Médecins*, vol. 1, 225. For more on the clinical method, see Foucault, *The Birth of the Clinic*; Ackerknecht, *Medicine at the Paris Hospital*, 32–33.

14. Léonard, *La Médecine entre les pouvoirs*, 44; Ramsey, *Professional and Popular Medicine*, 111.

15. Yves-Marie Bercé, *Le Chaudron et la lancette: Croyances populaires et médecine préventive, 1798–1830* (Paris, 1984), 63–98; Léonard, *La Médecine entre les pouvoirs*, 60–64; Ackerman, *Health Care in the Parisian Countryside*, 60–76.

16. To my knowledge, a close analysis of war's impact on French society and the medical profession remains to be written. I have pieced together my analysis based on almost passing references to the subject in Coleman, *Death Is a Social Disease*, 182–87; Léonard, *Les Médecins*, vol. 1, 221–22; Erwin H. Ackerknecht, "Hygiene in France, 1815–1848," *Bulletin of the History of Medicine* 22, no. 2 (March/April 1948): 119.

17. This was the title of the most conspicuous and impressive report describing the 1832 epidemic: *Rapport sur la marche et les effets du choléra-morbus*.

18. Ann F. La Berge, *Mission and Method: The Early Nineteenth-Century French Public Health Movement* (Cambridge, 1992); Ann F. La Berge, "The Early Nineteenth-Century French Public Health Movement: The Disciplinary Development and Institutionalization of *Hygiène publique*," *Bulletin of the History of Medicine* 58 (1984): 363–79; Ann F. La Berge, "Public Health in France and the French Public Health Movement, 1815–1848" (Ph.D. diss., University of Tennessee, 1974); Coleman, *Death Is a Social Disease*; Ackerknecht, *Medicine at the Paris Hospital*, 149–60; Ackerknecht, "Hygiene in France," 117–55; Léonard, *La Médecine entre les pouvoirs*, 149–59.

19. The Society sought to bypass the stodgy Paris Faculty of Medicine by bringing together physicians, surgeons, veterinarians, and pharmacists with the specific goal of preventing epidemics in crops and animals as well as in humans. Gillispie, *Science and Polity in France*, 194–256; Hannaway, "Medicine, Public Welfare, and the State."

20. La Berge, *Mission and Method*, 25. Among important hygienists who were not doctors, Léonard lists Moreau de Jonnés, Charles Dupin, Renoiston de Châteauneuf, Rambuteau, Watteville, Frégier, d'Augeville, Trébuchet, Moreau-Christophe, Belgrand, A. Husson, Haussmann, A. Durand Claye, and H. Monod. Léonard, *La Médecine entre les pouvoirs*, 182, n. 1.

21. La Berge, *Mission and Method*, 282–315. Ackerknecht also devotes a short chapter to discussing all of the foreigners drawn to study in Paris in the first half of the nineteenth century. Ackerknecht, *Medicine at the Paris Hospital*, 191–94. See also Russell M. Jones, "American Doctors and the Parisian Medical World, 1830–1840," *Bulletin of the History of Medicine* 47, no. 1 (1973): 40–65, and 47, no. 2 (1973): 177–204.

22. Ackerknecht, *Medicine at the Paris Hospital*, 149.

23. The vast collection of early-nineteenth-century popular literature that discusses the medical profession never uses the term *hygienist*. The various "physiognomies" of Parisian life popular in the early 1840s described the doctor, surgeon, and pharmacist, along with the journalist, bourgeois, artist, and *salonnière*, among others, but never the hygienist or

urban investigator. Since not even the hygienists of the 1820s and 1830s used this term to refer to themselves, it no doubt came into common usage only later in the century and was appropriated by subsequent historians. Perhaps if hygienists had investigated the dwellings of middle-class people with the same zeal they devoted to the lives of the poor, they may have emerged as a labeled sociocultural category sooner.

24. Ann F. La Berge, "The Paris Health Council, 1802–1848," *Bulletin of the History of Medicine* 49, no. 3 (1975): 339–52; Dora Weiner, "Public Health under Napoleon: The Conseil de Salubrité de Paris, 1802–1815," *Clio Medica* 9 (1974): 271–84.

25. J. F. Rameaux, *Appréciation des progrès de l'hygiène publique depuis le commencement du XIXᵉ siècle* (Strasbourg, 1839), quoted in Ackerknecht, "Hygiene in France," 134.

26. Moreau, *Histoire statistique du choléra-morbus,* 1–3.

27. By contrast, investigators later in the century would measure progress less exclusively in terms of mortality rates, adding employment rates, consumption habits, and literacy to their definition. See, for example, Robert Nye, *Crime, Madness, and Politics in Modern France: The Medical Concept of National Decline* (Princeton, 1984).

28. By studying the words most frequently used by hygienists, Léonard revealed that their approach to health was overwhelmingly negative. Léonard, *Les Médecins,* vol. 3, 1140–43.

29. Léonard, *La Médecine entre les pouvoirs,* 169.

30. Ackerman, *Health Care in the Parisian Countryside,* 88–89, brings up this point and notes that Coleman argues that the systematic search for cures comes only at the time of Pasteur. William Coleman, *Yellow Fever in the North: The Methods of Early Epidemiology* (Madison, 1987), xiv.

31. On Restoration policy regarding yellow fever, see Sussman, "From Yellow Fever to Cholera," particularly chaps. 2 and 3; E. A. Heaman, "Anticontagionism in France in the Nineteenth Century" (master's thesis, McGill University, 1990), 34–44. I thank George Weisz for this reference.

32. Ackerknecht, "Hygiene in France," 119–21. For a discussion of the doctors who took different sides, see Bourdelais and Raulot, *Une Peur bleue,* 67–75.

33. Sussman, "From Yellow Fever to Cholera," 149–50; Erwin H. Ackerknecht, "Anticontagionism between 1821 and 1867," *Bulletin of the History of Medicine* 22, no. 5 (1948): 570–75; Coleman, *Death Is a Social Disease,* 57.

34. For a thorough discussion of the intellectual origins of the concept, see Riley, *The Eighteenth-Century Campaign to Avoid Disease.*

35. For an account of the significance of odor in the hygienists' investigations, see Corbin, *The Foul and the Fragrant.*

36. On April 2, for example, the *Moniteur universel* printed a statement signed by all the doctors from the Hôtel Dieu, the capital's largest hospital: they had unanimously found cholera-morbus not to be contagious. *Moniteur universel,* 2 April 1832, 948. The paper published additional doctors'

statements to substantiate this view. See, for example, the issues of April 8, 9, and 13, 1832.

37. F.J.V. Broussais, *Le Choléra-morbus épidémique observé et traité selon la méthode physiologique* (Paris, 1832), quote from 9–13.

38. Quoted in Trolliet, Polinière, and Bottex, *Rapport*, 52.

39. Rostan, Roux, and Rousset, *Traité du choléra-morbus de 1849* (Paris, 1851), 12; emphasis in original.

40. While the conflict between contagionism and anticontagionism has ended, scholars continue a lively debate over its significance, as in the following: Ackerknecht, "Anticontagionism," 562–93; Pelling, *Cholera Fever and English Medicine*; Roger Cooter, "Anticontagionism and History's Medical Record," in *The Problem of Medical Knowledge: Examining the Social Construct of Medicine*, ed. Peter Wright and Andrew Treacher (Edinburgh, 1982), 87–108. Heaman examined the debate within the Paris Faculty of Medicine with particular subtlety in her "Anticontagionism in France."

41. Ackerknecht's "Anticontagionism" article launched this fundamental argument.

42. F. Foy, *Histoire médicale du choléra-morbus de Paris et des moyens thérapeutiques et hygiéniques* (Paris, 1832), 150.

43. Cooter, "Anticontagionism and History's Medical Record," 99.

44. This is one of Ackerknecht's main arguments in his article "Anticontagionism."

45. Ackerknecht, *Medicine at the Paris Hospital*, 183–88; Léonard, *La Médecine entre les pouvoirs*, 201–24; La Berge, *Mission and Method*, 23–24.

46. For a more detailed discussion, see Catherine J. Kudlick, "The Culture of Statistics and the Crisis of Cholera, 1830–1850," in *Recreating Authority in Revolutionary France*, ed. Bryant T. Ragan, Jr., and Elizabeth Williams (New Brunswick, 1992), 108–9.

47. Here, I am building on Cooter, "Anticontagionism and History's Medical Record," 94.

48. Most administrative histories date the birth of a modern bureaucracy to the middle of the eighteenth century. The literature concerned with the history of bureaucracy in France is sparse but fairly provocative, thanks in large part to the influence of Foucault. Guy Thuillier and Jean Tulard, *Histoire de l'administration française* (Paris, 1984); Guy Thuillier, *Bureaucratie et bureaucrates en France au XIXe siècle* (Geneva, 1980); Pierre Debofle, *L'Administration de Paris, 1789–1977* (Paris, 1979); Pierre Rosanvallon, *L'Etat en France de 1789 à nos jours* (Paris, 1990); Clive H. Church, *Revolution and Red Tape: The French Ministerial Bureaucracy, 1770–1850* (Oxford, 1981).

49. On reforms during the old regime, see Camille Bloch, *L'Assistance et l'état en France à la veille de la révolution* (Geneva, 1974), esp. book 2; Rosanvallon, *L'Etat en France*, 21–24, 61–62; Church, *Revolution and Red Tape*, 14–22. The classic study is, of course, Alexis de Tocqueville, *The Old Regime and the French Revolution*, trans. Stuart Gilbert (New York, 1955), which stresses the continuity between the periods before and after 1789.

50. Thuillier, *Bureaucratie et bureaucrates*, xi. Church contests the widely held view that Napoleon had such a large impact on the establishment of an administrative bureaucracy, arguing that the Directory went further in breaking with past recruitment and administrative practice, and that not until the July Monarchy did the structure become stable enough to be an important political force. Church, *Revolution and Red Tape*, 283.

51. Rosanvallon, *L'Etat en France*, 63.

52. On the culture of bureaucracy in France, see Thuillier and Tulard, *Histoire de l'administration*, 37–38; Rosanvallon, *L'Etat en France*, 51–55.

53. Thuillier and Tulard, *Histoire de l'administration*, 36. This figure includes Church functionaries.

54. Some examples of professional journals for administrators are: the *Bulletin administratif et judiciaire de la préfecture de police et de la ville de Paris* (begun in 1835), the *Bulletin officiel du ministère de l'Intérieur* (1838), and the *Revue administrative* (1839). At the same time, spoofs and outright attacks on bureaucratic efficiency began to appear in works such as Balzac's *L'Employé* (1837) and *Physiologie de l'employé* (1841), a further indication of bureaucracy's growing place in the Parisian popular imagination. List compiled by Rosanvallon, *L'Etat en France*, 58. The French term *bureaucratie* probably came into use at the time of the Revolution as a condemnation of any power that threatened to muffle the voice of the people. As the apparatus grew in prominence and weight, the critique shifted to one based on the cumbersome inefficiency of an entrenched institutional structure.

55. Church, *Revolution and Red Tape*, 215–20; Thuillier, *Bureaucratie et bureaucrates*, xiii.

56. The average wage of a Parisian worker during the first half of the nineteenth century was three francs a day, which amounts to approximately one thousand francs a year, while a low-level government employee made two to three thousand francs a year. Higher-level administrators earned even more: a *conseiller d'état* made twenty-five thousand; prefects, eight to twenty-four thousand; *chefs de division*, twelve thousand; and *chefs de bureau*, six thousand. Thuillier and Tulard, *Histoire de l'administration*, 20.

57. After the Revolution, the French administrative structure was essentially divided between *fonctionnaires*, who were elected, and *employés*, who were appointed. Under the Empire the election of *fonctionnaires* was abolished and was replaced by appointment. These people were considered much more political and earned a far better income than their *employé* counterparts, but their jobs were also more likely to be subject to the whims of changing political regimes. Apart from the prefects of police, most of the officials who documented the cholera epidemics were *employés*, a fact that created inevitable splits within the Parisian middle classes. On the distinction, see Thuillier and Tulard, *Histoire de l'administration*, 12; Thuillier, *Bureaucratie et bureaucrates*, x–xi; Church, *Revolution and Red Tape*, 286–93.

58. Reprinted in Thuillier, *Bureaucratie et bureaucrates*, 567.

59. The reality, of course, was often quite different, with employees complaining that they felt trapped in certain positions. Church, *Revolution and Red Tape*, 293; Thuillier and Tulard, *Histoire de l'administration*, 21–24, 39–47.

60. When Rosanvallon claims that "the state is not only an administrative apparatus, it is also an abstract political figure in the sense that it encapsulates the principle of sovereignty," he in fact underscores the idea that in France the state was philosophically conceived as being distinct from traditional party interests. Rosanvallon, *L'Etat en France*, 14; also see 139–40 for a discussion of philosophical considerations about the state. Max Weber established the terms of the debate in his classic essay, "Bureaucracy," in H. H. Gerth and C. Wright Mills, eds., *From Max Weber: Essays in Sociology* (New York, 1946), 196–244.

61. Louis Bergeron, *France under Napoleon*, trans. R. R. Palmer (Princeton, 1981), 52–62. It is significant that Napoleon made the claim to recruit personnel using objective criteria, even if actual practices fell short of this ideal.

62. Reprinted in Thuillier, *Bureaucratie et bureaucrates*, 567.

63. O'Brien, "Urban Growth and Public Order; Jean Tulard, *La Préfecture de police sous la monarchie de juillet.* . . . (Paris, 1964); Jacques Aubert, *L'Etat et la police en France, 1789–1914* (Geneva, 1979).

64. O'Brien, "Urban Growth and Public Order," 55.

65. Literary depictions of characters such as Hugo's rigid, literal-minded Javert in *Les Misérables* or the even more unflattering portraits of drunken, corrupt *sergeants de ville* by no means reassured respectable bourgeois Parisians that they were being fully protected, for until the second half of the century the police did not have a sound professional reputation. See O'Brien, "Urban Growth and Public Order," 5, 60–66.

66. Clarveau, quoted in Tulard, *La Préfecture de police*, 55.

67. Quoted in ibid., 56.

68. As proof of the significant administrative involvement of the police in both cholera epidemics, consider the fact that the bulk of the archival records about the outbreaks can be found in the Archives de la Préfecture de Police and in police documents contained in the Archives de Paris et du Département de la Seine, but very few records are in the Archives Nationales or the Archives de l'Assistance Publique.

69. On the city administrative structure during the July Monarchy, see Vigier, *Nouvelle histoire de Paris*, 125–57; Daumard, *Les Bourgeois de Paris*, 285–89.

70. Quoted in Tulard, *La Préfecture de police*, 40.

71. ADS VD^6 336, Arrêté du 20 August 1831.

72. ADS VD^4 3204, Epidémies, Préfecture de Police, Commission Centrale de Salubrité, "Instruction aux commissions d'arrondissements et de quartiers," 20 September 1831, 2.

73. ADS VD^6 336, Arrêté du 20 August 1831.

74. ADS VD^4 3204, Epidémies, Préfecture de Police, Commission Cen-

trale de Salubrité, "Instruction aux commissions d'arrondissements et de quartiers," 20 September 1831, 3.

75. *Journal des commissions sanitaires établies dans le département de la Seine contenant les travaux de ces commissions, les actes, décisions et instructions de l'administration qui leur sont relatifs*, published under the auspices of the Préfecture de Police, November 1831.

76. ADS VD⁴ 3204, Epidémies, Préfecture de Police, Commission Centrale de Salubrité, "Instruction aux commissions d'arrondissements et de quartiers," 20 September 1831, 2.

77. ADS VD⁶ 537 no. 1, Services Sanitaires, "Instruction de la Commission centrale de salubrité."

78. ADS VD⁶ 82 no. 1, Commissions Sanitaires, Préfecture de Police, to the members of the Commissions de Salubrité and to the mayors of the rural communes, 12 March 1832.

79. ADS VD⁶ 336, Arrêté du 20 August 1831.

80. Henri Boulay de la Meurthe, *Histoire du choléra-morbus dans le quartier du Luxembourg* (Paris, 1832), 4.

81. Poumiès de la Siboutie, *Souvenirs d'un médecin de Paris*, 235.

82. ADS VD⁴ 11, Hygiène publique, "Arrêté sur l'organisation de conseils d'hygiène publique et de salubrité," 18 December 1848.

83. "Une Correspondance," *L'Entracte*, 28 April 1832.

84. William M. Reddy, "Condottieri of the Pen: Journalists and the Public Sphere in Postrevolutionary France, 1815–1850," *American Historical Review* 99, no. 5 (December 1994): 1546–70; Theodore Zeldin, *France, 1848– 1945: Taste and Corruption* (Oxford, 1980), 144–63.

85. Because of space, the following narrative will appear somewhat schematic to anyone who specializes in the history of the French press. With a few notable exceptions, scholarship in the field is long on narrative and short on conceptualization. French studies have favored the multivolume approach, which stresses the battle for freedom between journalists and governments in which journalists emerge as business or political heroes. See, for example, Hatin, *Histoire politique et littéraire de la presse*; Bellanger et al., *Histoire générale de la presse*; René Livois, *Histoire de la presse française*, 2 vols. (Lausanne, 1965). The publisher Kiosque provided numerous small paperback volumes devoted specifically to the history of the press. In addition, Collins, *The Government and the Newspaper Press*, offers a concise, somewhat flat English version of the events. Despite increased critical awareness regarding the role of the press in the twentieth century, scholars have yet (to my knowledge) to write a truly critical history of the French press. In his *Structural Transformation*, Habermas explores the role of the press in a broad synthetic fashion, showing how the political and literary journalism once committed to the rational-critical thinking of the bourgeois public sphere eventually gave way to a press based on advertising, which ultimately destroys its political power, see esp. 181–95. Richard Terdiman, in *Discourse/Counter-Discourse: The Theory and Practice of Symbolic Resistance in Nineteenth-Century France* (Ithaca, 1985), devotes a chapter to "Newspa-

per Culture: Institution of Discourse; Discourse of Institutions." The chapter offers an intriguing look at the press as an artifact of the dominant bourgeois culture but without considering journalists' original oppositional (or "counter-discursive") stance, which profoundly influenced the nature of that domination. Scholars of American culture have been more attuned to this issue. See, for example, Michael Schudson, *Discovering the News* (New York, 1978), which raises the question of how objectivity became a goal in American journalistic practices over the course of the nineteenth century. I thank Roland Marchand for this reference, which has been invaluable in helping me think through the problem in France.

86. J.-P. Aguet, "Le Tirage des quotidiens de Paris sous la monarchie de juillet," *Schweizerische Zeitschrift für Geschichte* 10 (1960): 237; Bellanger et al., *Histoire générale de la presse*, vol. 2, 146; Allen, *In the Public Eye*, table A.3. When questioned by members of a parliamentary committee, the editors of Parisian newspapers estimated that it took eight thousand subscribers to keep a paper in business. Collins, *The Government and the Newspaper Press*, 72. For British figures, see Richard D. Altick, *The English Common Reader* (Chicago, 1957), 332–47.

87. Zeldin, *France, 1848–1945*, 146; Collins, *The Government and the Newspaper Press*, xi.

88. Allen, *In the Public Eye*, 65–68 and table A.7.

89. Quoted in Ledré, *La Presse à l'assaut de la monarchie*, 16.

90. Allen, *In the Public Eye*, 44–45. Allen makes a convincing case for the importance of a literary culture in France, particularly during the July Monarchy. He notes, for example, that most of the major publishing houses were founded between 1826 and 1851, 34.

91. *Physiologie de la presse: Biographie des journalistes et des journaux de Paris et de la province* (Paris, 1841), i–iii.

92. Muhammad As-Saffir, *Disorienting Encounters: Travels of a Moroccan Scholar in France in 1845–1846*, trans. Susan Gilson Miller (Berkeley and Los Angeles, 1992), 150–53.

93. The term and idea come from Benedict Anderson, *Imagined Communities: Reflections on the Origin and Spread of Nationalism* (London and New York, 1983), 74.

94. On print culture in the old regime, see Elizabeth Eisenstein, *The Printing Press as an Agent of Change: Communications and Cultural Transformations in Early-Modern Europe*, 2 vols. (Cambridge, 1979); Robert Darnton, *The Business of Enlightenment* (Cambridge, 1979); Jack R. Censer and Jeremy D. Popkin, eds., *Press and Politics in Pre-revolutionary France* (Berkeley and Los Angeles, 1987); Nina Rattner Gelbart, *Feminine and Opposition Journalism in Old Regime France: Le Journal des Dames* (Berkeley and Los Angeles, 1987).

95. Jeremy D. Popkin, *Revolutionary News: The Press in France, 1789–1977* (Durham and London, 1990); Hugh Gough, *The Newspaper Press in the French Revolution* (London, 1988). Figures are from Gough, 26.

96. Popkin, *Revolutionary News*, 170.

97. Ibid., 42, 78–82. Popkin points out that most revolutionary papers were not written to be read or heard aloud, readers could be unreliable, and a simple thing such as cold weather could prevent some impoverished readers from gaining access to the news, 81–82.

98. On the broader context of the relationship between government and the print trades, see Carla Hesse, *Publishing and Cultural Politics in Paris, 1789–1810* (Berkeley and Los Angeles, 1991).

99. Caution money for the Paris dailies during the first half of the nineteenth century ranged from six to ten thousand francs, approximately equivalent to twenty thousand U.S. dollars in 1989. Robert Justin Goldstein, *Political Censorship of the Arts and the Press in Nineteenth-Century Europe* (New York, 1989), 52–53.

100. Nettement, *Etudes critiques sur le feuilleton-roman*, vol. 2, 2.

101. Collingham, *The July Monarchy*, 173–74. Most standard histories of the French press, such as Hatin and Bellanger, discuss each newspaper almost solely in terms of its political affiliation. I suggest that scholars view the newspaper's role as "a flag" more critically because this perspective has made it too easy to treat two-dimensionally political discussions that took place at a time when the very idea of "politics" itself was undergoing much deeper changes.

102. Hesse, *Publishing and Cultural Politics*, 7.

103. Daniel L. Rader, *The Journalists and the July Revolution in France: The Role of the Political Press in the Overthrow of the Bourbon Restoration, 1827–1830* (The Hague, 1973), treats the subject in exhaustive chronological detail.

104. Quoted in Pilbeam, *The 1830 Revolution in France*, 60.

105. One journalist even had a special gift for designing strong barricades. Rader, *The Journalists and the July Revolution*, 237.

106. Ibid., 244–45; Collingham, *The July Monarchy*, 6–9; Ledré, *La Presse à l'assaut de la monarchie*, 116–23; Bellanger et al., *Histoire générale de la presse*, vol. 2, 99.

107. Collingham, *The July Monarchy*, 96. To get an idea of why Louis Philippe might have preferred *The Times*, see Cuno, "Charles Philipon and La Maison Aubert," 193–258, which discusses derogatory depictions of the king as a pear.

108. On the crackdown of 1835, see Ledré, *La Presse à l'assaut de la monarchie*, 150–75; Bellanger et al., *Histoire générale de la presse*, vol. 2, 111–14; Hatin, *Histoire politique et littéraire de la presse*, vol. 8, 563–69. Collins, *The Government and the Newspaper Press*, 82–85. On the ineffectiveness of François Guizot's press controls, see Collins, 99.

109. Bellanger et al., *Histoire générale de la presse*, vol. 2, 208–9.

110. A savvy publicist, Louis Napoleon used news stories, editorials, and other more blatant forms of advertising to create an image of himself as a man of the people as well as a defender of law and order. An interesting cultural history remains to be written of Louis Napoleon's election to power, in which the evolving modern press would play an important role. For a start, see Roger Price, *The French Second Republic: A Social History*

(London, 1972), 208–25. The silence of the Parisian press during the second outbreak will be taken up in the next chapter.

111. A mass press for the working classes would blossom only during the last quarter of the century. See Bellanger et al., *Histoire générale de la presse*, vol. 3; Zeldin, *France, 1848–1945*, 192–99.

112. Changes in scale and production capacity were already beginning to have an impact on publishing. Use of mechanical, steam-powered printing presses became increasingly widespread in Paris, and printing prices had declined considerably by the beginning of the July Monarchy, largely because France had begun to manufacture its own presses. At the same time, the desire to keep pace with the increasing number of readers generated by the expansion of suffrage in 1830 inspired ambitious entrepreneurs to broaden their use of steam power, to improve designs of parts such as rollers and paper feeders, as well as to develop cheaper ink and paper stock. By 1847 *La Presse* had dramatically increased its print runs by introducing a machine that printed simultaneously on both sides of the page. Bellanger et al., *Histoire générale de la presse*, vol. 2, 13–26.

113. On Girardin and his innovations, see Zeldin, *France, 1848–1945*, 146–49; Bellanger et al., *Histoire générale de la presse*, vol. 2, 113–33; Collins, *The Government and the Newspaper Press*, 88–91.

114. Reddy, "Condottieri of the Pen," 1556–70.

115. The decision to cut rates and rely on advertising is one of the great myths of modern journalism that needs to be explored more critically.

116. Nettement's *Etudes critiques sur le feuilleton-roman*, published in 1845, offered the first critical review of the genre. For information on where they appeared, see Bellanger et al., *Histoire générale de la presse*, vol. 2, 121–22. On the reception of Sue's *Les Mystères de Paris*, see Allen, *In the Public Eye*, 278–82. Throughout his study *Laboring Classes and Dangerous Classes*, Chevalier relies heavily on Sue's work to gauge the morbid fascination of the middle classes with the lives of the Parisian underworld.

117. Ledré, *La Presse à l'assaut de la monarchie*, 184–91; Collins, *The Government and the Newspaper Press*, 92–93.

118. Perhaps because of its apparent objectivity, the *Moniteur universel* has not inspired the same passionate biographies as other French newspapers published during the nineteenth century. In his *Bibliographie historique et critique de la presse périodique française* (Paris, 1866), 126, Eugène Hatin offers incorrect information. A better starting point might be the brief discussion in Bellanger et al., *Histoire générale de la presse*, vol. 1, 487–89.

119. Quoted in Hatin, *Bibliographie de la presse*, 125.

120. The *Moniteur* would continue in its capacity as official government organ into the twentieth century, while remaining under private ownership at least until 1866.

121. *Physiologie de la presse*, 1.

122. Victor Hugo, *Notre-Dame de Paris* (1836; Paris, 1959), 224. I thank Carla Hesse for this reference.

123. Most of the approximately two thousand copies of the *Moniteur* went to government employees free of charge. Collingham, *The July Monarchy,* 179.

124. Ibid., 169.

125. Zeldin points out that by the 1830s newspapers were in fact made up exclusively of several levels of advertisements because the contemporary ideal was to have virtually every column inch—from news stories to editorials to actual ads—paid for by some outside source. *France, 1848–1945,* 163–65.

126. Compiled from a list provided by Hatin, *Bibliographie de la presse,* 576–83. Of the 142 medical journals he lists from the old regime that were published through 1865, nearly half were begun in the period 1825–50. A fascinating study remains to be written on the role and development of the medical press as a genre. As a starting point, see Achille Chereau, "Essais sur l'origine du journalisme médical français," *L'Union médicale,* series that appeared in 1867, and Léonard, *La Médecine entre les pouvoirs,* 195–200.

127. Léonard, *La Médecine entre les pouvoirs,* 195–96, points out that some scholars have blamed the testy medical press for creating a kind of Balkanization within the profession by airing its dirty laundry in public and formalizing debates. I would argue that divisions within a profession suggest that it is sufficiently established to survive.

128. I am making this assumption based on the low circulation figures for papers generally. Even a general-interest paper such as the *Journal des débats* had under seven thousand *abonnements* in 1847. J.-P. Aguet, "Le Tirage," 216–86.

129. Hatin, *Bibliographie de la presse.*

130. Pinkney, *Decisive Years in France,* 75; Weisz, "The Politics of Medical Professionalization," 3–30.

131. *Gazette médicale de Paris,* 31 March 1832.

CHAPTER 3. INVENTING PERCEPTIONS OF DISEASE AND GOVERNMENT

1. ADS VD^4 3381, Département de la Seine, Commission Centrale de Salubrité, "Instruction populaire sur les principaux moyens à employer pour se garantir du choléra-morbus et sur la conduite à tenir lorsque cette maladie se déclare," 15 November 1831. Hereafter referred to as "Instruction, 1832."

2. *Moniteur,* 30 March 1832, 1.

3. Gisquet, *Mémoires de M. Gisquet,* vol. 1, 428; emphasis added.

4. "Instruction, 1832," 13.

5. Ibid., 14.

6. Ackerknecht, *Medicine at the Paris Hospital,* 129–38.

7. For examples of cholera cures hawked in the pages of the popular press, see *Le Journal des débats, La Quotidienne,* and *Le National* for the first two weeks of April 1832.

8. See, for example, the *istruzioni* reprinted in Carlo Cipolla's *Cristofano and the Plague: A Study in the History of Public Health in the Age of Galileo* (Berkeley, 1973), 166–70.

9. "Instruction, 1832," 9–10.

10. Red hot stones or bricks are placed under a chair along with a basin of water mixed with vinegar and camphor; the patient then sits on the chair surrounded by woolen sheets, which create a vaporous effect. Ibid., 11–13; all emphases in text.

11. Ibid., 6–8.

12. William Coleman, "Health and Hygiene in the *Encyclopédie*: A Medical Doctrine for the Bourgeoisie," *Journal of the History of Medicine and Allied Sciences* 29, no. 4 (October 1974): 399–421.

13. Blanc, ever vigilant regarding slights to the lower classes, noted that the *instruction* provided "recommendations that were probably wise but derisive for that portion of the people for whom unrighteous civilization portions out bread, shelter, clothing, and rest so sparingly." Blanc, *Histoire de dix ans,* vol. 3, 201.

14. "Instruction, 1832," 4.

15. Ibid., 4–5.

16. Rosenberg, *The Cholera Years*; also see Alan M. Kraut, *Silent Travelers: Germs, Genes, and the "Immigrant Menace"* (New York, 1994), 31–49. I thank James McCartin and Clarence Walker for reference to this book.

17. "Instruction, 1832," 8–9. Instead, it suggested substituting for the *eau de vie ordinaire* white wine or even bitters such as absinthe. In fact, "wine, in moderate quantities, is an appropriate *[convenable]* beverage for during and after a meal; but it must be of good quality. It would be better to drink half as much wine and to choose one of superior quality. Young and bitter wines are more dangerous than useful. Red wine is preferable to white. Those who have the means of mixing in bubbly water such as Seltzer water would do well to take advantage of this healthy and agreeable beverage."

18. "Instruction, 1832," 13.

19. Goubert, *The Conquest of Water*, 34–67. Reid, *Paris Sewers and Paris Sewermen*, 9–17.

20. "Instruction, 1832," 5. These ideas also came from "the doctrine of the non-naturals," a modernization of the ancient balance of elements that governed the functioning of all things in the universe. See Coleman, "Health and Hygiene in the *Encyclopédie*," 399–421.

21. "Instruction, 1832," 2.

22. Ibid., 3–4.

23. One word about the measures taken to publicize the *instruction*: unlike the case in 1832, several different versions appeared; although they all were based on the pamphlet discussed below, the offshoots seemed to be shorter, often appearing in an easy-to-read poster format. See, for example, ADS VI[5] no. 3, Hygiène et Travaux Publics, Préfecture de Police, "Avis," 6 June 1849. The National Academy of Medicine also released a much more detailed *instruction* that could be purchased for fifty centimes but generally

was not in wide circulation. For this analysis I have limited myself to the measures most widely publicized by the government in each epidemic. ADS VD⁶ 274 no. 5, Commissions Sanitaires, "Préfet de police, April 1849," hereafter "Instruction, 1849."

24. Significantly, the pamphlet did not mention Paris, where such improvements never advanced beyond the rhetoric used in political debates during the July Monarchy.

25. "Instruction, 1849," 2–3.

26. Ibid., 3–4.

27. *Moniteur*, 11 April 1849.

28. "Instruction, 1849," 3.

29. Ibid., 7–8.

30. Ibid., 5–6. In a footnote, the *instruction* refers interested readers to a more detailed pamphlet that describes provisions of the ordinance of November 30, 1848, concerning the cleanliness of dwellings.

31. Métral, *Description*, 39.

32. Trolliet, Polinière, and Bottex, *Rapport*, 48.

33. ADS VD⁶ 82 no. 1, Commissions Sanitaires, "Rapports de la commission chargée d'organiser le matériel et d'indiquer le personnel des bureaux de secours," 19 November 1831.

34. The prefect of police estimated that more than a thousand people worked in the city's medical stations. In addition to the unpaid doctors and pharmacists who had been drafted by the *commissions sanitaires* in each arrondissement, a large number of other volunteers, doctor's aides, medical students (who received one hundred francs a month and in some cases more) as well as paid stretcher bearers, custodians, and messengers manned the stations. See Gisquet, *Mémoires de M. Gisquet,* vol. 1, 430.

35. ADS VI⁵ 1 no. 7, daily log of the Bureau de Secours, Séminaire St. Sulpice, M. Boulay de la Meurthe to the mayor of the eleventh arrondissement, 2 April–12 May 1832, hereafter "Daily Log."

36. Magendie, *Leçons sur le choléra-morbus*, 235.

37. See, for example, the letter to the editor in *Le Courrier français,* 2 April 1832, 4, in which several doctors complained about the bad food during their service.

38. "Daily Log," 13 April 1832; emphasis in original.

39. *Gazette des hôpitaux civils et militaires,* 3 May 1832, 3.

40. ADS VD⁴ 3431, Epidémies, Préfecture de Police, "Etablissement d'un agent comptable dans chaque bureau de secours," 19 April 1832. This was the official, published announcement, but rumors had circulated about the accountants at least since April 13. See "Daily Log," 14 April 1832.

41. "Daily Log," 14 April 1832.

42. "Daily Log," 18 April 1832.

43. *Archives parlementaires: Recueil complet des débats législatifs de 1787 à 1860,* Paris, 2d series, vol. 77, 12 April 1832, 505–6.

44. ADS VI⁵ 1 no. 5, Choléra, "Arrêté de la préfecture de police aux maires des 12 arrondissements municipaux," 20 April 1832.

45. Poumiès de la Siboutie, *Souvenirs d'un médecin de Paris*, 239.

46. ADS VD⁶ 274 no. 5, Commissions Sanitaires, "Ordonnance concernant l'organisation des commissions de salubrité et des bureaux de secours," 13 May 1849.

47. Ibid.

48. ADS VI⁵ 1 no. 3, Choléra, Préfecture de Police to the mayor of the fourth arrondissement, 5 June 1849.

49. ADS VD⁶ 537 no. 5, Epidémies cholériques.

50. On the conference, see Weisz, "The Politics of Medical Professionalization," 3–30.

51. *L'Union médicale*, vol. 3, no. 69 (9 June 1849): 274.

52. E. A. Duchesne, *Histoire statistique du choléra-morbus dans le XI⁵ arrondissement de Paris* (Paris, 1851), 9.

53. Anaïs de Baucon Bazin, *L'Epoque sans nom: Esquisses de Paris*, vol. 2 (Paris, 1833), 266–67.

54. Before the cholera epidemic, the French press used tables to present qualitative data on trade and votes in the assembly, but these tables did not quantify an ongoing part of daily life in the same way as the *bulletins du choléra*. Moreover, such tables were much more common in the *Moniteur universel* as the official organ than they were in more popular papers such as the *Journal des débats, La Quotidienne*, and *Le National*.

55. Joshua Cole, "The Chaos of Particular Facts: Statistics, Medicine, and the Social Body in Early Nineteenth-Century France," *History of the Human Sciences* 7, no. 3 (1994): 1–27.

56. *Le Corsaire*, 4 April 1832.

57. *Le Globe*, 1 April 1832.

58. *L'Entracte*, 4 April 1832.

59. *Le National*, 2 April 1832.

60. *La Révolution*, reprinted in *La Quotidienne*, 3 April 1832.

61. *Le Bonhomme Richard*, 16 April 1832.

62. *Rapport sur la marche et les effets du choléra-morbus*, 43–44.

63. ADS VD⁶ 274, VD⁶ 354, VD⁶ 361, VD⁶ 537, VD⁶ 669, VD⁶ 689, VI⁵ 1.

64. *Journal des débats*, 30 March 1832.

65. *Le National*, 31 March 1832.

66. *Moniteur*, 9 April 1832.

67. See, for example, the Saint-Simonian paper, *Le Globe*, 1 April 1832.

68. Blanc, *Histoire de dix ans*, vol. 3, 202.

69. *Moniteur*, 2 April 1832.

70. *Moniteur*, 5 April 1832.

71. See, for example, *ibid.*, 14 May 1832.

72. *Le Corsaire*, 16 June 1832.

73. *Le Corsaire*, 22 June 1832.

74. Bazin, *L'Epoque sans nom*, vol. 2, 267.

75. *Moniteur*, 18 April 1832.

76. *Moniteur*, 22 March 1849.

77. See, for example, accounts on 28 March 1849, 29 March 1849, and 31 March 1849.

78. *L'Union médicale*, 13 March 1849, 121.

79. *L'Union médicale*, 15 May 1849, 231.

80. *Gazette médicale de Paris*, 19 May 1849, 375.

81. *Gazette des hôpitaux*, 26 June 1849. This move was somewhat arrogant, given the fact that the paper had been in the throes of a controversy with editors of *L'Union médicale*, who had criticized the *Gazette's* lack of accuracy and large number of typographical errors.

82. *L'Union médicale*, 15 May 1849, 231.

83. *Gazette des hôpitaux*, 3 April 1849.

84. Paul Caffe, *Notice sur le choléra* (Paris, 1849), 2–3.

85. Ibid.

86. For example, the medical press attempted to make up for the official silence by providing its own statistics with a rigor that challenged that of newspapers during the first outbreak, sometimes using the identical vocabulary of the political papers in 1832. On March 17, the day before officials declared the second epidemic, for example, the *Gazette médicale de Paris* promised its readers "a recapitulation as detailed as possible." The editors' main goal was to "furnish facts sufficient in number and detail for science and medicine, enabling a rigorous comparison between the current epidemic and that of 1832." Accordingly, the paper listed detailed points that it hoped to publish about as many patients as possible. *Gazette médicale de Paris*, 17 March 1849, 202.

87. *L'Union médicale*, 14 June 1849.

88. *Le Journal du peuple*, 18 July 1849.

89. *Journal des débats*, 8 June 1849. The *Moniteur universel* complained that the public imagination exaggerated figures, 8 June 1849 and 9 June 1849.

CHAPTER 4. CATHOLICISM AND CHOLERA

1. Even in more recent studies of cholera epidemics, religion either is ignored or assumes a predictable and unquestioned conservative role. Most scholarship follows Rosenberg's contention that religious ideas yielded to the secular influence of hygienists, an evaluation that may be more applicable to the United States than to nineteenth-century France. See Rosenberg, *The Cholera Years*.

2. Little work has been done on bourgeois piety during the first half of the nineteenth century. For this discussion I have relied upon Daumard, *Les Bourgeois de Paris*, 178–80, 326–27; René Rémond, *L'Anticléricalisme en France de 1815 à nos jours* (Paris, 1976), 64–66; Ralph Gibson, *A Social History of French Catholicism, 1789–1914* (London, 1989), 13–15, 195–200.

3. Yves Hilaire and Gérard Cholvy, eds., *Histoire religieuse de la France contemporaine*, 3 vols. (Paris, 1985–88); Adrien Dansette, *Histoire religieuse de la France contemporaine: L'Eglise catholique dans la mêlée politique et sociale* (Paris, 1961); François Lebrun, ed., *Histoire des catholiques en France du XVe*

siècle à nos jours (Toulouse, 1980); Philip Spencer, *The Politics of Belief in Nineteenth-Century France: Lacordaire, Michon, Veuillot* (New York, 1954).

4. I am well aware that the above narrative is somewhat schematic, but, given the constant changes in the social and political position of the Church after the Revolution, it proves difficult to pinpoint its influence on the development of the French state. Moreover, even at the institutional level, the Catholic Church meant many things to many people, a fact that makes it difficult to speak of Catholicism in any monolithic way. Finally, a word about sources. Because many Church records either were destroyed by the Commune fire in 1871 or were lost in the subsequent consolidation of parish records, I have been forced to rely heavily on official documentation such as *mandements* and newspapers. These sources have no doubt shaped my predominantly institutional approach to the problems of religious and secular culture.

5. For an excellent discussion of this complexity during an earlier period, see Suzanne Desan, *Reclaiming the Sacred: Lay Religion and Popular Politics in Revolutionary France* (Ithaca and London, 1990).

6. Chateaubriand, *Mémoires*, vol. 4, 62–63.

7. Paul Caffe, *Paris vue dans ses causes* (Paris, 1835), 6.

8. *Mémorial catholique* quoted in Paul Christophe, *Les Choix du clergé dans les révolutions de 1789, 1830 et 1848*, vol. 2 (Lille, 1976), 41.

9. Felix Pyat, "Les Cultes," in *Nouveau tableau de Paris au XIXᵉ siècle*, vol. 6 (Paris, 1834–35), 1.

10. The archbishop of Sens, quoted in Bourdelais and Raulot, *Une Peur bleue*, 193.

11. Bellemare, *Le Fléau de Dieu*.

12. Exodus 8: 1–13; Bellemare, *Le Fléau de Dieu*, 35.

13. Shortly after the publication of *Le Fléau de Dieu* at the end of April, *La Quotidienne* called the book "a most remarkable writing on choleramorbus" and reprinted lengthy excerpts. *La Quotidienne*, 4 May 1832. Meanwhile, *L'Ami de la religion* printed a long review praising the book's intelligence and courage. "The author's reflections, always solemn and solid," the review proclaimed, "are most developed in the firmest and frankly Christian language." *L'Ami de la religion*, 3 May 1832.

14. *L'Ami de la religion*, 7 April 1832; II Chronicles 12.

15. Roch, *Paris malade*, vol. 1, 260.

16. François René Chateaubriand, "Courtes explications sur les 12,000 francs offerts par Mme la duchesse de Berry aux indigents attaqués de la contagion" (Paris, 1832), 42–43, Bibliothèque Historique de la Ville de Paris.

17. *La Quotidienne*, 5 April 1832.

18. *L'Ami de la religion*, 14 April 1832.

19. Hugues de Changy, *Le Soulèvement de la duchesse de Berry, 1832* (Paris, 1986), 82–100; Rémond, *L'Anticléricalisme en France*, 64–66.

20. Christophe, *Les Choix du clergé*, vol. 2, 88. Moreover, fears of a Catholic conspiracy linked to freemasonry persisted from the final years of the Restoration. Rémond, *The Right-Wing in France*, 74–75.

21. Figures compiled by Sussman, "From Yellow Fever to Cholera," 261.

22. *Le Corsaire*, 4 April 1832.

23. Letter to the editor in *Le National*, 18 April 1832.

24. Roch, *Paris malade*, vol. 1, 403.

25. AA 1D IV 10 no. 9, Gisquet to Quélen, 31 March 1832.

26. AA 1D IV 10 no. 12, chief of the Bureau Sanitaire de la Préfecture de Police to Archbishop Quélen, 1 April 1832.

27. Spencer, *The Politics of Belief in Nineteenth-Century France*, 30.

28. *La Quotidienne*, 17 April 1832, 4.

29. *Le Corsaire*, 7 May 1832.

30. I thank Herbert Sloan for bringing this point to my attention.

31. Deville, *Histoire médicale du choléra-morbus*, 20–21.

32. *Rapport sur la marche et les effets du choléra-morbus*, 141.

33. *Le Corsaire*, 28 April 1832.

34. Archbishop Quélen, *Mandement* #109831, 30 March 1832, Bibliothèque Historique de la Ville de Paris.

35. Archbishop Quélen, *Mandement* #109832, 18 April 1832, Bibliothèque Historique de la Ville de Paris.

36. Ibid.

37. J. Gerlitt, "The Development of Quarantine," *Ciba Symposia* 2 (1940): 566–80; David Musto, "Quarantine and the Problem of AIDS," in *AIDS: The Burdens of History*, ed. Elizabeth Fee and David Fox (Berkeley and Los Angeles, 1988), 67–84. The term *quarantaine* is also invested with a highly charged (if unconscious) social significance, for at the time of the first epidemic it loosely referred to the period of time that had elapsed between the revolutions in 1789 and 1830.

38. Ramsey, *Professional and Popular Medicine*.

39. Goldstein, *Console and Classify*, ch. 3.

40. *Gazette des hôpitaux*, 12 June 1832.

41. *Gazette médicale de Paris*, 12 June 1832.

42. Bazin, *Epoque sans nom*, vol. 2, 264–66.

43. For a discussion of the budget of the first epidemic, see Sussman, "From Yellow Fever to Cholera," 238–39, and Gisquet, *Mémoires de M. Gisquet*, vol. 1, 451–53.

44. Jones, *Charity and Bienfaisance*, esp. parts 3 and 4; Olwen Hufton, *The Poor of Eighteenth-Century France* (Oxford, 1974), 131–93; Norberg, *Rich and Poor in Grenoble*, esp. part 3; Christophe, *Les Choix du clergé*, vol. 2, 24–44.

45. Pierre Marie Bondy, quoted in Chateaubriand, *Mémoires*, vol. 4, 68.

46. Ibid.

47. ADS VD⁶ 82 no. 1, "Bureaux de secours, 1832," prefecture of the Seine to the mayor of the first arrondissement, 20 April 1832.

48. Chateaubriand, *Mémoires*, vol. 4, 74.

49. *Le Bonhomme Richard*, 19 April 1832.

50. *Journal de Paris*, quoted in *La Quotidienne*, 19 April 1832.

51. *Le Bonhomme Richard*, 20 April 1832, 2.

52. Blanc, *Histoire de dix ans,* vol. 3, 212; Apponyi, *Vingt-cinq ans à Paris,* vol. 2, 178.

53. Quoted in *Le Corsaire,* 2 May 1832.

54. *Le National,* 27 April 1832.

55. *La Quotidienne,* 19 April 1832.

56. Reprinted in *Le Bonhomme Richard,* 5 May 1832. The same letter also appeared in *La Quotidienne* with an editor's introduction explaining that "normally a somewhat serious journal, in this instance *Le Courrier* has been the victim of a hoax."

57. Chateaubriand, "Courtes explications." Unfortunately, there is no way of knowing whether Chateaubriand truly believed his own story or whether he simply wrote the pamphlet to soothe public opinion.

58. Ibid., 14–15.

59. Ibid., 13.

60. Ibid., 15.

61. Changy, *Le Soulèvement.*

62. *La Quotidienne,* 5 April 1832, 1.

63. *L'Ami de la religion,* 5 April 1832, 441.

64. Letter to the editor from the prefect of the Seine, *La Quotidienne,* 6 April 1832.

65. Both newspapers and archives are filled with records of charitable donations. On April 19, for example, the head administrator of the Halles aux Grains, Farines et de la Boulangerie wrote to the prefecture of police announcing subscriptions collected on behalf of cholera patients. APP D/A 134, "Choléra, 1832."

66. *Moniteur,* 2 April 1832.

67. "La Corbeille des noces," *Le Bonhomme Richard,* 12 April 1832.

68. *La Quotidienne,* a staunch defender of Chateaubriand's contribution, for example, immediately questioned the political nature of the royal family's own donations as well as the whole system of relief being put into place by the administration. *La Quotidienne,* 20 April 1832, 1–2.

69. François Isambert, "L'Attitude religieuse des ouvriers français au milieu du XIXe siècle," *Archives de la sociologie des religions* 6 (July-December 1958): 7.

70. Edward Berenson, *Populist Religion and Left-Wing Politics in France, 1830–1852* (Princeton, 1984); Christophe, *Les Choix du clergé,* vol. 2; Marcel Dion, *Etat, église et luttes populaires* (Paris, 1980); Jean Baptiste Duroselle, *Les Débuts du catholicisme social en France, 1822–1870* (Paris, 1951); Isambert, "L'Attitude religieuse des ouvriers"; François Isambert, *Christianisme et classe ouvrière: Jalons pour une étude de sociologie historique* (Paris, 1961); Pierre Pierrard, *L'Eglise en France face aux crises révolutionnaires: 1789–1871* (Lyon, 1974); Pierre Pierrard, *L'Eglise et les ouvriers en France, 1840–1940* (Paris, 1984); Pierre Pierrard, *1848: Les Pauvres, l'évangile et la révolution* (Paris, 1977); Paul Thureau-Dangin, *L'Eglise et l'état sous la monarchie de juillet* (Paris, 1880).

71. I thank Edward Berenson for calling my attention to this issue. See his "A New Religion of the Left: Christianity and Social Radicalism in France, 1815–1848," in *The Transformation of Political Culture, 1789–1848,* edited by François Furet and Mona Ozouf, vol. 3 of *The French Revolution and the Creation of Modern Political Culture,* ed. Keith Michael Baker (Oxford, 1989).

72. Quoted in Gibson, *A Social History of French Catholicism,* 200.

73. The disputes over the changing attitude toward religion during the July Monarchy begin at the most fundamental level of how the change was defined. Tocqueville, for example, perceived it as early as 1835 but saw it more in terms of declining anticlericalism than as a positive rise in religious fervor or the product of a Catholic revival; quoted in Thureau-Dangin, *L'Eglise et l'état,* 13.

74. Ibid., 15.

75. Ibid., 56; Christophe, *Les Choix du clergé,* vol. 2, 84.

76. Collingham, *The July Monarchy,* 385–415.

77. This is Berenson's term. Berenson, "A New Religion of the Left."

78. Hufton, *The Poor of Eighteenth-Century France,* 3; Pierrard, *1848,* 211–12.

79. L'abbé F. Roy, quoted in Christophe, *Les Choix du clergé,* vol. 2, 34.

80. These potential alliances will be discussed in Chapter 5.

81. Pierrard, *1848,* 180.

82. See Berenson's discussion of the July Monarchy in *Populist Religion,* 36–73. Although his study concerns rural France, limited evidence suggests similar mechanisms at work in Paris.

83. Pierrard, *1848,* 177.

84. J. Brugerette, *Le Prêtre français et la société contemporaine* (Paris, 1933), vol. 1, 142; Pierrard, *1848,* 185.

85. Reprinted in Yvan Daniel, ed., *La Religion est perdue à Paris; lettres d'un vicaire parisien à son archevêque en date de 1849* (Paris, 1978), 32.

86. *La Démocratie pacifique,* 9 June 1849, 4.

87. Unfortunately, neither reliable nor impressionistic figures exist to provide a concrete measure of church attendance at the time of either epidemic.

88. *L'Union,* 7 April 1849, 3.

89. L. F. Guérin, *Le Dévouement catholique pendant le choléra de 1849,* vol. 1 (Lille, 1852), 10.

90. *La Bonne Foi,* 13 June 1849, 3; *L'Union,* 13 June 1849, 4; *Moniteur universel,* 13 June 1849.

91. *La Démocratie pacifique,* 13 June 1849, 3.

92. *L'Opinion publique,* 11 June 1849, 2.

93. The constitution of the Second Republic explicitly stated that the French government should aid revolutionary movements elsewhere in Europe. When Bonaparte ordered French troops to fight with the Pope against the nationalist forces in Rome, it prompted groups on the left to declare that the constitution had been violated. These groups called upon the peo-

ple of Paris to revolt—coincidentally just at the moment when the second cholera epidemic reached its peak, prompting the insurrection of June 13. See Chapter 5, pp. 202–3.

94. AN F^{19} 6434, "Cultes," Frédéric Falloux to the bishops of France, 28 April 1849.

95. Marie-Dominique-Auguste Sibour, *Mandements, lettres et instructions pastorales* (Paris, 1856), letter of 2 May 1849, 75.

96. The Church and government did not enjoy flawless cooperation however. The two battled much as they had in 1832 over the issue of cholera orphans, for example. In a bishop's letter, Sibour took the government to task for false reports in the press that exaggerated the city administration's success in finding homes, especially for boys. Despite all its impressive talk, the city had managed to place only one hundred while the Church could claim four hundred; Sibour, *Mandements*, letter of 10 September 1849, 95–97.

97. *La Bonne Foi*, 31 May 1849, 3.

98. AA 1D VI 1, "Lettre de monseigneur l'archevêque de Paris et Réglement pour l'association générale de charité," Paris, 1849.

99. *Gazette médicale de Paris*, 30 June 1849, 425.

100. Société des Traités Religieux de Paris, *Instructions à la portée de tout le monde sur le choléra-morbus* (Paris, 1849).

101. Ibid.

102. *L'Union médicale*, 9 June 1849, 274.

103. *L'Union médicale*, 14 June 1849, 282.

104. *Gazette des hôpitaux*, 22 May 1849, 3.

105. *Rapport sur les épidémies cholériques*, 159.

106. *Le Journal du peuple*, 17 June 1849, 1.

107. *Le Journal du peuple*, 24 June 1849, 1.

CHAPTER 5. DISEASE AND SOCIAL UNREST

1. *Le Crédit*, 11 June 1849, 2.

2. Sussman offers a detailed analysis of the disturbances in each location, concluding that they were inspired mostly by outside political agitators. While this may have been true, the provocateurs would have had little or no success if underlying tensions had not already existed. Sussman, "From Yellow Fever to Cholera," 294–303. *Gazette des tribunaux*, 2 and 3 April 1832, 1; Gisquet, *Mémoires de M. Gisquet*, vol. 1, 469–70.

3. The secondary literature is surprisingly sparse. Alain Faure, "Classe malpropre, classe dangereuse? Quelques remarques à propos des chiffonniers parisiens au XIXe siècle et leurs cités," *Recherches* 29 (1978): 79–102; Ratcliffe, "Perception and Realities of the Urban Margin," 198–233, argues that the portrait created by elite Parisians served "less to reveal rag pickers than to reinforce the identity of the centre, to explain away differences and inequalities, to impose an identity and personal responsibility on those deemed marginal," 233. In taking on "elite discourse," he did not take up the particular "bourgeois" component of the problem. John M. Merri-

man considers related theoretical issues in his study *The Margins of City Life: Explorations on the French Urban Frontier, 1815–1851* (New York, 1991).

4. The ranks of *chiffonniers*, for example, contained an especially large number of older workers who had presumably been forced into retirement. Faure, "Classe malpropre," 84–85.

5. Fanfan Lallumette, "Protestation adressée par les chiffonniers de Paris à M. Gisquet, préfet de police" (Paris, 1832), 5, Bibliothèque Nationale. This is a strange little document allegedly written by an extremely articulate ragpicker who had the presence of mind to anticipate that readers might find his eloquence suspect. Formerly a clerk to a *notaire,* Lallumette apparently found himself on the streets after his employer went bankrupt. The name, the author's gross exaggeration of the number of signatures he could have obtained from ragpickers, the absence of the signatures, as well as the very fact of the pamphlet's publication (which Lallumette clearly tried to market), all make the document interesting yet problematic as the voice of a ragpicker.

6. Heine, *Saemtliche Werke,* vol. 6, 181.

7. William Pitt Byrne, *Realities of Paris Life: Paris and the Parisians,* vol. 1 (London, 1859), 302.

8. H. A. Frégier, *Des Classes dangereuses de la population dans les grandes villes et des moyens de les rendre meilleures,* vol. 1 (Paris, 1840), 104–10.

9. APP D/A 122, "Choléra, 1832," Affiche, 2 April 1832.

10. Lallumette, "Protestation adressée par les chiffonniers," 5.

11. Ratcliffe cites examples of bourgeois Parisians collecting knick-knacks, such as mantelpiece clocks and candelabra, depicting ragpickers. "Perception and Realities of the Urban Margin," 206.

12. Though it would be impossible to arrive at an accurate figure, contemporary estimates placed the number of ragpickers between two thousand and six thousand men, women, and children. Frégier suggested eighteen hundred in his *Classes dangereuses,* vol. 1, 105, while Métral placed the figure between five thousand and six thousand in *Description,* 24. Chevalier estimated eighteen hundred in *Le Choléra,* 21, while Ratcliffe projected twenty-two hundred actual ragpickers supporting some nine thousand dependents in "Perception and Realities of the Urban Margin," 216. While written after the first cholera epidemic, several literary accounts recapture the world of the *chiffonniers.* Throughout the nineteenth century a tension existed within this literary tradition. Counterbalancing the stories of *chiffonniers* as threatening transgressors, there was always a moralizing streak that made them "the salt of the earth" or fallen aristocrats lured by the freedom of being outside social restraints. See, for example, Félix Pyat's *Le Chiffonnier de Paris* (Paris, 1847), which was rewritten several times over the course of the century and which subsequently appeared as a silent movie under the same title in 1929. Peter Petrov, *Les Chiffonniers de la Butte aux Cailles* (Paris, 1983), reprints a Russian traveler's glorification of the ragpicker as the true proletarian in the 1870s. Ragpickers also have prominent roles in Eugène Sue, *Les Mystères de Paris* (Paris, 1842); Eugène Sue, *Le*

Juif errant (Paris, 1844). Also, the famous caricaturist Honoré Daumier made several noted drawings. For an analysis of the literary tradition, see Faure, "Classe malpropre," 86–90.

13. Moreau, *Histoire statistique du choléra-morbus*, 2.

14. Quoted in Chevalier, *Le Choléra*, 21.

15. For a related, intriguing theoretical discussion of cultural boundaries between the middle and lower classes, primarily in England, see Stallybrass and White, *The Politics and Poetics of Transgression*, 125–48.

16. Métral, *Description*, 24.

17. Byrne, *Realities of Paris Life*, vol. 1, 300.

18. For a discussion of the history of this obsession with sexual difference, see Thomas Laqueur, *Making Sex: Body and Gender from the Greeks to Freud* (Cambridge, 1990); Foucault, *History of Sexuality*; Michel Foucault, *Herculine Barbin, Being the Recently Discovered Memoirs of a Nineteenth-Century French Hermaphrodite*, trans. Richard McDougall (New York, 1980). The major nineteenth-century French text was published only in 1874 by Ambroise Tardieu, *Questions médico-légales de l'identité dans les rapports avec les vices de conformation des organes sexuels* (Paris, 1874).

19. Frégier, *Des Classes dangereuses*, vol. 1, 107. "It is [within a single room] that [the ragpickers] put the filthy product they seek; it is here that they do the sorting, amidst, and with the help of, their children." Over the course of the century, the ragpickers were housed in *cités* on the periphery of the city, which inspired further critiques. For a description of the new dwellings and how *chiffonniers* lived in them, see Faure, "Classe malpropre," 95–98.

20. Frégier, *Des Classes dangereuses*, vol. 1, 105.

21. Roger-Henri Guerrand, "Private Spaces," in *A History of Private Life: From the Fires of Revolution to the Great War*, ed. Michelle Perrot, trans. (Cambridge, 1990), esp. 359–69.

22. Byrne, *Realities of Paris Life*, vol. 1, 306.

23. I have taken some liberties in this translation based on the context in which it appeared. Explaining the three shifts when the ragpickers could collect garbage, Frégier notes: "Le chiffonnier adulte . . . est obligé de faire communément trois rondes, deux de jour, et une de nuit; les deux premières ont lieu de cinq heures du matin à neuf heures, et de onze heures à trois heures, et la troisième, dans la soirée, de cinq à onze heures et quelquefois minuit. Le chiffonnier déjeune à neuf heures et dine à trois heures." Frégier, *Des Classes dangereuses*, vol. 1, 105.

24. Anne Martin-Furgier, "Bourgeois Rituals," in *A History of Private Life: From the Fires of Revolution to the Great War*, ed. Michelle Perrot, trans. (Cambridge, 1990), esp. 268–77. Martin-Furgier dates the earliest manuals to the 1820s and links them to urbanization, 268. Intriguing connections exist between the hygienists' exploration and understanding of lower-class domestic space, on the one hand, and the manuals published for members of the middle classes on the other.

25. This ordinance was the third major attempt to regulate the "profession" since the late seventeenth century. See APP DB 194, police ordinances of 9 August 1698, 10 June 1701, and 6 February 1756. It is important to note that none of the earlier ordinances seemed quite as preoccupied with establishing such systematic conformity.

26. APP DB 194, *Chiffonniers*, ordinance from the prefect of police, 1 September 1828, art. 4.

27. Ibid., preamble.

28. Frégier, *Des Classes dangereuses*, vol. 1, 108.

29. Chevalier, *Laboring Classes and Dangerous Classes*, 181–85; Chevalier, *La Formation de la population parisienne*, 45–50. Between the two books, Chevalier shows how the population of the capital increased dramatically during the first half of the nineteenth century, while the percentage of nonnative Parisians remained fairly constant, between 50 and 60 percent; even so, contemporaries *perceived* a sizable gain in the number of immigrants. The Paris population was 546,856 in 1801, 785,866 in 1831, and 1,053,897 in 1846. Chevalier, *Laboring Classes and Dangerous Classes*, 182.

30. By the early twentieth century both sides would be most conscious of the *opposition*. "Questions of hygiene are totally disregarded among this population [of ragpickers]," Joseph Durien wrote in *Les Parisiens d'aujourd'-hui*, published in 1910. "The very word is a scarecrow for them. In it, they see a sort of evil Goddess who is given the task of persecuting poor ragpickers; it is in the name of hygiene that the police hassle them [*tracasse*] to get them to clean up their dwellings and limit the number of pigs they are allowed to raise. Quite often . . . I have heard this exclamation: 'You see, our greatest enemy is hygiene.'" Quoted in Faure, "Classe malpropre," 94.

31. *Le Bonhomme Richard*, 6 April 1832, 2.

32. René Baehrel, "Epidémie et terreur: Histoire et sociologie," *Annales historiques de la révolution française* 23 (1951): 119–21. For a long-term history, see Jean Delumeau, *La Peur en Occident, XIVᵉ–XVIIIᵉ siècle: Une Cité assiégée* (Paris, 1978). On scapegoating during the plague, see Jean-Noel Biraben, *Les Hommes et la peste en France et dans les pays européens et méditerranéens*, vol. 1 (Paris, 1975), 57–65; Ernest Wickensheimer, *Les Accusations d'empoisonnement portées pendant la première moitié du XIVᵉ siècle contre les lépreux et les juifs, leurs relations avec les épidémies de peste* (Antwerp, 1927). Biraben points out that the persecution of Jews had less to do with the plague itself than with broader ongoing tensions between Christians and Jews during the fourteenth century. Western countries seemed to be more likely to create scapegoats. See R. I. Moore, "Lepers," in his *Foundations of a Persecuting Society* (New York, 1987), 45–65; Michael Dols, "The Comparative Communal Response to the Black Death in Muslim and Christian Societies," *Viator* 5 (1974): 269–87.

33. Pelling, *Cholera Fever and English Medicine*, 113–20.

34. Links between cholera and poison existed from the time cholera began its journey from India to the European continent. In 1817, one of the disease's first victims was a Hindu man scheduled to testify as a witness in

a criminal case. Rumors quickly spread that he had been poisoned by those who feared his revelations at the trial. Auguste Cabanés, *Moeurs intimes du passé* (Paris, 1920), 246–47. For a discussion of unrest and cholera more generally, see Evans, "Epidemics and Revolutions," 123–45.

35. Michael Durey, *The Return of the Plague: British Society and Cholera, 1831–32* (London, 1979), 158–59; R. J. Morris, *Cholera: 1832* (London, 1976), 101–14; Ruth Richardson, *Death, Dissection and the Destitute* (London and New York, 1988), 222–30; Evans, *Death in Hamburg*, 243–45; Theodore Friedgut, "Labor Violence and Regime Brutality in Tsarist Russia: The Iuzovka Cholera Riots of 1891," *Slavic Review* 46, no. 2 (summer 1987): 245–65 (I thank Glennys Young for this reference); Chevalier, *Le Choléra*, xv.

36. Roch, *Paris malade*, quoted in Chevalier, *Le Choléra*, 22; A. Pontmartin quoted in René Baehrel, "La Haine de classe en temps d'épidémie," *Annales: Economies, sociétés, civilisations* 7, no. 3 (July/September 1952): 356–57. M. Gisquet remembered fearing for the lives of the "honest citizens of Paris." Gisquet, *Mémoires de M. Gisquet*, vol. 1, 464–65.

37. *Le Courrier français*, 5 April 1832; *Le Messager* reprinted in *La Quotidienne*, 5 April 1832; Roch, *Paris malade*, vol. 1, 106–7. There were, for example, no derogatory cartoons or diatribes against the presence of Jews in the capital. In the context of cholera, I suspect that Jews were singled out in large part because of a longstanding epidemic tradition that linked them with the poisoning of wells. It is also possible that the rhetoric was directed more toward Jews as *merchants* in the context of expanding capitalism in Paris. For what it's worth, Chevalier does not mention Jews in his study of marginal Parisians, *Laboring Classes and Dangerous Classes*.

38. *La Quotidienne*, 6 April 1832.

39. See Chapter 2. Physicians were threatened throughout Europe. See Evans, "Epidemics and Revolutions," 137–39; Baehrel, "La Haine de classe," 351–60. Delaporte, *Disease and Civilization*, argues that doctors also had a reputation for "studying the diseases of the poor to save the rich," 55.

40. Magendie, *Leçons sur le choléra-morbus*, 232–33.

41. Poumiès de la Siboutie, *Souvenirs d'un médecin de Paris*, 236.

42. On hospitals in nineteenth-century Paris, see *Les Machines à guérir* (Brussels, 1979), a collection of essays by Michel Foucault, Blandine Barret Kriegel, Anne Thalamy, François Beguin, and Bruno Fortier.

43. *La Quotidienne* reported rumors that typhus had also broken out in the Hôtel Dieu, 13 April 1832. After the epidemic, officials confirmed that these rumors had been true. *Rapport sur la marche et les effets du choléramorbus*, 45.

44. Métral, *Description*, 49.

45. Rosen, *A History of Public Health*, 126–27. A fascinating study remains to be written on the hospital in nineteenth-century France along the lines of Charles E. Rosenberg, *The Care of Strangers: The Rise of America's Hospital System* (New York, 1987). Much of the ample literature on the development of the medical profession mentions the hospital only in passing or in regard to the practice of clinical medicine developed there. See, for

example, Ackerknecht, *Medicine at the Paris Hospital*, 15–22. For the eighteenth century, see Foucault, *The Birth of the Clinic*. Giorgio Pons's work *Essai de sociologie des malades dans les hôpitaux de Paris pendant les années 1815 à 1848* (Zurich, 1969) is thin in every respect.

46. Métral, *Description*, 21.

47. ADS VD⁶ 682 no. 5, Rapports de santé du XIIe arrondissement, 9 April 1832.

48. AAP #210, Correspondence of the Hôtel Dieu, January 1826–December 1833, letter to M. le Major de la Place de Paris, 27 April 1832; Magendie, *Leçons sur le choléra morbus*, 232–33.

49. A considerable amount of anti-Russian feeling emerged during the 1832 epidemic. Frequently, as in this example, the French equated Russians (particularly the Cossacks) with the lowest level of humans. Thus, the upper-class Parisians whom so many Russians sought to emulate condemned the behavior of the French lower classes by comparing them to Russians.

50. *Journal des débats*, 4 April 1832. The story probably originated in an article in the *Gazette des tribunaux*, 3 April 1832. In one edition of Blanc's memoirs, for example, there is even a lithograph depicting the scene. Blanc, *Histoire de dix ans*, vol. 3, 200–201.

51. *Gazette médicale de Paris*, quoted in Delaporte, *Disease and Civilization*, 207. Delaporte gives no date for this quote, but it seems to have appeared much later than the actual uprisings, thus providing an example of medical authority drawing information from popular accounts.

52. Heine, *Saemtliche Werke*, vol. 6, 181–82. Newspapers also printed the story but with less graphic detail. See *Le Journal du commerce*, 6 April 1832, reprinted in *La Quotidienne*, 7 April 1832.

53. Heine's account raises the obvious question about whether responses to cholera had a gendered dimension. In many ways Heine's women—bare-breasted Marianne-type figures and violent old hags—conformed to stereotypes of women in the era of the French Revolution and its aftermath. But in most of the literature cholera remained distinctly unfeminized for two reasons. First, the noun is masculine in French, thus explaining the depictions of the disease as a male vagabond in much of the literature. Second, mortality rates remained almost equal for men and women in the 1832 epidemic. See the *Rapport sur la marche et les effets du choléra-morbus*, 63. In the Hamburg outbreak of 1892 mortality rates differed substantially, thus provoking an intriguing discourse on gender. See Evans, *Death in Hamburg*, 450–65.

54. Apponyi, *Vingt-cinq ans à Paris*, vol. 2, 169.

55. Janin, *Paris depuis la révolution*, 8–9.

56. Blanc, *Histoire de dix ans*, vol. 3, 211; emphasis added for clarification.

57. *L'Ami de la religion*, 5 April 1832, 443–44.

58. *Journal des débats*, 3 April 1832.

59. *Le Courrier français*, 5 April 1832.

60. Circular from the mayor of the fourth arrondissement, reprinted in *Le Courrier français*, 5 April 1832, 2.

61. ADS VD^6 537, Correspondence pertaining to the tenth arrondissement. (Unfortunately, the employee at the archives who copied the manuscript did not include the file number.)

62. AN F^7 3886, "Police générale—Bulletin de Paris," 5 April 1832.

63. Gisquet, quoted in Blanc, *Histoire de dix ans*, vol. 3, 211.

64. It is worth noting that two days later the prefect tried to explain that opponents spread the rumor and not the substance, but the damage had already been done. ADS VD^4 3204, Circular of 4 April 1832. Gisquet's action met with universal criticism. In May the *Gazette des tribunaux* reported the trial of two hawkers who allegedly peddled Gisquet's circular as "the latest details on the poisoning, . . . the names of victims, . . . and the formalities they must go through." The court ultimately dismissed the case, finding that the document had already generated considerable controversy on its own. *Gazette des tribunaux*, 13 May 1832, 708, quoted in Sussman, "From Yellow Fever to Cholera," 280–81.

65. *Moniteur*, 8 April 1832, 1002; see also "La Vérité toute entière sur les empoisonnements. Cruautés exercées sur les malheureuses victimes. Sanglant excès de la fureur populaire" (Paris, n.d.), Bibliothèque Nationale; "Brutalité des bruits d'empoisonnement," *Gazette des hôpitaux*, week of 1 April 1832, 8; *Journal des commissions sanitaires établies dans le département de la Seine*, no. 16, 7 April 1832, 218; *Le Bonhomme Richard*, 8 April 1832, 1; *La Quotidienne*, 6 April 1832, 2.

66. *Moniteur*, 3 April, 953; 5 April, 973; 6 April, 983; 8 April, 1002—all in 1832.

67. Métral, *Description*, 131.

68. *Moniteur*, 6 June 1832, 1291.

69. Daumard, *Les Bourgeois de Paris*, 307, 310.

70. AN F^7 3886, "Bulletin de Paris," 3 June 1832.

71. AN F^7 3886, "Bulletin de Paris," 4 June 1832.

72. Accounts taken from points of agreement in the *Moniteur*, 6 June 1832, 1291; 7 June 1832, 1295–96; 8 June 1832, 1299–1300; *Le Bonhomme Richard*, 7 June 1832, 1–3; *La Quotidienne*, 6 June 1832, 1–2; *Le Corsaire*, 6 June 1832, 1–2; *Le Courrier français*, 6 June 1832, 1–2; Métral, *Description*, 133–41; Blanc, *Histoire de dix ans*, vol. 3, 272–315; Louis Ledieu, *A ces concitoyens sur les événements des 5 et 6 juin* (Paris, 1832); Noël Parfait, *L'Aurore d'un beau jour: Episodes des 5 et 6 juin 1832* (Paris, 1833), a narrative poem nearly eighty pages long that glorifies the insurgents; L. G. Pelissier, *Procès relatifs aux journées des 5 et 6 juin 1832* (Paris, 1893); Jean Lucas-Dubreton, *La Grande Peur de 1832: Le Choléra et l'émeute*, 4th ed. (Paris, 1932), an account sometimes lifted directly from Blanc, *Histoire de dix ans*, vol. 3, 144–203.

73. Karol Forster, *Quinze ans à Paris: Paris et les parisiens*, vol. 1 (Paris, 1848), 41.

74. In the fighting around these barricades a young boy and an old man were reportedly killed while hoisting the tricolor flag, a scene that allegedly served as the model for Gavroche's death in *Les Misérables* by Victor Hugo.

75. AN F⁷ 3886, "Bulletin de Paris," 6 June 1832; Métral, *Description*, 142.

76. *Le Corsaire*, 6 June 1832.

77. *Le Corsaire*, 6 June 1832, 2. According to Chateaubriand, "La Parisienne" was written in 1832 as a government-sponsored song to celebrate the glory of the 1830 revolution. Chateaubriand, *Mémoires*, vol. 4, 64, n. 3.

78. *Le Bonhomme Richard*, 7 June 1832, 1; *Moniteur*, 6 June 1832, 1291.

79. APP D/A A^A 421, "Troubles des 5 et 6 juin."

80. *Procès des vingt-deux accusés du cloître St. Méry* (Paris, 1832), 12.

81. *Rapport sur la marche et les effets du choléra-morbus*, 140.

82. *Rapport sur les épidémies cholériques*, 14.

83. *Rapport sur la marche et les effets du choléra-morbus*, 140. Chevalier lists ten streets around the church that had deaths ranging from thirty-four to seventy-five per thousand. Chevalier, *Le Choléra*, 44.

84. ADS VD⁶ 175, "Blessés de 5 et 6 juin," letter from the prefect of the Seine to the mayor of the second arrondissement, 6 June 1832.

85. Métral, *Description*, 141.

86. *Gazette des hôpitaux*, 12 June 1832, 1. It is interesting to note that the doctors appealed their case by invoking both the Code Pénal and traditional Catholic authority, comparing their role to that of a priest; see Chapter 4.

87. *Gazette médicale de Paris*, 12 June 1832.

88. Forster, *Quinze ans à Paris*, vol. 1, 43.

89. *Le Bonhomme Richard*, 6 June 1832, 1.

90. "Sur les blessés reçus dans les hôpitaux de Paris," *Gazette médicale de Paris*, reprinted in *La Quotidienne*, 6 June 1832, 2.

91. *Le Corsaire*, 14 June 1832, 4; *Le Corsaire*, 21 June 1832, 3. Also see Chapter 2, pp. 129–31.

92. *Rapport sur la marche et les effets du choléra-morbus*, 140.

93. Ibid., 141.

94. Rostan, Roux, and Rousset, *Traité du choléra-morbus*, 31.

95. *L'Union*, 12 June 1849, 4.

96. *Le Crédit*, 25 June 1849, 2.

97. F. J. D____ , "Le Choléra-morbus asiatique n'a jamais existé dans Paris, ou un mot sur l'épidémie régnante" (Paris, 1849), Bibliothèque Nationale.

98. *Le Courrier français*, 23 March 1849, 1.

99. Much of the literature in 1849 actually juxtaposed the arrival of cholera with the California gold rush.

100. Interestingly, I first found this image at the Bibliothèque Nationale misfiled among those for the 1832 outbreak.

101. Because of the limited sources, I will focus primarily on government interpretations of the events. A more complete study of the June 13 insurrection remains to be written, especially in light of the increasingly conservative swing of the Second Republic. Maurice Agulhon's *1848 ou l'apprentissage de la République* (Paris, 1973), 90–96, and Price, *The French Second Republic*, 246–49, offer a good starting point. For official primary accounts of these events, see *Moniteur*, 14 June 1849, 1; *Le Journal des débats*,

14 June 1849, 1; AN F⁷ 12178, "Surveillance légale, 1848–51"; APP A/A 432, "Affaire du 13 juin 1849."

102. This includes figures for deaths in private homes as well as in the hospitals. Compiled from the *Rapport sur les épidémies cholériques*, table 6, and *Rapport sur l'épidémie cholérique de 1853–54*, table 40.

103. The higher estimate is from Karl Marx, the lower one from the historian Philippe Vigier, cited in Price, *The French Second Republic*, 249.

104. Like the district surrounding the Cloître St. Méry in the first outbreak, the neighborhood around the June 13 insurrection had a mortality rate higher than that for the city as a whole. The city average of home deaths per arrondissement was approximately 481 for the month of June while that for the sixth arrondissement, in which the Conservatoire des Arts et Métiers was located, was 615. *Rapport sur les épidémies cholériques*, table 6.

105. Given the paucity of documentation on the June 13 uprising, it is unfortunately impossible to verify this claim. *Le Journal du peuple*, 1 July 1849, 2. Also see *L'Union*, which noted that "the Paris population responded to the provocations of the socialist press with calm." *L'Union*, 12 June 1849, 1.

106. *Rapport sur les épidémies cholériques; Rapport sur la marche et les effets du choléra-morbus*, 140–41.

107. "Les deux fléaux," *Le Journal du peuple*, 9 June 1832, 1.

108. *Le Courrier français*, 16 June 1832, 1.

109. Marx, *Class Struggles in France*, 93.

110. *Le Dix décembre*, 15 June 1849, 1.

111. *Le Courrier français*, 16 June 1849, 1.

112. *La Bonne Foi*, 16 June 1849, 3, and *Le Corsaire*, 16 June 1849, 2, printed the same article.

113. *Le Corsaire*, 11 April 1849, 1; *Le Journal du peuple*, 22 June 1849, 2. Also see *Le Corsaire*, 2 April 1849, 1; *L'Union*, 12 April 1849, 1; *L'Opinion publique*, 18 June 1849, 1; *Le Dix décembre*, 12 June 1849, 1; "Sur les neuf représentants socialistes médecins," *Le Corsaire*, 5 June 1849, 1.

114. *Le Journal du peuple*, 22 June 1849, 2.

115. *Le Corsaire*, 19 May 1849, 3.

116. Apponyi, *Vingt-cinq ans à Paris*, vol. 4, 283–84.

117. E.V.E.B. Castellane, *Journal du maréchal de Castellane*, vol. 4 (Paris, 1895–97), 165.

118. *L'Opinion publique*, 18 June 1849, 1. This opinion, incidentally, is shared by all the historians who mention the 1849 cholera epidemic at all. See, for example, Price, *The French Second Republic*, 248.

119. *Rapport sur les épidémies cholériques*, 153.

120. "Les ouvriers et le 13 juin," *La Bonne Foi*, 17 June 1849, 3. Also printed in *L'Union*, 17 June 1849, 1.

121. *Journal des débats*, 14 June 1849, 1.

122. *La Bonne Foi*, 13 June 1849, 2; Janin, *Paris depuis la révolution*, 8–9.

123. Louis François Lélut, *De la Santé du peuple* (Paris, 1849), 8–9.

124. *Le Corsaire*, 11 June 1849, 2.

125. See Chapter 2. For specific figures, see Aguet, "Le Tirage," 216–86.

126. Emphasis added. F.-A. Poujol, "Dictionnaire de médecine pratique," in vol. 17 of *Nouvelle encyclopédie théologique*, ed. Abbé Jacques-Paul Migne (Paris, 1852), 344–45. See, for example, "L'Urgence pour les améliorations populaires," *Le Crédit*, 16 June 1849, 1. Echoing the cries of 1848, the editors called for jobs, public instruction, care for the elderly and infirm as well as for public works projects in order to clean up poor neighborhoods in the battle against "the two hideous armies of insurrection and death."

127. *Gazette des hôpitaux*, 16 June 1849, 1.

128. Rostan, Roux, and Rousset, *Traité*, 132.

129. See Chapter 3; ADS VD^6 274 no. 5, Commissions Sanitaires, Préfet de Police, "Instruction," April 1849, 3.

130. *Rapport sur les épidémies cholériques*, 25, 87. In fact an article entitled "La Mortalité par suite du choléra, est-elle plus grande dans la classe pauvre que dans la classe aisée?" in the *Gazette des hôpitaux* demonstrated that mortality rates ran lower among prisoners and indigents; prisoners, the editors of the reputable medical journal concluded, were more likely to eat regular, balanced meals and were restricted from *les excès*, while indigents could get doctors' services more promptly than others through relief organizations. *Gazette des hôpitaux*, 12 May 1849, 1; see also Dr. Lanessan, *Rapport statistique sur le choléra épidémique à Bercy pendant les mois de mars, avril, mai, juin et juillet 1849* (Paris, 1849), 3.

131. Given the strict censorship of the press and probable destruction of inflammatory back issues, it is difficult to gain an accurate understanding of how the opposition may have used the epidemic to criticize the government or incite revolution. Limited evidence from columns such as "Revue des journaux socialistes," in *Le Journal du peuple*, offers some insight into this area. The regular column responded to attacks against the government within the socialist press, but, judging from the paper's discussions, the socialist press used the epidemic only rarely as a political weapon. One notable exception appeared just as cholera deaths began to climb and was probably reprinted for sensationalist purposes: "They say that cholera continues its *assassinations* [emphasis in original] with increasing intensity. Malthus need no longer worry; cholera is the scythe, the ladle, the rope, the weapon, and the cannon that divides the workers according to the wishes of the royalists and the aristocrats." *La Vraie république*, reprinted in *La Bonne Foi* as a "tasty morsel." *La Bonne Foi*, 7 June 1849, 4.

132. Louis Canler, *Mémoires de Canler: Ancien chef du service de la sûreté* (Paris, 1832), 268–72.

CONCLUSION

1. P. Barthélemy, trans., *Report on the Cholera in Paris Published by Authority of the French Government* (New York, 1849), v–vi.

Selected Bibliography

ARCHIVES

Archives de la Préfecture de Police de Paris
Archives de l'Archevêché de Paris
Archives de l'Assistance Publique
Archives du Département de la Seine et de la Ville de Paris
Archives Nationales de France

CONTEMPORARY NEWSPAPERS AND PERIODICALS
(ALL PUBLISHED IN PARIS)

L'Ami de la religion
Annales d'hygiène publique et de médecine légale
Le Bonhomme Richard
La Bonne Foi: Journal des intérêts populaires
Le Charivari
Le Constitutionnel
Le Corsaire
Le Courrier français
Le Crédit
La Démocratie pacifique
Le Dix décembre: Journal de l'ordre
L'Entracte
Gazette des hôpitaux civils et militaires
Gazette des tribunaux: Journal de jurisprudence et des débats judiciaires
Gazette médicale de Paris: Journal de médecine et sciences accessoires
Le Globe: Journal philosophique et littéraire
Journal des commissions sanitaires établies dans le département de la Seine
Journal des débats politiques et littéraires
Le Journal du peuple: Amélioration morale et matérielle de la condition des classes populaires
Moniteur universel
Le National
L'Opinion publique
Le Peuple: Journal de la république démocratique et sociale
La Quotidienne
L'Union
L'Union médicale

PUBLISHED PRIMARY SOURCES

Administration Générale de l'Assistance Publique. *Rapport sur les épidémies cholériques de 1832 et 1849*. Paris, 1850.

————. *Rapport sur l'épidémie cholérique de 1853–54, dans les établissements dependant de l'administration générale de l'assistance publique de la ville de Paris*. Paris: Dupont, 1855.

Apponyi, Radolphe. *Vingt-cinq ans à Paris: Journal du comte*. 4 vols. Paris, 1913.

Bazin, Anais de Baucon. *L'Epoque sans nom: Esquisses de Paris*. 2 vols. Paris, 1833.

Bellemare, M. *Le Fléau de Dieu en 1832*. Paris, 1832.

Béranger, Charles. "Le Choléra, Napoléon, l'ordre légal." Saint-Simonian pamphlet, Bibliothèque Nationale. Paris, 1832.

Blanc, Louis. *Histoire de dix ans, 1830–1840*. 5 vols. Paris, 1867.

Boisseau, F. G. *Traité du choléra considéré sous le rapport médical et administratif*. Paris, 1832.

Bouchardat, A. *Sur la nature, le traitement et les préservatifs du choléra-morbus*. Paris, 1832.

Boucher de Crevecour de Perthes, Jacques. *Sous dix rois: Souvenirs*. 8 vols. Paris, 1863–68.

Boulay de la Meurthe, Henri. *Histoire du choléra-morbus dans le quartier de Luxembourg*. Paris, 1832.

Bourdelais, Patrice, and André Dodin, eds. *Visages du choléra*. Paris, 1987.

Broussais, F.J.V. *Le Choléra-morbus épidémique observé et traité selon la méthode physiologique*. Paris, 1832.

Byrne, William Pitt. *Realities of Paris Life: Paris and the Parisians*. 2 vols. London, 1859.

Caffe, Paul. *Considération sur l'histoire médicale et statistique du choléra-morbus de Paris*. Paris, 1832.

————. *Notice sur le choléra*. Paris, 1849.

————. *Paris vu dans ses causes*. Paris, 1835.

Candy, Dr. Camille. *Rapport sur le choléra-morbus de Paris présenté à M. le maire de Lyon*. Lyon, 1849.

Castellane, E.V.E.B. *Journal du maréchal de Castellane*. 5 vols. Paris, 1895–97.

Chateaubriand, François René de. "Courtes explications sur les 12,000 francs offerts par Mme la duchesse de Berry aux indigents attaqués de la contagion." Pamphlet, Bibliothèque Historique de la Ville de Paris. Paris, 1832.

————. *Mémoires d'outre tombe*. 4 vols. 1849–50. Reprint, Paris, 1968.

Chaumette, M. *Résumé du système de nettoiement de la ville de Paris*. Paris, 1830.

Comité Consultatif d'Hygiène Publique, Académie Nationale de Médecine. "Instructions conçernant les mesures générales à prendre à l'occasion de l'épidémie du choléra." In *Instructions sanitaires et les moyens préservatifs du choléra-morbus*. Paris, 1849.

Commission Centrale de Salubrité. *Rapport sur la salubrité des habitations.* Paris, 1832.

D——, F. J. "Le Choléra-morbus asiatique n'a jamais existé dans Paris, ou un mot sur l'épidémie régnante." Pamphlet, Bibliothèque Nationale. Paris, 1849.

Delarue, Dr. François. *De la peur et de la folie des gouvernements de l'Europe au sujet du choléra.* Paris, 1831.

Deville, Jean. *Compte-rendu des travaux de la Commission centrale de salubrité du quartier de l'Hôtel de Ville depuis son installation jusqu'à l'invasion du choléra-morbus et depuis cette époque jusqu'au 30 août 1832.* Paris, 1832.

———. *Histoire médicale du choléra-morbus dans le quartier de l'Hôtel de Ville.* Paris, 1833.

Dictionnaire d'hygiène publique et de salubrité, ou Répertoire de toutes les questions relatives à la santé publique. Paris, 1862–64.

Duchesne, E. A. *Histoire statistique du choléra-morbus dans le XIe arrondissement de Paris.* Paris, 1851.

Dudon, Dr. *Recherches sur le siège, les causes et le traitement du choléra-morbus épidémique observé en avril et en mai 1832.* Paris, 1832.

Forster, Karol. *Quinze ans à Paris: Paris et les parisiens.* 3 vols. Paris, 1848–49.

Foy, F. *Histoire médicale du choléra-morbus de Paris et des moyens thérapeutiques et hygiéniques.* Paris, 1832.

Frégier, H. A. *Des Classes dangereuses de la population dans les grandes villes et des moyens de les rendre meilleures.* 2 vols. Paris, 1840.

Gardner, Augustus. *Old Wine in New Bottles, or Spare Hours of a Student in Paris.* Dublin, 1849.

Gisquet, Henri. *Mémoires de M. Gisquet, ancien préfet de police, écrites par lui-même.* 4 vols. Paris, 1840.

Gonneau. *Vocabulaire ou nouvel indicatif sur les rues de Paris.* Paris, 1839.

Haspot, Emile. "Les Médecins." Saint-Simonian pamphlet, Bibliothèque Nationale. Paris, 1832.

Heine, Heinrich. *Saemtliche Werke in zehn Baenden,* unter Mitwirkung von Jonas Fraenkel, Ludwig Kraehe, Albert Leitzmann und Julius Petersen herausgegeben von Oskar Walzel. 10 vols. Leipzig, 1912.

Henry, Napoléon. *Le Choléra-morbus, sa nature, son siège et son traitement.* Paris, 1832.

Janin, Jules. *Paris depuis la révolution de 1830.* Brussels, 1832.

Journal des commissions sanitaires établies dans le département de la Seine contenant les travaux de ces commissions, les actes, décisions et instructions de l'administration qui leur sont relatifs. Published under the auspices of the Préfecture de Police. [Paris,] November 1831.

Lallumette, Fanfan. "Protestation adressée par les chiffonniers de Paris à M. Gisquet, préfet de police." Pamphlet, Bibliothèque Nationale. Paris, 1832.

Lanessan, Dr. *Rapport statistique sur le choléra épidémique à Bercy pendant les mois de mars, avril, mai, juin et juillet 1849.* Paris, 1849.

Lélut, Louis François. *De la Santé du peuple.* Paris, 1849.

Le Livre des cent-et-un. 15 vols. Paris, 1831–34.

Lurine, Louis. *Les Rues de Paris, Paris ancien et moderne.* Paris, 1844.

Magendie, M. F. *Leçons sur le choléra-morbus.* Paris, 1832.

Métral, Antoine. *Description naturelle, morale et politique du choléra-morbus à Paris.* Paris, 1833.

Moreau, François Marc. *Histoire statistique du choléra-asiatique de 1849.* Paris, 1850.

———. *Histoire statistique du choléra-morbus dans le quartier du faubourg St.-Denis.* Paris, 1833.

Moreau de Jonnès, Alexandre. *Rapport au conseil supérieur de santé sur le choléra-morbus pestilentiel.* Paris, 1831.

Moulin, E. *Hygiène et traitement du choléra-morbus: Coup d'oeil historique sur l'épidémie de Paris de 1832.* Paris, 1832.

Nettement, Alfred. *Etudes critiques sur le feuilleton-roman.* 2 vols. Paris, 1845–46.

Nouveau tableau de Paris au XIXᵉ siècle. 7 vols. Paris, 1834–35.

Parfait, Noël. *L'Aurore d'un beau jour: Episodes des 5 et 6 juin 1832.* Paris, 1833.

Pelissier, L. G. *Pièces relatives aux journées des 5 et 6 juin 1832.* Paris, 1893.

Petit, C. F. *Rapport sur le choléra-morbus observé à Paris.* Paris, 1832.

Physiologie de la presse: Biographie des journalistes et des journaux de Paris et de la province. Paris, 1841.

Pontmartin, Armand. *Mes mémoires d'enfance et de jeunesse.* Paris, 1885.

Pouillet, M. *Le Conservatoire des arts et métiers pendant la journée du 13 juin 1849.* Paris, 1849.

Poujol, F.-A. "Dictionnaire de médecine pratique." In vol. 17 of *Nouvelle encyclopédie théologique,* edited by Abbé Jacques-Paul Migne. Paris, 1852.

Poumiès de la Siboutie, F. L. *Souvenirs d'un médecin de Paris.* Paris, 1910.

Préfecture de Police, Commission Centrale de Salubrité. *Préservatif contre le choléra-morbus: Rapports de la commission chargé d'organiser et d'indiquer le personnel des bureaux de secours.* Paris, 1832.

———. *Rapport sur la surveillance des établissements publiques.* Paris, 1831.

Procès des vingt-deux accusés du cloître St. Méry. Paris, 1832.

Rapport au conseil supérieur de la santé sur un rapport de son secrétaire relatif aux modifications à apporter dans les règlements sanitaires. Paris, 1840.

Rapport sur la marche et les effets du choléra-morbus dans Paris et les communes rurales de la Seine, année 1832. Paris, 1834.

Rapports généraux des travaux du conseil de salubrité. Paris, 1829–43.

Rapports généraux sur la salubrité publique, ville de Paris et département de la Seine. Paris, 1802–39.

Rémusat, Charles. *Mémoires de ma vie.* 5 vols. Paris, 1960.

Rey-Dusseuil, A.F.M. *Le Cloître St. Méry.* Paris, 1832.

Roch, Eugène. *Paris malade: Esquisses du jour.* 2 vols. Paris, 1832.

Rostan, Roux, and Rousset. *Traité du choléra-morbus de 1849.* Paris, 1851.

Société des Traités Religieux de Paris. *Instructions à la portée de tout le monde sur le choléra-morbus.* Paris, 1849.

Tacheron, C. P. *Statistique médicale de la mortalité du choléra-morbus dans le 11ᵉ arrondissement de Paris.* Paris, 1832.

Tardieu, Ambroise. *Treatise on Epidemic Cholera.* Trans. Boston, 1849.

Trébuchet, Adolphe. *Le Rapport général sur les travaux du conseil d'hygiène et de salubrité du département de la Seine pour la période 1849–1858.* Paris, 1861.

Trolliet, Louis François, Augustin Pierre Isidore Polinière, and Alexandre Bottex. *Rapport sur le choléra-morbus de Paris.* Lyon, 1832.

"La Vérité toute entière sur les empoisonnements. Cruautés exercées sur les malheureuses victimes. Sanglant excès de la fureur populaire." Pamphlet, Bibliothèque Nationale. Paris, n.d.

SECONDARY SOURCES

Ackerknecht, Erwin H. "Anticontagionism between 1821 and 1867." *Bulletin of the History of Medicine* 22, no. 5 (1948): 562–93.

———. "Hygiene in France, 1815–1848." *Bulletin of the History of Medicine* 22, no. 2 (March/April 1948): 117–55.

———. *Medicine at the Paris Hospital, 1794–1848.* Baltimore: Johns Hopkins University Press, 1967.

Ackerman, Evelyn. *Health Care in the Parisian Countryside, 1800–1914.* New Brunswick: Rutgers University Press, 1990.

Aguet, J.-P. "Le Tirage des quotidiens de Paris sous la monarchie de juillet." *Schweizerische Zeitschrift für Geschichte* 10 (1960): 216–86.

Agulhon, Maurice. *Marianne into Battle: Republican Imagery and Symbolism in France, 1789–1880.* Translated by Janet Lloyd. Cambridge: Cambridge University Press, 1981.

Allen, James Smith. *In the Public Eye: A History of Reading in Modern France, 1800–1940.* Princeton: Princeton University Press, 1991.

Allison, John. *Church and State in the Reign of Louis-Philippe, 1830–1848.* Princeton: Princeton University Press, 1916.

Baehrel, René. "Epidémie et terreur: Histoire et sociologie." *Annales historiques de la révolution française* 23 (1951): 113–46.

———. "La Haine de classe en temps d'épidémie." *Annales: Economies, sociétés, civilisations* 7, no. 3 (July/September 1952): 351–60.

Beauchamp, Chantal. *Délivrez-nous du mal!: Epidémies, endémies, médecine, et hygiène au XIXᵉ siècle dans l'Indre, l'Indre-et-Loire et le Loir-et-Cher.* Maulevrier: Editions Hérault, 1990.

Bellanger, Claude, et al. *Histoire générale de la presse française.* 5 vols. Paris: Presses Universitaires de France, 1969–76.

Berenson, Edward. "A New Religion of the Left: Christianity and Social Radicalism in France, 1815–1848." In *The Transformation of Political Culture, 1789–1848,* edited by François Furet and Mona Ozouf. Vol. 3

of *The French Revolution and the Creation of Modern Political Culture,* edited by Keith Michael Baker. Oxford: Pergamon Press, 1989.

———. *Populist Religion and Left-Wing Politics in France, 1830–1852.* Princeton: Princeton University Press, 1984.

Bezine, B. "Le Choléra à Paris de 1849." Thesis, Faculté de Médecine (Paris), 1921.

Bourdelais, Patrice. "Le Choléra en France, 1832 et 1854: Essai d'épistémologie historique." Thesis, Ecole des Hautes Etudes en Sciences Sociales (Paris), 1979.

Bourdelais, Patrice, and Jean-Yves Raulot. "La Marche du choléra en France, 1832 et 1854." *Annales: Economies, sociétés, civilisations* 33, no. 1 (January-February 1978): 125–42.

———. *Une Peur bleue: Histoire du choléra en France, 1832–1854.* Paris: Payot, 1987.

Briggs, Asa. "Cholera and Society in the Nineteenth Century." *Past and Present* 19 (1961): 76–96.

Chevalier, Louis, ed. *Le Choléra: La Première épidémie du XIXᵉ siècle.* La Roche-sur-Yon: Imp. Centrale de l'Ouest, 1958.

———. *Classes laborieuses et classes dangereuses à Paris pendant la première moitie du XIXᵉ siècle.* Paris: Plon, 1958. Translated by Frank Jellinek under the title *Laboring Classes and Dangerous Classes in Paris during the First Half of the Nineteenth Century.* Princeton: Princeton University Press, 1973.

———. *La Formation de la population parisienne au XIXᵉ siècle.* Paris: Presses Universitaires de France, 1950.

Christophe, Paul. *Les Choix du clergé dans les révolutions de 1789, 1830 et 1848.* 2 vols. Lille: P. Christophe, 1975–76.

Church, Clive H. *Revolution and Red Tape: The French Ministerial Bureaucracy, 1770–1850.* Oxford: Oxford University Press, Clarendon Press, 1981.

Clark, T. J. *The Absolute Bourgeois: Artists and Politicians in France, 1848–1851.* Princeton: Princeton University Press, 1982.

Cole, Joshua. "The Chaos of Particular Facts: Statistics, Medicine, and the Social Body in Early Nineteenth-Century France." *History of the Human Sciences* 7, no. 3 (1994): 1–27.

Coleman, William. *Death Is a Social Disease: Public Health and Political Economy in Early-Industrial France.* Madison: University of Wisconsin Press, 1982.

———. "Health and Hygiene in the *Encyclopédie:* A Medical Doctrine for the Bourgeoisie." *Journal of the History of Medicine and Allied Sciences* 29, no. 4 (October 1974): 399–421.

———. *Yellow Fever in the North: The Methods of Early Epidemiology.* Madison: University of Wisconsin Press, 1987.

Collingham, H.A.C. *The July Monarchy: A Political History of France, 1830–1848.* London: Longman, 1988.

Collins, Irene. *The Government and the Newspaper Press in France, 1814–1881.* London: Oxford University Press, 1959.

Cooter, Roger. "Anticontagionism and History's Medical Record." In *The Problem of Medical Knowledge: Examining the Social Construct of Medicine*, ed. Peter Wright and Andrew Treacher. Edinburgh: Edinburgh University Press, 1982.

Corbin, Alain. *The Foul and the Fragrant: Odor and the French Social Imagination.* Translation. Cambridge: Harvard University Press, 1986.

Costanzo, Dennis Paul. "Cityscape and the Transformation of Paris during the Second Empire." Ph.D. diss., University of Michigan, 1981.

Cuno, James. "Charles Philipon and La Maison Aubert: The Business, Politics, and Public of Caricature in Paris, 1820–1840." Ph.D. diss., Harvard University, 1985.

Daumard, Adeline. *Les Bourgeois de Paris au XIXe siècle.* Paris: Flammarion, 1970.

———. *La Bourgeoisie parisienne de 1815 à 1848.* Paris: S.E.V.P.E.N., 1963.

Delaporte, François. *Disease and Civilization: The Cholera in Paris, 1832.* Translated by Arthur Goldhammer. Cambridge: MIT Press, 1986.

Droulers, Paul. "L'Episcopat devant la question ouvrière en France sous la monarchie de juillet." *Revue historique,* no. 466 (1963): 335–62.

Duby, Georges, ed. *Histoire de la France urbaine.* 5 vols. Paris: Seuil, 1980–85.

Duroselle, Jean Baptiste. *Les Débuts du catholicisme social en France, 1822–1870.* Paris: Presses Universitaires de France, 1951.

"En feuilletant les archives de la préfecture de police: L'Epidémie du choléra à Paris en 1832." *Liaisons,* no. 173 (October 1970): 28–32.

Evans, Richard J. *Death in Hamburg: Society and Politics in the Cholera Years, 1830–1910.* London: Oxford University Press, 1987; New York: Penguin Books, 1990.

———. "Epidemics and Revolutions: Cholera in Nineteenth-Century Europe." *Past and Present* 120 (August 1988): 123–45.

Faure, Alain. "Classe malpropre, classe dangereuse? Quelques Remarques à propos des chiffonniers parisiens au XIXe siècle et leurs cités." *Recherches* 29 (1978): 79–102.

Ferguson, Priscilla Parkhurst. *Paris as Revolution: Writing the Nineteenth-Century City.* Berkeley and Los Angeles: University of California Press, 1994.

Foucault, Michel. *The Birth of the Clinic: An Archaeology of Medical Perception.* Translated by A. M. Sheridan Smith. New York: Pantheon Books, 1973.

———. *Discipline and Punish: The Birth of the Prison.* Translated by Alan Sheridan. New York: Pantheon Books, 1977.

———. *The History of Sexuality.* Vol. 1: *An Introduction.* Translated by Robert Hurley. New York: Vintage Books, 1980.

———. *Power/Knowledge: Selected Interviews and Other Writings, 1972–1977.* Edited and translated by Colin Gordon, Leo Marshall, John Mepham, and Kate Soper. New York: Pantheon Books, 1980.

Friedgut, Theodore. "Labor Violence and Regime Brutality in Tsarist Russia: The Iuzovka Cholera Riots of 1891." *Slavic Review* 46, no. 2 (summer 1987): 245–65.

Furet, François. *Revolutionary France, 1770–1880.* Translated by Antonia Nevill. Oxford: Oxford University Press, 1992.

Furet, François, and Jacques Ozouf, eds. *Lire et écrire: L'Alphabétisation des français de Calvin à Jules Ferry.* 2 vols. Paris: Editions de Minuit, 1978.

Furet, François, and Mona Ozouf, eds. *The Transformation of Political Culture, 1789–1848.* Vol. 3 of *The French Revolution and the Creation of Modern Political Culture,* edited by Keith Michael Baker. Oxford: Pergamon Press, 1989.

Gelfand, Toby. *Professionalizing Modern Medicine: Paris Surgeons, Medical Science, and Institutions in the 18th Century.* Westport, Conn.: Greenwood Press, 1980.

Gerlitt, J. "The Development of Quarantine." *Ciba Symposia* 2 (1940): 566–80.

Gibson, Ralph. *A Social History of French Catholicism, 1789–1914.* London: Routledge, 1989.

Gillispie, Charles Coulston. *Science and Polity in France at the End of the Old Regime.* Princeton: Princeton University Press, 1980.

Goldstein, Jan. *Console and Classify: The French Psychiatric Profession in the Nineteenth Century.* Cambridge: Cambridge University Press, 1987.

———. "Moral Contagion: A Professional Ideology. . . ." In *Professions and the French State, 1700–1900,* edited by Gerald Geison. Philadelphia: University of Pennsylvania Press, 1984.

Gonnet, P. "Esquisse de la crise économique en France de 1827–32." *Revue d'histoire économique et sociale* 33 (1955).

Goubert, Jean-Pierre. *The Conquest of Water: The Advent of Health in the Industrial Age.* Translated by Andrew Wilson. Princeton: Polity Press, 1989.

Habermas, Jürgen. *The Structural Transformation of the Public Sphere: An Inquiry into a Category of Bourgeois Society.* Translated by Thomas Burger, with the assistance of Frederick Lawrence. Cambridge: MIT Press, 1989.

Hannaway, Caroline. "Medicine, Public Welfare, and the State in Eighteenth-Century France: The Société Royale de Médecine of Paris, 1776–1793." Ph.D. diss., Johns Hopkins University, 1974.

Hartmann, Georges. "Les Ravages du choléra dans le quartier de l'Hôtel de Ville en 1832." *La Cité* (January 1933): 293–96.

Hatin, Eugène. *Bibliographie historique et critique de la presse périodique française.* Paris, 1866.

———. *Histoire politique et littéraire de la presse en France.* 8 vols. Paris: Poulet-Malassis et de Broise, 1859–61.

Heaman, E. A. "Anticontagionism in France in the Nineteenth Century." Master's thesis, McGill University, 1990.

Hesse, Carla. *Publishing and Cultural Politics in Paris, 1789–1810.* Berkeley and Los Angeles: University of California Press, 1991.

Hilaire, Yves, and Gérard Cholvy, eds. *Histoire religieuse de la France contemporaine.* 3 vols. Toulouse: Privat, 1985–88.

Hugo, Victor. *Notre-Dame de Paris.* 1836. Reprint, Paris: Editions Garnier Frères, 1959.

Hunt, Lynn, ed. *The New Cultural History*. Berkeley and Los Angeles: University of California Press, 1988.

———. *Politics, Culture, and Class in the French Revolution*. Berkeley and Los Angeles: University of California Press, 1984.

Isambert, François. "L'Attitude religieuse des ouvriers français au milieu du XIXe siècle." *Archives de sociologie des religions* 6 (July-December 1958): 7–35.

———. *Christianisme et classe ouvrière: Jalons pour une étude de sociologie historique*. Paris: Casterman, 1961.

Jardin, A., and A.-J. Tudesq. *La France des notables: L'Evolution générale, 1815–1848*. 2 vols. Paris: Editions du Seuil, 1973.

Jones, Colin. *Charity and Bienfaisance: The Treatment of the Poor in the Montpellier Region, 1740–1815*. Cambridge: Cambridge University Press, 1982.

Jones, Russell M. "American Doctors and the Parisian Medical World, 1830–1840." *Bulletin of the History of Medicine* 47, no. 1 (1973): 40–65, and 47, no. 2 (1973): 177–204.

Kudlick, Catherine J. "The Culture of Statistics and the Crisis of Cholera, 1830–1850." In *Recreating Authority in Revolutionary France*. Ed. Bryant T. Ragan, Jr., and Elizabeth Williams. New Brunswick: Rutgers University Press, 1992.

La Berge, Ann F. "A.J.B. Parent-Duchâtelet: Hygienist of Paris, 1821–36." *Clio Medica* 12, no. 4 (1977): 279–301.

———. "The Early Nineteenth-Century French Public Health Movement: The Disciplinary Development and Institutionalization of *Hygiène publique*." *Bulletin of the History of Medicine* 58 (1984): 363–79.

———. *Mission and Method: The Early Nineteenth-Century French Public Health Movement*. Cambridge: Cambridge University Press, 1992.

———. "The Paris Health Council, 1802–1848." *Bulletin of the History of Medicine* 49, no. 3 (1975): 339–52.

———. "Public Health in France and the French Public Health Movement, 1815–1848." Ph.D. diss., University of Tennessee, 1974.

Laporte, Dominique. *Histoire de la merde: Prologue*. Paris: C. Bourgeois, 1978.

Leca, Ange-Pierre. *Et le choléra s'abattit sur Paris, 1832*. Paris: A. Michel, 1982.

Ledré, Charles. *La Presse à l'assaut de la monarchie, 1815–1848*. Paris: A. Colin, 1960.

Le Mée, R. "Les Villes de France et leurs populations de 1806 à 1851." *Annales de démographie historique* (Paris) (1989): 321–93.

Léonard, Jacques. *La Médecine entre les pouvoirs et les savoirs: Histoire intellectuelle et politique de la médecine française du XIXe siècle*. Paris: Aubier-Montaigne, 1981.

———. *Les Médecins de l'Ouest au XIXe siècle*. 3 vols. Paris: H. Champion, 1978.

Lucas-Dubreton, Jean. *La Grande Peur de 1832: Le Choléra et l'émeute*. 4th ed. Paris: Gallimard, 1932.

Lynch, Katherine A. *Family, Class, and Ideology in Early Industrial France: Social Policy and the Working-Class Family, 1825–1848.* Madison: University of Wisconsin Press, 1988.

McGrew, Rodrick. "The First Cholera Epidemic and Social History." *Bulletin of the History of Medicine* 36 (1966).

Marx, Karl. *The Class Struggles in France, 1848–1850.* Trans. New York: International Publishers, 1964.

———. *The Eighteenth Brumaire of Louis Bonaparte.* Trans. New York: International Publishers, 1963.

Mayer, Arno J. "The Lower-Middle Class as Historical Problem." *Journal of Modern History* 47 (September 1975): 409–36.

Merriman, John M. *The Margins of City Life: Explorations on the French Urban Frontier, 1815–1851.* New York: Oxford University Press, 1991.

Murphy, T. D. "Medical Knowledge and Statistical Method in Early Nineteenth-Century France." *Medical History* 25, no. 4 (1981): 301–19.

Musto, David. "Quarantine and the Problem of AIDS." In *AIDS: The Burdens of History,* edited by Elizabeth Fee and David Fox. Berkeley and Los Angeles: University of California Press, 1988.

Norberg, Kathryn. *Rich and Poor in Grenoble, 1600–1814.* Berkeley and Los Angeles: University of California Press, 1985.

O'Brien, Patricia Ann. "Urban Growth and Public Order: The Development of a Modern Police in Paris, 1829–1854." Ph.D. diss., Columbia University, 1973.

Pelling, Margaret. *Cholera Fever and English Medicine, 1825–1865.* Oxford: Oxford University Press, 1978.

Pierrard, Pierre. *L'Eglise en France face aux crises révolutionnaires, 1789–1871.* Lyon: Le Chalet, 1974.

———. *L'Eglise et les ouvriers en France, 1840–1940.* Paris: Hachette Littérature, 1984.

———. *1848: Les Pauvres, l'évangile et la révolution.* Paris: Desclée, 1977.

Pilbeam, Pamela M. *The 1830 Revolution in France.* London: Macmillan, 1991.

Pinkney, David H. "The Crowd in the French Revolution of 1830." *American Historical Review* 70 (October 1964): 1–17.

———. *Decisive Years in France, 1840–1847.* Princeton: Princeton University Press, 1986.

———. *The French Revolution of 1830.* Princeton: Princeton University Press, 1972.

———. *Napoleon III and the Rebuilding of Paris.* Princeton: Princeton University Press, 1958; reprint, 1972.

Piquemal, Jacques. "Le Choléra en France et la pensée médicale." Thesis, Institut de l'Histoire des Sciences et Technologies, Université de Paris, 1959.

Pollitzer, Robert. *Cholera.* Geneva: World Health Organization, 1959.

Porter, Theodore M. *The Rise of Statistical Thinking, 1820–1900.* Princeton: Princeton University Press, 1986.

Preston, S. H. "Urban French Mortality in the Nineteenth Century." *Population Studies* (Great Britain) 32, no. 2 (1978): 275–98.

Price, Roger. *The French Second Republic: A Social History.* London: Batsford, 1972.

Rader, Daniel L. *The Journalists and the July Revolution in France: The Role of the Political Press in the Overthrow of the Bourbon Restoration, 1827–1830.* The Hague: Nijoff, 1973.

Ramsey, Matthew. *Professional and Popular Medicine in France, 1770–1830: The Social World of Medical Practice.* Cambridge: Cambridge University Press, 1988.

Ratcliffe, Barrie. "Perception and Realities of the Urban Margin: The Rag Pickers of Paris in the First Half of the Nineteenth Century." *Canadian Journal of History/Annales canadiennes d'histoire* 27 (August 1992): 198–233.

Reddy, William M. "Condottieri of the Pen: Journalists and the Public Sphere in Postrevolutionary France, 1815–1850." *American Historical Review* 99, no. 5 (December 1994): 1546–70.

Reid, Donald. *Paris Sewers and Sewermen: Realities and Representations.* Cambridge: Harvard University Press, 1991.

Rémond, René. *L'Anticléricalisme en France de 1815 à nos jours.* Paris: Fayard, 1976.

———. *The Right-Wing in France from 1815 to de Gaulle.* 1954. Trans. James M. Laux. Philadelphia: University of Pennsylvania, 1966.

Rigaudias-Weiss, Hilde. *Les Enquêtes ouvrières en France entre 1838 et 1848.* Paris: Presses Universitaires de France, 1936.

Riley, James C. *The Eighteenth-Century Campaign to Avoid Disease.* Houndmills, England: Macmillan, 1987.

Roche, Daniel. *The People of Paris: An Essay in Popular Culture in the Eighteenth Century.* Trans. Marie Evans and Gwynne Lewis. Berkeley and Los Angeles: University of California Press, 1987.

Rollet, Catherine, and Agnès Sauriac. "Epidémies et mentalités: Le Choléra de 1832 en Seine-et-Oise." *Annales: Economies, sociétés, civilisations* 29 no. 4 (July/August 1974): 935–66.

Rosanvallon, Pierre. *L'Etat en France de 1789 à nos jours.* Paris: Editions du Seuil, 1990.

Rosen, George. *From Medical Police to Social Medicine: Essays on the History of Health Care.* New York: Science History Publications, 1974.

———. *A History of Public Health.* New York: MD Publications, 1958; reprint, with an introduction by Elizabeth Fee and a biographical essay and bibliography by Edward T. Morman, Baltimore: Johns Hopkins University Press, 1993.

———. "Problems in the Application of Statistical Analysis to Questions of Health." *Bulletin of the History of Medicine* 29, no. 1 (1955): 27–45.

Rosenberg, Charles E. "Cholera in Nineteenth-Century Europe." *Comparative Studies in Society and History* 8, no. 4 (July 1966): 452–63.

———. *The Cholera Years: The United States in 1832, 1849, and 1866.* Chicago: University of Chicago Press, 1962; reprint, with an afterword, 1987.

Sellier, Jacques. "Le Choléra à Paris au XIXe siècle: Essai de topographie biologique." Thesis, Académie de Médecine de Paris, 1979.

Sewell, William H., Jr. *Work and Revolution in France: The Language of Labor from the Old Regime to 1848.* Cambridge: Cambridge University Press, 1980.

Stallybrass, Peter, and Allon White. *The Politics and Poetics of Transgression.* Ithaca: Cornell University Press, 1986.

Stearns, Peter N. "The Middle Class: Toward a Precise Definition." *Comparative Studies in Society and History* 21 (1979): 377–96.

Sussman, George David. "Carriers of Cholera and Poison Rumors in France in 1832." *Societas* 3, no. 3 (1973): 233–51.

———. "From Yellow Fever to Cholera: A Study of French Government Policy, Medical Professionalism and Popular Movements in the Epidemic Crises of the Restoration and the July Monarchy." Ph.D. diss., Yale University, 1971.

———. "The Glut of Doctors in Mid-Nineteenth-Century France." *Comparative Studies in Society and History* 19, no. 3 (July 1977): 287–304.

Terdiman, Richard. *Discourse/Counter-Discourse: The Theory and Practice of Symbolic Resistance in Nineteenth-Century France.* Ithaca: Cornell University Press, 1985.

Thuillier, Guy. *Bureaucratie et bureaucrates en France au XIXe siècle.* Geneva: Droz, 1980.

Thullier, Guy, and Jean Tulard. *Histoire de l'administration française.* Paris: Presses Universitaires de France, 1984.

Thureau-Dangin, Paul. *L'Eglise et l'Etat sous la monarchie de juillet.* Paris: E. Plon, 1880.

———. *Histoire de la monarchie de juillet.* 7 vols. Paris: E. Plon, Nourrit, 1884–92.

Traugott, Mark. *Armies of the Poor: Determinants of Working-Class Participation in the Parisian Insurrection of June 1848.* Princeton: Princeton University Press, 1985.

Tufte, Edward R. *The Visual Display of Quantitative Information.* Cheshire, Conn.: Graphics Press, 1983.

Tulard, Jean. *La Préfecture de police sous la monarchie de juillet. . . .* Paris: Imp. Municipale, 1964.

Vigarello, Georges. *Le Propre et le sale: L'Hygiène du corps depuis le Moyen Age.* Paris: Editions du Seuil, 1985.

Vigier, Philippe. *Nouvelle histoire de Paris: Paris pendant la monarchie de juillet.* Paris: Hachette, 1991.

Weiner, Dora. "Public Health under Napoleon: The Conseil de Salubrité de Paris, 1802–1815." *Clio Medica* 9 (1974): 271–84.

Weisz, George. "The Politics of Medical Professionalization in France, 1845–1848." *Journal of Social History* 12, no. 1 (fall 1978): 3–30.

Index

Absolutism, 33, 219; health policies under, 230n5

Accountants, at first-aid stations, 119–20, 121, 138, 250n40

Administrators, government, 81–89; in Affair of the Twelve Thousand Francs, 156, 157–58; agency in epidemics, 11, 26, 30, 81–89; attacks on Catholic Church, 174; authority in epidemics, 120, 121–23, 138; autonomy of physicians under, 154; bourgeoisie among, 25, 83–84, 103; Catholic press on, 147; conflict with Catholic Church, 142, 143–54, 159, 163; conflict with medical professionals, 117, 118–21, 123, 137, 138, 197; control of first-aid stations, 117, 118–21; cooperation with Catholic Church, 170, 174–75, 257n96; cooperation with medical professionals, 88, 89, 104–5, 138, 140, 175, 216; cultural authority of, 159, 164; dissemination of information, 64, 81–89, 104; elected, 242n57; in epidemic of 1832, 40, 81–88, 104, 124, 154–56; in epidemic of 1849, 88–89, 115, 138, 216; and flight from cholera, 62; funding of epidemic of 1832, 154–55; hygienists among, 71; improvement of urban environment, 27, 88; in literature, 242n54, 243n65; of old regime, 34; professional literature for, 83, 242n54; relations with print trades, 93, 246n98; role in policy making, 66–67; shaping of perception of cholera, 4, 52, 62, 63, 208–9, 210, 215; upward mobility of, 84, 243n59; use of statistical reports, 132, 135–37, 138; wages of, 83, 242n56. *See also* Bureaucracy; Public health officials; Professionals

Advertisements, newspaper, 97, 100, 150, 151, 244n85, 247n115, 248n125; for cholera remedies, 20–21, 69, 106, 107, 248n7; for physicians, 238n10

Affair of Rome (1849), 170, 202, 256n93

Affair of the Twelve Thousand Francs, 156–59, 162–63, 255n57; newspaper comment on, 255n56

AIDS epidemic, 10, 11, 219

Alcohol, in treatment of cholera, 111, 249n17

Alms, distribution of, 142–43, 155, 163, 173. *See also* Charity

L'Ami de la religion (periodical), 2, 221n6; under July Monarchy, 147; on poison riots, 190; on secular authority, 146–47, 148, 159, 163

L'Ami du peuple (periodical), 98

Ancien régime. *See* Old regime

Annales d'hygiène publique et de médecine légale (periodical), 72, 101. *See also* Public health

Anticlericalism: of July Monarchy, 49, 141, 146, 147–48, 159–60, 165, 256n73; of newspapers, 148, 162, 168–69

Anticontagionism, 14, 75; bourgeois support of, 78–79, 80; in epidemic of 1832, 117, 213; in epidemic of 1849, 115; influence of Napoleonic wars on, 76; in *instructions populaires*, 112, 113, 138; official support of, 78, 79; role of class in, 80; in study of urban environment, 77; support of medical professionals for, 77, 78, 137. *See also* Contagionism

Anti-Semitism, 184, 186, 260n32, 261n37

Antisepsis, 72

Apponyi, Rudolphe, 61; on Affair of the Twelve Thousand Francs, 158; on June 13 insurrection, 205; on poison riots, 189

Aristocracy: decline of, 23–24, 26; excesses of, 51; overlap with bourgeoisie, 227n65; and practice of medicine, 68; religious beliefs of, 140

Artisans, 87. *See also* Working classes

L'Atelier (periodical), 98

Auvergne, cholera refugees in, 61

Compositor:	Braun-Brumfield, Inc.
Text:	10/13 Palatino
Display:	Palatino
Printer:	Braun-Brumfield, Inc.
Binder:	Braun-Brumfield, Inc.